FRONTIERS IN HEADACHE RESEARCH

Volume 7

Headache Pathogenesis
Monoamines, Neuropeptides, Purines, and Nitric Oxide

Frontiers in Headache Research Series

Volume 1: Migraine and Other Headaches: The Vascular Mechanisms
J. Olesen, editor; 384 pp.; 1991.
Volume 2: 5-Hydroxytryptamine Mechanisms in Primary Headaches
J. Olesen and P.R. Saxena, editors; 384 pp.; 1992.
Volume 3: Tension-Type Headache: Classification, Mechanisms, and Treatment
J. Olesen and J. Schoenen, editors; 314 pp.; 1993.
Volume 4: Headache Classification and Epidemiology
J. Olesen, editor; 416 pp.; 1994.
Volume 5: Experimental Headache Models in Animal and Man
J. Olesen and M.A. Moskowitz, editors; 384 pp.; 1995.
Volume 6: Headache Treatment: Trial Methodology and New Drugs
J. Olesen and P. Tfelt-Hansen, editors; 363 pp.; 1996.
Volume 7: Headache Pathogenesis: Monoamines, Neuropeptides, Purines, and Nitric Oxide
J. Olesen and L. Edvinsson, editors; 336 pp.; 1997.

FRONTIERS IN HEADACHE RESEARCH SERIES

Volume 7

Headache Pathogenesis
Monoamines, Neuropeptides, Purines, and Nitric Oxide

Editors

Jes Olesen, M.D.

Professor of Neurology
University of Copenhagen
Chairman, Department of Neurology
Glostrup Hospital
Copenhagen, Denmark

Lars Edvinsson, M.D., Ph.D.

Professor of Neurology
Department of Internal Medicine
Lund University Hospital
Lund, Sweden

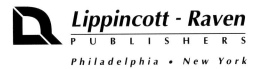

Philadelphia • New York

Acquisitions Editor: Mark Placito
Manufacturing Manager: Dennis Teston
Associate Managing Editor: Kathleen Bubbeo
Production Services: Colophon
Cover Designer: Patricia Gast
Indexer: Beta Computer Indexing
Compositor: Eastern Compositon
Printer: Quebecor Kingsport

© 1997, Lippincott–Raven Publishers. All rights reserved. This book is protected by copyright. No part of it may be reproduced, stored in a retrieval system, or transmitted, in any form or by any means—electronic, mechanical, photocopy, recording, or otherwise—without the prior written consent of the publisher, except for brief quotations embodied in critical articles and reviews. For information write **Lippincott–Raven Publishers, 227 East Washington Square, Philadelphia, PA 19106-3780.**

Materials appearing in this book prepared by individuals as part of their official duties as U.S. government employees are not covered by the above-mentioned copyright.

Printed in the United States of America

9 8 7 6 5 4 3 2 1

Library of Congress Cataloging-in-Publication Data

Headache pathogenesis : monoamines, neuropeptides, purines, and nitric
  oxide / editors, Jes Olesen, Lars Edvinsson.
     p. cm. — (Frontiers in headache research ; v. 7)
  Includes bibliographical references and index.
  ISBN 0-7817-1208-4
  1. Headache—Pathogenesis. 2. Biogenic amines—Pathophysiology.
  3. Neuropeptides—Pathophysiology. 4. Nitric oxide—Pathophysiology.
  5. Second messengers (Biochemistry)—Pathophysiology. I. Olesen,
  Jes. II. Edvinsson, Lars. III. Series
     [DNLM: 1. Headache—physiopathology. 2. Headache—etiology.
  3. Neurotransmitters—physiology. 4. Central Nervous System—
  physiopathology. W1 FR945YD v.7 1997 / WL 342 H4319 1997]
  RB128.H4448   1997
  616.8'49107—dc21
  DNLM/DLC
  for Library of Congress   97-8666
                                                                CIP

Care has been taken to confirm the accuracy of the information presented and to describe generally accepted practices. However, the authors, editors, and publisher are not responsible for errors or omissions or for any consequences from application of the information in this book and make no warranty, express or implied, with respect to the contents of the publication.

The authors, editors, and publisher have exerted every effort to ensure that drug selection and dosage set forth in this text are in accordance with current recommendations and practice at the time of publication. However, in view of ongoing research, changes in government regulations, and the constant flow of information relating to drug therapy and drug reactions, the reader is urged to check the package insert for each drug for any change in indications and dosage and for added warnings and precautions. This is particularly important when the recommended agent is a new or infrequently employed drug.

Some drugs and medical devices presented in this publication have Food and Drug Administration (FDA) clearance for limited use in restricted research settings. It is the responsibility of the health care provider to ascertain the FDA status of each drug or device planned for use in their clinical practice.

Contents

Contributing Authors xi
Preface to the Series xix
Preface xx

Section I. General Aspects of Messenger Molecules: Localization, Methods for Measurement, Receptors, and Second Messengers

1. Migraine Pain Originates from Blood Vessels 3
   James W. Lance

2. Neuropeptide Analysis: Past, Present, and Future 11
   Rolf Ekman

3. Discussion Summary: General Aspects of Messenger Molecules: Localization, Methods for Measurement, Receptors, and Second Messengers 17
   Peter J. Goadsby

Section II. Messenger Molecules in Cranial Blood Vessels

4. Messenger Molecules in the Cranial Sympathetic Nervous System 21
   Lars Edvinsson

5. Messenger Molecules in the Cranial Parasympathetic Nervous System 37
   Rolf Uddman and Anders Luts

6. Messenger Molecules in the Cranial Sensory Nervous System 47
   Norihiro Suzuki

7. Endothelial Messengers and Cerebral Vascular Tone Regulation 61
   Tony J-F. Lee

8. Discussion Summary: Messenger Molecules in Cranial Blood Vessels 73
   Patrick P. A. Humphrey

Section III. Role of Messenger Molecules in Pain Processing

9. Messenger Molecules Involved in Sensitization of
   Peripheral Nerve Endings 79
   Stephen B. McMahon

10. Messenger Molecules Involved in Central
    Sensitization 89
    Clifford J. Woolf

11. Messenger Molecules Involved in Sensitization at
    Supraspinal Levels 99
    Mary M. Heinricher

12. An Epidemiological Study on the Activity of
    Cannabis in Idiopathic Headache 107
    *V. Amenta, G. M. Pitari, M. Caff, D. Impellizzieri,
    F. Giuliano, R. Costa, I. Sapuppo, and A. Bianchi*

13. Activation of Cutaneous Afferent Neurons by
    Adenosine Triphosphate in the Neonatal Rat Tail-Spinal
    Cord Preparation in Vitro 111
    Derek J. Trezise and Patrick P. A. Humphrey

14. Cortical Spreading Depression Does Not Activate
    Trigeminal C Fibers 117
    *Bente Krag Ingvardsen, Henning Laursen, Uffe B. Olsen, and
    Anker Jon Hansen*

15. Systemic Nitroglycerin Activates Catecholaminergic,
    Neuropeptidergic, and Nitric Oxide Pathways in the
    Rat Brain 123
    *Cristina Tassorelli, Shirley Anne Joseph, G. Sandrini,
    Alfredo Costa, and Giuseppe Nappi*

16. Discussion Summary: Role of Messenger Molecules
    in Pain Processing 131
    Clifford J. Woolf

Section IV. Involvement of Amines and Amino Acids in Primary Headache

17. Amines and Amino Acids in Migraine 139
    Vivette A.S. Glover

18. Amines, Purines, and Amino Acids in Tension-Type
    Headache and Cluster Headache 145
    László Vécsei, János Tajti, and Délia Szok

19. Effects of Migraine Treatments on Amines and Amino Acid
    Messenger Molecules 153
    Helen E. Connor

20. Systemic Administration of *m*-Chlorophenylpiperazine Does
    Not Induce Fos Expression in the Rat Trigeminal Nucleus
    Caudalis 161
    Renée S. Martin and Graeme R. Martin

21. Release of Histamine from Dural Mast Cells by Substance
    P and Calcitonin Gene-Related Peptide and Effect of
    Sumatriptan 167
    Anders Ottosson and Lars Edvinsson

22. Variability of Vascular Receptors on the Human Cerebral
    Arteries as Determined in Vitro 173
    *Peer Tfelt-Hansen, Inger Jansen-Olesen, A. Mortensen,
    and Lars Edvinsson*

23. Variability of the Vascular α-Adrenoceptor on Human
    Omental Vessels: An in Vitro Study 177
    Peer Tfelt-Hansen and Lars Edvinsson

24. A Study on Hormonal Responses and Painful Attacks
    Induced by *m*-Chlorophenylpiperazine in Cluster Headache
    Patients during Cluster Period 181
    *Massimo Leone, Domenico D'Amico, Licia Grazzi,
    Angelo Attanasio, Danilo Croci, Giuseppe Libro,
    Angelo Nespolo, and Gennaro Bussone*

25. Discussion Summary: Involvement of Amines and Amino
    Acids in Primary Headache 187
    James W. Lance

Section V. Involvement of Neuropeptides in Primary Headaches

26. Opioid Peptides in Primary Headaches 193
    Flemming W. Bach

27. Nonopioid Peptides in Migraine and Cluster Headache 201
    Peter J. Goadsby

28. Increased Plasma Level of Endothelin-1 in Cluster
    Headache 211
    *Linda R. White, Maurice B. Vincent, Helene M. G. Arcanjo,
    Paulo L. M. Araujo, Lars J. Stovner, and Jan Aasly*

29. Plasma Homocysteine Levels in Primary Headache 215
    Stefan Evers, Hans Georg Koch, and Ingo-Wilhelm Husstedt

30. Endothelin-B Receptors in Human Temporal Artery 219
    *Linda R. White, Roar Juul, Guilherme A. Lucas,
    Knut H. Leseth, Jan Aasly, Johan Cappelen, and
    Lars Edvinsson*

31. Presence of Contractile Endothelin-A and Dilatory
    Endothelin-B Receptors in Human Cerebral Arteries 223
    *Torun Nilsson, Leonor Cantera, Mikael Adner, and
    Lars Edvinsson*

32. Evidence for Calcitonin Gene-Related Peptide-1
    Receptors in Human Cranial Arteries 229
    *Inger Jansen-Olesen, Sergio Gulbenkian, Leonor Cantera, and
    Lars Edvinsson*

33. Discussion Summary: Involvement of Neuropeptides in Primary
    Headaches 235
    Lars Edvinsson

Section VI. Involvement of Nitric Oxide–Cyclic GMP Products in Primary Headache

34. Nitroxidergic Nerve in Cranial Arteries 241
    Noboru Toda

35. Nitric Oxide Synthase Activation and Inhibition
    in Migraine 247
    Lisbeth H. Lassen and Jes Olesen

36.	The Nitric Oxide Hypothesis of Migraine and Other Vascular Headaches .... *Jes Olesen, Lars L. Thomsen, Lisbeth H. Lassen, and Inger Jansen-Olesen*	255
37.	Normal Radial Artery Dilation during Reactive Hyperemia in Migraine without Aura .... *Lars L. Thomsen, Dorthe Daugaard, Helle K. Iversen, and Jes Olesen*	267
38.	Effect of the Nitric Oxide Donor Glyceryl Trinitrate on Nociceptive Thresholds in Humans .... *Lars L. Thomsen, Jannick Brennum, Helle K. Iversen, and Jes Olesen*	273
39.	Nitric Oxide as the Final Mediator of Headaches Induced by Central and Peripheral Serotoninergic Mechanisms .... *Richard Peatfield, N. Jarrett, F. Ahmed, and Vivette A. S. Glover*	279
40.	Spreading Depression Evokes a Quantity of Release of Cortical Nitric Oxide Not Correlated to a Change in Pial Artery Diameter or Regional Pial Cerebral Blood Flux .... *Simon J. Read, M. I. Smith, and A. A. Parsons*	283
41.	Nitric Oxide Synthesis in Nitric Oxide Donor Migraine .... *Paolo Martelletti, Simona D'Aló, Giuseppe Stirparo, Cristina Rinaldi, Maria Grazia Cifone, and Mario Giacovazzo*	287
42.	Endothelium-Dependent Mechanics of Nitric Oxide Donor Migraine .... *Paolo Martelletti and Mario Giacovazzo*	291
43.	5-Hydroxytryptamine$_1$ Agonists Inhibit the Activity of Constitutive Nitric Oxide Synthase in Guinea Pig Cerebral Vessels .... *Bertel Rüdinger and Inger Jansen-Olesen*	297
44.	Discussion Summary: Involvement of Nitric Oxide-Cyclic GMP Pathway Products in Primary Headaches .... *Jes Olesen*	303
Subject Index		307

Contributing Authors

Jan Aasly, M.D., Ph.D.
Head
Department of Neurology
University Hospital
Olav Kyrres Gt. 17
N-7006 Trondheim
Norway

Mikael Adner, B.M.
Division of Experimental Vascular Research
Department of Internal Medicine
Lund University Hospital
S-221 85 Lund
Sweden

F. Ahmed, M.B., M.R.C.P.
Princess Margaret Migraine Clinic
Charing Cross Hospital
Fulham Palace Road
London W6 8RF
United Kingdom

V. Amenta, M.D.
Department of Pharmacology and Toxicology
University of Catania Medical School
Viale Andrea Doria, 6
95125 Catania
Italy

Paulo L.M. Araujo
Faculdad de Medicina
Universidade Federal do Rio de Janeiro
21949-590 Rio de Janeiro
Brazil

Helene M. G. Arcanjo
Faculdad de Medicina
Universidade Federal do Rio de Janeiro
21949-590 Rio de Janeiro
Brazil

Angelo Attanasio, M.D.
Headache Center
Neurological Institute "C. Besta"
Via Celoria 11
20133 Milan
Italy

Flemming W. Bach, M.D.
Associate Professor
Department of Neurology
The National University Hospital
Rigshospitalet
Blegdamsvej 9
DK-2100 Copenhagen
Denmark

Alfredo Bianchi
Professor
Department of Pharmacology and Toxicology
University of Catania Medical School
Viale Andrea Doria, 6
95125 Catania
Italy

Jannick Brennum
Department of Neurosurgery
University Hosptial
Rigshospitalet
Blegdamsvej
DK-2100 Copenhagen
Denmark

Gennaro Bussone, M.D.
Headache Center
Neurological Institute "C. Besta"
Via Celoria, 11
20133 Milan
Italy

M. Caff, M.D.
Department of Pharmacology and
    Toxicology
University of Catania Medical School
Viale Andrea Doria, 6
95125 Catania
Italy

Leonor Cantera
Division of Experimental Vascular
    Research
Department of Internal Medicine
Lund University Hospital
S-221 85 Lund
Sweden

Johan Cappelen, M.D.
Consultant Neurosurgeon
Department of Neurosurgery
University Hospital
Olave Kyrres Gt. 17
N-7006 Trondheim
Norway

Maria Grazia Cifone, Ph.D.
Associate Professor of Immunopathology
Department of Experimental Medicine
University of L'Aquila
I-6700 L'Aquila
Italy

Helen E. Connor,
Glaxo-Wellcome Research and
Development
Gunnel's Wood Road
Stevenage, Herts SG1 2NY
United Kingdom

Alfredo Costa, M.D.
Research Assistant
Neurological Institute "C. Mondino"
University of Pavia
Via Palestro, 3
I-27100 Pavia
Italy

R. Costa, M.D.
Department of Pharmacology and
    Toxicology
University of Catania Medical School
Viale Andrea Doria, 6
95125 Catania
Italy

Danilo Croci, M.D.
Biochemistry and Pharmacology
    Laboratory
Neuroligical Institute "C. Besta"
Via Celoria, 11
20133 Milan
Italy

Simona D'Alò, M.D.
Department of Experimental Medicine
University of L'Aquila
I-67100 L'Aquila
Italy

Domenico D'Amico, M.D.
Headache Center
Neurological Institute "C. Besta"
Via Celoria, 11
20133 Milan
Italy

Dorthe Daugaard, M.D.
Department of Neurology
Glostrup Hospital
University of Copenhagen
Ndr. Ringvej, 57
DK-2600 Glostrup, Copenhagen
Denmark

Lars Edvinsson, M.D., Ph.D.
Professor
Department of Internal Medicine
Lund University Hospital
S-221 85 Lund
Sweden

Rolf Ekman, M.D., Ph.D.
Professor of Neurochemistry
Institute of Clinical Neuroscience
Department of Psychiatry and
    Neurochemistry
Göteborg University
Sahlgrenska University
Hospital/Mölndal
S-431 80 Mölndal
Sweden

Stefan Evers, M.D.
Department of Neurology
University of Münster
Albert Schweitzer Str. 33
D-48129 Münster
Germany

Mario Giacovazzo, M.D.
Full Professor of Internal Medicine
Department of Clinical Medicine
University "La Sapienza"
Viale del Policlinico
I-10061 Rome
Italy

F. Giuliano, M.D.
Biologist
Department of Pharmacology and
Toxicology
University of Catania Medical School
Viale Andrea Doria, 6
95125 Catania
Italy

Vivette A.S. Glover, M.A., Ph.D., D.Sc.
Department of Pediatrics
Queen Charlotte's Hospital
Goldhawk Road
London W6 0XG
United Kingdom

Peter J. Goadsby, M.D., Ph.D., D.Sc., F.R.C.P.
Reader in Clinical Neurology
Institute of Neurology
The National Hospital for Neurology
    and Neurosurgery
Queen Square
London WC1N 3BG
United Kingdom

Licia Grazzi, M.D.
Headache Center
Neurological Institute "C. Besta"
Via Celoria, 11
20133 Milan
Italy

Sergio Gulbenkian, Ph.D.
Gulbenkian Institute of Science
Oeiras
Portugal 2781

Anker Jon Hansen, M.D., D.Sc.
Senior Research Scientist
Department of Neuropharmacology
Novo Nordisks A/S
Novo Nordisk Park
DK-2760 Maaloev
Denmark

Mary M. Heinricher, Ph.D.
Associate Professor
Division of Neurosurgery
Oregon Health Sciences University
3181 S.W. Sam Jackson Park Road
Portland, Oregon 97201

Patrick P. A. Humphrey, B.Pharm., Hons., Ph.D., D.Sc., F.R.Pharm. S.
Glaxo Institute of Applied Pharmacology
Department of Pharmacology
University of Cambridge
Tennis Court Road
Cambridge CB2 1QJ
United Kingdom

Ingo-Wilhelm Husstedt, M.D.
Department of Neurology
University of Münster
Albert Schweitzer Str. 33
D-48129 Münster
Germany

D. Impellizzieri, M.D.
Department of Pharmacology and Toxicology
University of Catania Medical School
Viale Andrea Doria, 6
95125 Catania
Italy

Bente Krag Ingvardsen, B.S, M.S.
Department of General Pharmacology
Novo Nordisk A/S
Novo Nordisk Park
DK-2760 Maaloev
Denmark

Helle K. Iversen
Department of Neurology
Glostrup Hospital
University of Copenhagen
Ndr. Ringvej 57
DK-2600 Glostrup, Copenhagen
Denmark

Inger Jansen-Olesen, Ph.D., D.Sc.
Associate Professor of Pharmacology
Department of Biological Sciences
The Royal Danish School of Pharmacy
Universitetsparken 2
DK-2100 Copenhagen Ø
Denmark

N. Jarrett, M.Sc.
Department of Biochemistry
Queen Charlotte's Hospital
Goldhawk Road
London W6 0XG
United Kingdom

Shirley Anne Joseph, Ph.D.
Associate Professor of Anatomy and Neurobiology
Division of Neurological Surgery
Strong Memorial Hospital
601 Elmwood Avenue
Rochester, New York 14642

Roar Juul, M.D., Ph.D.
Consultant Neurosurgeon
Department of Neurosurgery
University Hospital
Olave Kyrres Gt. 17
N-7006 Trondheim
Norway

Hans Georg Koch, M.D.
Department of Pediatrics
University of Münster
Albert Schweitzer Str. 33
D-48129 Münster
Germany

James W. Lance, M.D., Hon. D.Sc.
Emeritus Professor of Neurology and Consultant Neurologist
Institute of Neurological Sciences
Wales Medical Center
66 High Street
Randwick, New South Wales 2031
Australia

Lisbeth H. Lassen, M.D.
Department of Neurology
Glostrup Hospital
University of Copenhagen
Ndr. Ringvej 57
DK-2600 Glostrup, Copenhagen
Denmark

Henning Laursen, M.D., Dr. Med. Sci.
Head of Clinical Neuropathology
Laboratory of Neuropathology
University Hospital
Biegdamsvej
DK-2100 Copenhagen
Denmark

Tony J-F. Lee, Ph.D.
Professor
Department of Pharmacology
Southern Illinois University
801 North Rutledge, P.O. Box 19230
Springfield, Illinois 62794-1222

Massimo Leone, M.D.
Headache Center
Neurological Institute "C. Besta"
Via Celoria, 11
20133 Milan
Italy

Knut H. Leseth
Department of Neurology
University Hospital
Olave Kyrres Gt. 17
N-7006 Trondheim
Norway

Giuseppe Libro, M.D.
Headache Center
Neurological Institute "C. Besta"
Via Celoria, 11
20133 Milan
Italy

Guilherme A. Lucas, M.D., M.Sc.
Research Fellow
Department of Neurology
University Hospital
Olave Kyrres Gt. 17
N-7006 Trondheim
Norway

Anders Luts
Departments of Physiology and Neurscience, and Psychiatry
University of Lund
S-221 85 Lund
Sweden

Paolo Martelletti, M.D.
Researcher Associate of Internal Medicine
Department of Clinical Medicine
University "La Sapienza"
Viale de Policlinico
I-10061 Rome
Italy

Graeme R. Martin, Ph.D.
Head
Department of Molecular Pharmacology
Roche Bioscience
Center for Biological Research
3401 Hillview Avenue
Palo Alto, California 94304

Renée S. Martin, M.Sc.
Department of Molecular Pharmacology
Roche Bioscience
Center for Biological Research
3401 Hillview Avenue
Palo Alto, California 94304

Stephen B. McMahon, B.Sc., Ph.D.
Professor
Department of Physiology
St. Thomas' Hospital Medical School
Lambeth Palace Road
London SE1 7EH
United Kingdom

A. Mortensen
Department of Neurosurgery
Glostrup Hospital
Ndr. Ringvej 57
DK-2600 Glostrup, Copenhagen
Denmark

Giuseppe Nappi, M.D.
Professor
Neurological Institute "C. Mondino"
University of Pavia
Via Palestro, 3
I-27100 Pavia
Italy

Angelo Nespolo, M.D.
Chief
Biochemistry and Pharmacology
 Laboratory
Neurological Institute "C. Besta"
Via Celoria, 11
20133 Milan
Italy

Torun Nilsson, M.D.
Division of Experimental Vascular
 Research
Department of Internal Medicine
Lund University Hospital
S-221 85 Lund
Sweden

Jes Olesen, M.D.
Profesor
Department of Neurology
Glostrup Hospital
University of Copenhagen
Ndr. Ringvej 57
DK-2600 Glostrup, Copenhagen
Denmark

Uffe B. Olsen, Ph.D.
Senior Principal Scientist
Department of Neuropharmacology
Novo Nordisk A/S
Novo Nordisck Park
DK-2760 Maaloev
Denmark

Anders Ottosson, M.D., Ph.D.
Department of Forensic Medicine
University of Lund
S-221 85 Lund
Sweden

A. A. Parsons
SmithKline Beecham Pharmaceuticals
Neurology Branch
New Frontier Science Park (N)
Third Avenue
Harlow, Essex CM19 5AW
United Kingdom

Richard Peatfield,
Princess Margaret Migraine Clinic
Charing Cross Hospital
Fulham Palace Road
London W6 8RF
United Kingdom

G. M. Pitari, M.D.
Department of Pharmacology and
 Toxicology
University of Catania Medical School
Viale Andrea Doria, 6
95125 Catania
Italy

Simon J. Read, B.Sc., M.Sc.
Research Scientist
Department of Neuroscience
SmithKline Beecham Pharmaceuticals
New Frontiers Science Park (N)
Third Avenue
Harlow, Essex CM19 5AW
United Kingdom

Cristina Rinaldi, Ph.D.
Associate Professor of Immunology
Department of Experimental Medicine
and Pathology
University "La Sapienza"
Viale del Policlinico
I-10061 Rome
Italy

Bertel Rüdinger
Department of Biological Sciences
The Royal Danish School of Pharmacy
Universitetsparken 2
DK-2100 Copenhagen
Denmark

G. Sandrini, M.D.
Associate Professor of Neurology
Neurological Institute "C. Mondino"
University of Pavia
Via Palestro, 3
I-27100 Pavia
Italy

I. Sapuppo
Department of Pharmacology and Toxicology
University of Catania Medical School
Viale Andrea Doria, 6
95125 Catania
Italy

M.I. Smith
SmithKline Beecham Pharmaceuticals
Neurology Research
New Frontiers Science Park (N)
Third Avenue
Harlow, Essex CM9 5AW
United Kingdom

Giuseppe Stirparo, Ph.D.
Institute of Biomedical Technologies
National Council of Research
I-10061 Rome
Italy

Lars J. Stovner, M.D., Ph.D.
Professor
Department of Neurology
University Hospital
Olave Kyrres Gt. 17
N-7006 Trondheim
Norway

Norihiro Suzuki, M.D., Ph.D.
Assistant Professor
Department of Neurology
Keio University
35 Shinanomachi
Shinjuku-ku
Tokyo 160
Japan

Délia Szok, M.D.
Assistant Professor of Neurology
Department of Neurology
Szent-Györgyi University Medical School
Semmelweis St. 6
Steged 6725
Hungary

János Tajti, M.D., Ph.D.
Assistant Professor of Neurology
Department of Neurology
Szent-Györgyi University Medical School
Semmelweis St. 6
Steged 6725
Hungary

Cristina Tassorelli, M.D., Ph.D.
Research Assistant
Neurological Institute "C. Mondino"
University of Pavia
Via Palestro, 3
I-27100 Pavia
Italy

Peer Tfelt-Hansen, M.D., Ph.D.
Department of Neurology
Bispebjerg Hospital
Bispebjerg Bakke
DK-2400 Copenhagen
Denmark

Lars L. Thomsen, M.D., Ph.D.
Department of Neurology
Glostrup Hospital
University of Copenhagen
Ndr. Ringvej 57
DK-2600 Glostrup, Copenhagen
Denmark

Noboru Toda, M.D., Ph.D.
Professor of Medicine
Department of Pharmacology
Shiga University of Medical Science
Ohtsu/Shiga 520-21
Japan

Derek J. Trezise, B.Sc., Ph.D.
*Glaxo Institute of Applied
    Pharmacology
Department of Pharmacology
University of Cambridge
Tennis Court Road
Cambridge CB2 1QJ
United Kingdom*

Rolf Uddman, M.D., Ph.D.
*Assistant Professor
Department of Otorhinolaryngology
Malmö University Hospital
S-205 02 Malmö
Sweden*

László Vécsei, M.D., Ph.D., D.Sc.
*Professor and Head
Department of Neurology
Szent-Györgyi University Medical
    School
Semmelweis St. 6
Steged 6725
Hungary*

Maurice B. Vincent, M.D., Ph.D
*Serviço de Neurologia
Hospital Universitário Clementino
    Fraga Filho
Rio de Janeiro
Brazil*

Linda R. White, B.Sc., Ph.D.
*Laboratory Leader
Department of Neurology
University Hospital
Olave Kyrres Gt. 17
N-7006 Trondheim
Norway*

Clifford J. Woolf, M.D., Ph.D.
*Professor of Neurobiology
Department of Anatomy and
    Developmental Biology
University College London
Gower Street
London WC1E 6BT
United Kingdom*

Preface to the Series

Among the adult population, 16% are migraine sufferers, and 71% have had tension-type headache. The burden on society in terms of work days lost and health care costs and the amount of suffering by the victims are enormous. Headache disorders have not been taken seriously, however. Patients try to hide their suffering because they are afraid of being accused of faking or because the disorders are often regarded as more or less psychiatric. Lack of knowledge and inconsistencies in published research work have turned many medical scientists away from the study of these disorders. Over the last decade, however, headache research has been burgeoning. Unfortunately, this has not yet had significant impact on general medicine or the neurological disciplines. It is the aim of this series of books, entitled *Frontiers in Headache Research,* to demonstrate the major advances made in our understanding of headache.

Each book in this series focuses on a major field of headache research. The scope is multidisciplinary, involving both the medical and the basic sciences. Each chapter is introduced by one or more overview papers by leading experts. Thereafter, the newest developments are presented in short articles. Finally, each chapter closes with a summary of the discussions by the chairpersons. The books in this series are the result of international headache research seminars held each year in late November. The meetings are organized according to a rigorously structured program with a view to generating the best possible books. The publication time has been kept to a minimum to ensure timeliness.

Jes Olesen

Preface

The mechanisms of headache attacks can be viewed from many different perspectives. Nosographic studies are important to delineate the major disease entities, epidemiological studies characterize their frequency and socioeconomic impact, and pathophysiological studies help to clarify the nature of diseases. The topic of this book—studies of messenger molecules involved in headache—is of critical importance for future drug development targeted to specific receptors. This book brings together available knowledge about messenger molecules involved in primary headaches and their receptors. The first messenger molecule to be implicated, and still an extremely important one, is 5-hydroxytryptamine (5-HT). Blood 5-HT decreases during a migraine attack, thus prompting the search for 5-HT receptor antagonists and agonists as possible therapeutic agents. This was successful because antagonists were proven effective in migraine prophylaxis, and agonists at the $5\text{-HT}_{1B/1D}$ receptors have revolutionized the treatment of the acute migraine attack. Other molecules have now been implicated in the mechanisms of vascular headaches. The concentration of calcitonin gene–related peptide in external jugular venous blood is increased during migraine attacks, and the mechanisms for this have been dissected out in a series of elegant experiments in animals and humans. The freely diffusible messenger molecule nitric oxide (NO) seems to be even more important. Intravenous infusion of glyceryl trinitrate, a NO donor or "pro-drug," causes a vascular headache in nonmigraine sufferers and a more intense headache as well as a real migraine attack in migraine sufferers. Furthermore, the NO synthase inhibitor N^G-monomethylarginine (L-NMMA) has a significant therapeutic effect on acute migraine attacks. Further messenger molecules are involved in the modulation of peripheral sensitization of nociceptors. Central sensitization to painful and nonpainful stimuli may occur at the level of the trigeminal nucleus caudalis and at higher levels of the neuraxis. The present volume brings the reader up to date on these exciting developments.

Jes Olesen
Lars Edvinsson

SECTION I

General Aspects of Messenger Molecules: Localization, Methods for Measurement, Receptors, and Second Messengers

1
Migraine Pain Originates from Blood Vessels

James W. Lance

Institute of Neurological Sciences, Wales Medical Center, Randwick, New South Wales 2031, Australia

Why is migraine often referred to as a "vascular headache"? In 1684, *Dr. Willis's Practice of Physicke*, published in London 9 years after the death of Thomas Willis (1621–1675), included two chapters on headaches (1,2). Willis pointed out that the source of pain was not the brain, cerebellum, or medulla "because they want sensible fibres" but distension of the vessels, which "pulls the nervous fibres one from another and so brings to them painful corrugations or wrinklings." Erasmus Darwin, the grandfather of Charles Darwin, suggested in 1796 a trial of centrifugal force for the relief of headache "so as to force the blood from the brain into other parts of the body." He added, unnecessarily, that this "cannot be done in private practice, and which I would therefore recommend to some hospital physician." Harold G. Wolff took up this challenge 150 years later when he used a man-carrying centrifuge to ease the pain of migraine headache (3).

PAIN SENSITIVITY OF CRANIAL VESSELS

Wolff and his colleagues (3) studied the reaction of conscious subjects to probing, stimulation, or distension of intracranial and extracranial blood vessels. Distension of the middle meningeal artery caused pain in the ipsilateral retro-orbital area and temple. Stimulation of the intracranial segment of the internal carotid artery and the proximal 2 cm of the middle and anterior cerebral arteries produced pain in the eye, forehead, and temple on that side. The vertebral artery referred pain to the occiput. Pain elicited from the superior sagittal sinus was less intense than arterial pain and was felt diffusely over the frontotemporal region (Fig. 1).

Cerebral infarction or transient ischemic attacks are usually painless. Fisher (4) has described the referral pattern of headache in those in whom headache accompanied the event. The most common sites of headache were ipsilateral frontal for the internal carotid artery, frontal and retro-orbital for the middle cerebral artery, and frontal or occipital for the posterior cerebral, posterior inferior cerebellar (PIC), vertebral, and basilar arteries.

Inflation of a balloon in the internal carotid and middle cerebral arteries during

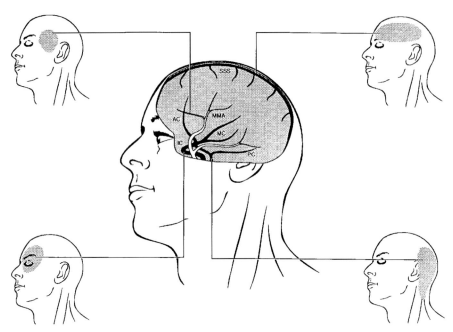

FIG. 1. Referral of pain from intracranial vessels, based on Wolff (3). AC, anterior cerebral artery; IC, internal carotid artery; MC, middle cerebral artery; MMA, middle meningeal artery; PC, posterior cerebral artery; SSS, superior sagittal sinus. From Lance (31).

embolization of arteriovenous malformations has given additional localizing information (5). The distal internal carotid artery and proximal part of the middle cerebral artery cause discomfort or pain lateral to the eye, whereas the middle third of the middle cerebral artery induces retro-orbital pain and the distal third refers pain above the ipsilateral eye.

Martins et al. (6) used the same technique to plot pain referral from Heubner's artery, the anterior choroidal artery, and branches of the posterior cerebral artery as well as the middle cerebral artery. Curiously, pain from the superior cerebellar and PIC arteries was felt in the periorbital and frontal areas. With the exception of the PIC artery, which gave rise to bifrontal pain, the referral pattern was ipsilateral. Pain reached maximum intensity rapidly, was initially severe, and declined over 10 minutes or less.

CLINICAL OBSERVATIONS

Patients with severe migraine headache often describe it as throbbing (pulsatile), i.e., increasing with each heart beat; they may notice that pressure on a prominent temporal artery eases ipsilateral headache. Graham and Wolff (7) demonstrated that the pulsation of branches of the superficial temporal artery diminished as migraine headache was relieved by the injection of ergotamine tartrate. The concept of migraine being an "extracranial vascular headache" appeared to be strengthened by Tunis and Wolff (8), who reported that the mean amplitude of temporal artery pulsation was greater during headache than in periods of freedom. This conclusion may have been biased by their selection of 10 patients for detailed study after examining 5,000 recordings from 75 patients.

Blau and Dexter (9) occluded the scalp circulation by means of a sphygmomanometer cuff in 50 patients suffering from migraine headache to assess the importance of extracranial vasodilation in the production of pain. In only 21 patients did the pain decrease. Of the 50 patients, 49 stated that their headache increased on coughing, head jolting, or breath holding, indicative of an intracranial vascular component. Drummond and Lance (10) examined 66 patients during unilateral migraine headache by recording the pulse amplitude of the superficial temporal artery and its frontal branches, facial thermographs, and compression of the temporal and common carotid arteries. In 39 patients with frontotemporal headache, the amplitude of the frontal branch of the superficial temporal artery increased significantly, whereas that of the main trunk remained unaltered. Thermography showed that the affected side was warmer in 11 of 18 patients whose headaches had been eased by compression of the superficial temporal artery. From the result of compression tests they concluded that extracranial vasodilation contributed substantially to headache in about one-third of patients and that another third responded to carotid compression but that the remaining third were not eased by either maneuver. There have been two reports of a skull defect bulging at the height of migraine headache, consistent with intracranial vasodilation or cerebral edema (11,12).

The evidence thus supports the involvement of both extracranial and intracranial vessels in most, if not all, attacks of migraine headache. Vasodilator agents are a potent trigger for migraine. Bonuso et al. (13) found that the local application of a nitroglycerine ointment to the frontotemporal region induced a headache in seven of ten migrainous patients, whereas no patient experienced headache after a placebo ointment. Vasodilators often induce migraine. Vasoconstrictors usually relieve it.

TRANSCRANIAL DOPPLER STUDIES

Cerebral vascular studies using transcranial Doppler ultrasound assume that changes in blood flow velocity indicate arterial dilation or constriction, providing that regional cortical blood flow remains constant. Comparison of velocities in major cerebral arteries in and out of migraine attacks have given conflicting results. Thie et al. (14) reported that flow velocity diminished in one or more of the three arteries studied (middle, anterior, and posterior cerebral) in 13 patients during migraine without aura but increased in 5 patients with aura. No correlation with the side of headache was found. By contrast, no flow change could be found in the internal or external carotid arteries or middle and anterior cerebral arteries of 27 migraineurs without aura during attacks studied by Zwetsloot et al. (15) or in a later study from the same center (16) of the middle cerebral, vertebral, or basilar arteries in 23 patients with migraine headache.

Two studies from the Copenhagen group compared flow velocities on headache and nonheadache sides, both showing a lower value in the middle cerebral artery on the affected side. The first, involving six patients with and four without aura, demonstrated a change corresponding to a mean increase in arterial diameter of 20% (17). The second, on 25 patients without aura, correlated with a mean increase in cross-sectional area of the middle cerebral artery of 9% (18). Although this was statistically significant, 7 of the 25 patients had a higher or unchanged velocity on the affected side. No velocity asymmetry was found in the anterior or posterior cerebral arteries.

EFFECT OF INJECTED SUMATRIPTAN AND SEROTONIN ON CRANIAL ARTERIES

In the study by Friberg et al. (17), sumatriptan 2 mg was administered by intravenous infusion, causing relief of headache within 30 minutes without affecting regional cerebral blood flow. As the headache subsided, flow in the middle cerebral artery returned to normal. Diener et al. (19) were unable to find any flow changes in the middle cerebral or basilar arteries of five subjects given 2 or 3 mg of sumatriptan s.c. for the treatment of headache induced by drug withdrawal, although headache was relieved for 8 hours. In a later study of the middle meningeal artery, sumatriptan 2 mg delivered into the arterial lumen in six patients and 6 mg s.c. in two patients induced vasoconstriction imaged by arteriography (20). This is consistent with the increase in flow velocity demonstrated in the internal carotid and middle cerebral arteries in 67 patients with migraine after the injection of sumatriptan 4 to 12 mg s.c., in parallel with the improvement in headache (21).

The slow IV injection of sumatriptan's parent substance 5-hydroxytryptamine (5-HT) 2 to 7.5 mg relieved migraine headache on six occasions in four patients at the expense of side effects such as hyperpnea, nausea, faintness, restlessness, the sensation of facial flushing, and paresthesias (22). The injection of 5-HT 40 to 160 µg into the common carotid artery produced a marked diminution of the amplitude of the superficial temporal artery, lasting 3 to 8 minutes, in five of seven migrainous subjects (23) (Fig. 2). Carotid angiograms carried out before and after the injection of 5-HT 100 and 150 µg into the common carotid artery of two patients confirmed the constriction of extracranial arteries with equivocal changes in the intracranial circulation in one patient and slight diminution of caliber of the anterior and middle cerebral arteries in the other (23).

CENTRAL FACTORS

The extent of vasodilation observed in the extracranial and intracranial circulations in migraine would not be sufficient to cause headache in nonmigrainous pa-

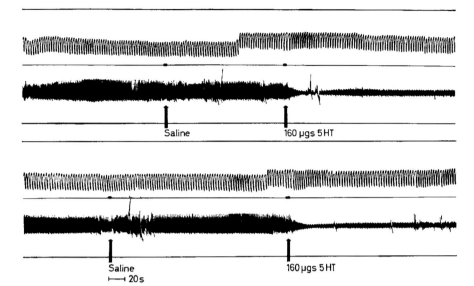

FIG. 2. Vasoconstrictor response of the superficial temporal artery to the intracarotid injection of serotonin (5-HT) on two occasions without any change after control injections of normal saline. *Upper traces*, respiratory excursion; *lower traces*, pulse amplitude. From Lance et al. (23), by permission of *Archives of Neurology*.

tients, during body heating or exercise, for example. There must be some source of amplification of visceral afferent input from those vessels in migraine. This process may take place peripherally as a "sterile inflammatory response" in and around the dilated arteries or centrally because of failure of the endogenous pain control system.

Migraine headache can be triggered from the periphery by vasodilator agents or by local irritation such as the injection of a contrast medium in angiography. More often it arises as the result of stress, overload of the special senses (by flickering light, noise, or strong smells), or changes in the internal milieu (hypoglycemia, the cyclical fall in estradiol levels in women). It is evident that migraine headache involves an interaction between the brain and the blood vessels that supply it and its encasing framework.

Pain fibers from all three divisions of the trigeminal nerve descend to the second cervical cord segment, where they converge with input from the occipital region on cells in the spinal nucleus of the trigeminal nerve. Second-order neurons ascend through the brain stem as the quintothalamic tract. Studies in cats have demonstrated that the third-order neurons mediating cerebral vascular pain originate in the periphery of the ventroposteromedial and other posterior nuclei of the thalamus and the intralaminar complex (24). Afferent input is regulated by the endogenous pain control pathway, which arises in the periaqueductal gray matter and locus coeruleus in the midbrain. Headache may result from a lesion in this area (25–27), which has been shown to increase in metabolic activity during and after migraine headaches (28).

Activation of locus coeruleus and nucleus raphe dorsalis in the same area has been shown in experimental animals to cause dilation of cerebral and extracranial vessels (29,30). It is therefore possible for a discharge of midbrain nuclei to generate headache and the vascular changes that follow and augment it, thus adding a pulsatile quality to severe migraine headache.

CONCLUSION

The dilation of cerebral, dural, and extracranial arteries, sensitized to originate painful impulses by some mechanism yet to be determined, plays an important role in the pathophysiology of migraine headache. Some evidence shows that the migrainous process is generated centrally in the brain and brain stem, with vasodilation being a secondary phenomenon but one responsible for many of the characteristics of severe migraine headache.

REFERENCES

1. Knapp RDJ. Reports from the past. 2. *Headache* 1963;3:112.
2. Knapp RDJ. Reports from the past. 3. *Headache* 1964;3:143.
3. Wolff HG. *Headache and other head pain*. New York: Oxford University Press, 1963.
4. Fisher CM. Headaches in cerebrovascular disease. In: Vinken PJ, Bruyn GW, eds. *Handbook of clinical neurology*, vol 5. Amsterdam: North Holland, 1968;124–151.
5. Nichols FT, Mawad M, Mohr JP, Stein B, Hilal S, Michelsen WJ. Focal headache during balloon inflation in the internal carotid and middle cerebral arteries. *Stroke* 1990;21:555–559.
6. Martins IP, Baeta E, Paiva T, Campos J, Gomes L. Headaches during intracranial endovascular procedures: a possible model of vascular headache. *Headache* 1993;33:227–233.
7. Graham JR, Wolff HG. Mechanism of migraine headache and action of ergotamine tartrate. *Arch Neurol Psychiatry* 1938;39:737–763.
8. Tunis MM, Wolff HG. Long term observations of the reactivity of the cranial arteries in subjects with vascular headache of the migraine type. *Arch Neurol Psychiatry* 1953;70:551–557.
9. Blau JN, Dexter SL. The site of pain origin during migraine attacks. *Cephalalgia* 1981;1:143–147.
10. Drummond PD, Lance JW. Extracranial vascular changes and the source of pain in migraine headache. *Ann Neurol* 1983;13:32–37.
11. Goltman AM. The mechanism of migraine. *J Allergy* 1935;36:351–355.
12. Lance JW. Swelling at the site of a skull defect during migraine headache. *J Neurol Neurosurg Psychiatry* 1995;59:641.
13. Bonuso S, Marano E, Di Stasio E, Sorge F, Barbieri F, Ullucci EA. Source of pain and primitive dysfunction in migraine: an identical site? *J Neurol Neurosurg Psychiatry* 1989;52:1351–1354.
14. Thie A, Fuhlendorf A, Spitzer K, Kunze K. Transcranial Doppler evaluation of common and classic migraine. Part II. Ultrasonic features during attacks. *Headache* 1990;30:209–215.
15. Zwetsloot CP, Caekebeke JFV, Jansen JC, Odink J, Ferrari MD. Blood flow velocity changes in migraine attacks—a transcranial Doppler study. *Cephalalgia* 1991;11:103–107.
16. Zwetsloot CP, Caekebeke JFV, Jansen JC, Odink J, Ferrari MD. Blood flow velocities in the vertebrobasilar system during migraine attacks—a transcranial Doppler study. *Cephalalgia* 1992;12:29–32.
17. Friberg L, Olesen J, Iversen HK, Sperling B. Migraine pain associated with middle cerebral artery dilatation reversed by sumatriptan. *Lancet* 1991;338:13–17.
18. Thomsen LL, Iversen HK, Olesen J. Cerebral blood flow velocities are reduced during attacks of unilateral migraine without aura. *Cephalalgia* 1995;15:109–116.
19. Diener HC, Haab J, Peters C, Ried S, Dichgans J, Pilgrim A. Subcutaneous sumatriptan in the treatment of headache during withdrawal from drug-induced headache. *Headache* 1991;31:205–209.

20. Henkes H, May A, Kuhne JD, Berg-Dammer E, Diener HC. Sumatriptan: vasoactive effect on human dural vessels, demonstrated by subselective angiography. *Cephalalgia* 1996;16:224–230.
21. Caekebeke JFV, Ferrari, MD, Zwetsloot CP, Jansen J, Saxena PR. Antimigraine drug sumatriptan increases blood flow velocity in large cerebral arteries during migraine attacks. *Neurology* 1992;42:1522–1526.
22. Anthony M, Lance JW. Plasma serotonin in migraine and stress. *Arch Neurol* 1967;16:544–552.
23. Lance JW, Anthony M, Gonski A. Serotonin, the carotid body and cranial vessels in migraine. *Arch Neurol* 1967;16:553–558.
24. Goadsby PJ, Zagami AS, Lambert GA. Neural processing of craniovascular pain: a synthesis of the central structures involved in migraine. *Headache* 1991;31:365–371.
25. Haas DC, Kent PF, Friedman DI. Headache caused by a single lesion of multiple sclerosis in the periaqueductal gray area. *Headache* 1993;33:452–455.
26. Raskin NH, Hosobuchi Y, Lamb S. Headache may arise from perturbation of the brain. *Headache* 1987;27:416–420.
27. Veloso F, Kumar K. Deep brain implant migraine. *Neurology* 1996;46[suppl]:A168–169.
28. Weiller C, May A, Limmroth V, et al. Brainstem activation in spontaneous human migraine attacks. *Nature Med* 1995;1:658–660.
29. Goadsby PJ, Piper RD, Lambert GA, Lance JW. The effect of activation of the nucleus raphe dorsalis (DRN) on carotid blood flow. I. The monkey. *Am J Physiol* 1985;248:257–262.
30. Lance JW, Lambert GA, Goadsby PJ, Duckworth JW. Brainstem influences on the cephalic circulation: experimental data from cat and monkey of relevance to the mechanism of migraine. *Headache* 1983;23:258–265.
31. Lance, JW. *Mechanism and management of headache*, 5th ed. Portsmouth, NH: Butterworth-Heinemann, 1993.

Headache Pathogenesis: Monoamines, Neuropeptides, Purines, and Nitric Oxide, edited by J. Olesen and L. Edvinsson.
Lippincott–Raven Publishers, Philadelphia © 1997.

2

Neuropeptide Analysis

Past, Present, and Future

Rolf Ekman

Institute of Clinical Neuroscience, Department of Psychiatry and Neurochemistry, Göteborg University, Sahlgrenska University Hospital/Mölndal, S-431 80 Mölndal, Sweden

Over the past 25 years, a large number of biological active peptides have been recognized to exist within biological tissues and fluids. The biosynthesis of bioactive peptides starts from large preprohormones. In response to various stimuli, these undergo several transformation steps during biomaturation to active peptide before final degradation and inactivation (1). Neuropeptides are known to play important roles in brain function and may serve as a category of neurotransmitters and/or neuromodulators (2). Futhermore, they are also known to serve as messenger molecules in both the nervous and immune systems through specific receptors common to both systems (3). It is also conceivable that some peptides in the central nervous system are not only transmitters, but also control metabolism and critical functions in the brain. Although the role of the peptides in cellular communication/regulation is not well understood, they represent the most diverse class of transmitter molecules (4). Several recent studies have indicated an internalization and nuclear localization of neuropeptides (5–7). Because of these interesting observations, it is tempting to speculate (even though it may be too soon) that the nuclear peptides are involved in the regulation of transcription and/or that they may have a direct influence on the regulation of DNA (8,9).

RADIOIMMUNOASSAY OF NEUROPEPTIDES

After more than 20 years of experience, the standard method for the quantitative determination of neuropeptides is still radioimmunoassay (RIA) (10). Over the years numerous innovations and refinements have emerged. Each has advantages and disadvantages and may reflect to some extent a somewhat immature technology (11). Despite the obvious power of RIA, it is also clear from many reports in the literature that determination of neuropeptides in tissue extracts and body fluids presents many unresolved problems: (a) neuropeptides may be lost or altered by degradation during sampling; and (b) fragmentation, oxidation, etc., may occur either during storage before extraction, during extraction, or during storage following extraction. Different molecular forms of a neuropeptide may be differentially recovered during the extraction or differentially measured in the subsequent RIA (12). The problems outlined above are inherent in any test situation when one relies on one antiserum only. These problems can to some extent be restricted employing several region-specific antisera (13).

The levels of neuropeptides in tissue and body fluids are in the low pico- to femtomolar range. The peptides appear in several modified forms, which may cross-react to an unknown degree in the RIA. Hence, because of truncation, deamidation, oxidation, and many other chemical modifications, the heterogeneity of peptides is derived in vivo from native processing, while those derived in vitro from preparation artifacts raise problems in the interpretation of the results.

Leaving aside the obvious requirement of sensitivity, which tends to be an assay-specific issue, as well as specificity, the possibilities for separating various peptide fragments and structurally modified forms of the native peptide have been markedly improved by the introduction of reverse-phase, high-performance liquid chromatography (RP HPLC) (14–17). Nowdays RIA is almost exclusively used after prior separation of biological extracts by HPLC. However, the results from this technique are affected by the specificity of the antibody and thus yield an incomplete picture of the processing and chemical modifications of the neuropeptide.

For quantitative determinations of a neuropeptide, a standard curve using a reference calibrator is required. However, this method yields only semiquantitative results unless the cross-reactions of the whole entity of the neuropeptide-like peptides relative to the reference standard are known. Despite this drawback, the HPLC-RIA procedure still remains the method of choice for the "quantitation" of small amounts of peptide material in biological samples (18). Although this technology has enhanced our knowledge, a more specific assay system is needed providing structural information of the actual neuropeptide under investigation.

COMBINATION OF RADIOIMMUNOASSAY AND MASS SPECTROMETRY

Mass spectrometric techniques have long played an important role in the analysis of biological materials. Mass spectrometry (MS) linked to different chromatographic or electrophoretic techniques is the method of choice in up-to-date neurochemistry. It will reduce identification problems due to cross-reactions of structural, modified, peptide-like material frequently emerging in the RIAs. Characterization of neuropeptides in human cerebrospinal fluid using fast atom bombardment MS, for fractions separated by HPLC, has been reported (19,20).

Matrix-assisted laser desorption/ionization time-of-flight mass spectrometry (MALDI-TOF MS) is a relatively new technique and has been demonstrated to be a powerful analytical method for studying peptides and proteins. The strengths of MALDI-TOF MS include high sensitivity (picomole to low femtomole) and the ability to examine complex samples without requirement for extensive purification. It can be used without any sample pretreatment to study the in vitro processing of peptides directly in biological fluids, reflecting in vivo conditions during different pathological conditions. We have recently studied the processing of neuropeptide Y (NPY) in cerebrospinal fluid from patients with depression using MALDI-TOF MS. The results provide direct support for a phenotypic and selective processing rate of NPY, whereas other peptides do not evidence such proteolysis (21) (Fig. 1).

Using an approach based on microscale immunoaffinity, capture of target peptides in combination with MALDI-TOF MS followed by mass-specific identification and quantitation has recently been demonstrated (22). The most important as-

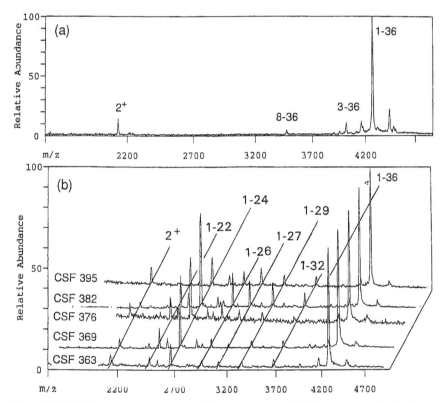

FIG. 1. MALDI-TOF mass spectra acquired for cerebrospinal (CSF) samples spiked with neuropeptide Y (NPY) (2.5 pmol/µl, 10 mM buffer, pH 7, after 18-hour incubation. **a:** Normal control. **b:** Five patients with the diagnosis of major depression. Numerical intervals above the peaks indicate amino acids residues retained from the original NPY sequence.
Reprinted from "Novel Neuropeptide Processing in Human Cerebrospinal Fluid from Depressed Patients," Rolf Ekman, in *Peptides* vol. 17, #7, p. 1107 (1996), with kind permission from Elsevier Science-NL, Sara Burgerhartstraat 25, 1055 KV Amsterdam, The Netherlands.

pect of such mass-specific detection is the ability to use a single assay to screen biological systems for the presence of multiple, mass-resolved antigens. Quantitation is possible by using a single antibody to capture both the intact peptide as well as different peptide variants that have been chemically modified.

CONCLUSIONS

It is too early to stop using sequence-specific RIA employing two antibodies directed to different epitopes as well as the combination of RP HPLC and subsequent RIA with different antibodies as a tool in clinical research as well as in some routine analysis. However, direct detection using MS offers several advantages over the indirect detection methods of conventional immunoassays. The most significant advantage of mass-resolved detection is the ability to analyze simultaneously for multiple peptides and their chemically modified versions in a single assay. MALDI-TOF MS will facilitate extensive investigations of neuropeptide metabolism that could provide the basis for clinical assays and could reflect new aspects of the pathophysiology of many diseases/disturbances related to the central nervous system as well as the peripheral nervous system. Finally, knowledge of the chemical structure of the peptide in cerebrospinal fluid could provide the basis for future attempts to develop improved clinical routine analysis.

ACKNOWLEDGMENTS

These studies were supported by the Swedish MRC (21X-07517), the Bank of Sweden Tercentenary Foundation (94-0388), and Eivind & Elsa K:son Sylvans Stiftelse.

REFERENCES

1. Hökfelt T. Neuropeptides in perspective: the last ten years. *Neuron* 1991;7:867–879.
2. Brownstein MJ. Neuropeptides. In: Siegel GJ, Agranoff BW, Albers WR, Molinoff PB, eds. *Basic neurochemistry: molecular, cellular, and medical aspects*. Lippincott–Raven, Philadelphia, 1994; 341–365.
3. Weigent DA, Blalock JE. Interaction between the neurocrine and immune system: common hormones and receptors. *Immunol Rev* 1987;100:79–108.
4. Hökfelt TGM, Castel M-N, Morino P, Zhang X, Dagerlind Å. General overview of neuropeptides. In: Bloom FE, Kupper DJ, eds. *Psychopharmacology: the fourth generation of progress*. Lippincott–Raven, Philadelphia, 1995;483–492.
5. Faure M-P, Shaw I, Gaudreau P, Cashman N, Beaudet A. Binding and internalization of neurotensin in hybrid cells derived from septal cholinergic neurons. In: Kitabgi P, Nemeroff CB, eds. *The neurobiology of neurotensin*. New York: The New York Academy of Science, 1992;668:345–347.
6. Ekman R, Servenius B, Castro MG, Lowry PJ, Cederlund A-S, Bergman O, Sjögren HO. Biosynthesis of corticotropin-releasing hormone in human T-lymphocytes. *J Neuroimmunol* 1993; 44:7–14.
7. Morel G. Internalization and nuclear localization of peptide hormones. *Biochem Pharmacol* 1994;47:63–76.
8. Tjian R. Molecular machines that control genes. *Sci Am* 1995;272:38–45.

9. Stanojeic D, Verdine GL. Deconstruction of GCN/4GCRE into a monomeric peptide-DNA complex. *Nature Struct Biol* 1995;2:450–457.
10. Rehfeld JF, Bardram L, Cantor P, Hilsted L, Johnsen AH. The unique specifity of antibodies in modern radioimmunochemistry—an essay on assay. *Scand J Clin Lab Invest* 1989; 49[Suppl 194]:41–44.
11. Hage DS. Immunoassays. *Anal Chem* 1995;67:455R–462R.
12. Ekman R. Radioimmunoassay of neuropeptides in the CSF. Problems and pitfalls. *Nord Pskiatr Tidsskr* 1985;Suppl 11:31–34.
13. Rehfeld JF. How to measure cholecystokinin in plasma? *Gastroenterology* 1984;87:434–438.
14. Bach FW, Ekman R, Jensen FM. β-Endorphin-immunoreative components in human cerebrospinal fluid. *Regul Pept* 1986;16:189–198.
15. Widerlöv E, Heilig M, Ekman R, Wahlestedt C. Neuropeptide Y—possible involvement in depression and anxiety. In: Mutt V, Hökfelt T, Fuxe K, Lundberg JM, eds. *Neuropeptide Y*. Lippincott–Raven, Philadelphia, 1989;331–342.
16. Edvinsson L, Ekman R, Thulin T. Increased plasma levels of neuropeptide Y-like immunoreactivity and catecholamines in severe hypertension remain after treatment to normotension in man. *Regul Pept* 1991;32:279–287.
17. Nilsson C, Karlsson G, Blennow K, Heilig M, Ekman R. Differences in the neuropeptide Y-like immunoreactivity of the plasma and platelets of human volunteers and depressed patients. *Peptides* 1996;17:359–362.
18. Toresson G, Brodin E, Wahlström A, Bertilsson L. Detection of N-terminally extended substance P but not of substance P in human cerebrospinal fluid: quantitation with HPLC-radioimmunassay. *J Neurochem* 1988;50:1701–1707.
19. Glämsta E-L, Nyberg F, Silberring J. Application of fast-atom bombardment mass spectrometry for sequencing of hemoglobin fragment, naturally occurring in human cerebrospinal fluid. *Rapid Commun Mass Spectrom* 1992;6:777–780.
20. Eriksson U, Andrén P, Silberring J, Nyberg F, Wiessel FA. Characterization of neurotensin-like immunoreactivity in human cerebrospinal fluid by high-performance liquid chromatography combined with mass spectrometry. *Biol Mass Spectrom* 1994;23:225–229.
21. Ekman R, Juhasz P, Heilig M, Ågren H, Costello CE. Novel neuropeptide Y processing in human cerebrospinal fluid from depressed patients. *Peptides* 1996;17:1107–1111.
22. Nelson RW, Krone JR, Bieber AL, Williams P. Mass spectrometric immunoassay. *Anal Chem* 1995;67:1153–1158.

3

Discussion Summary: General Aspects of Messenger Molecules—Localization, Methods for Measurement, Receptors, and Second Messengers

Peter J. Goadsby

Institute of Neurology, The National Hospital for Neurology and Neurosurgery, London WC1N 3BG, United Kingdom

Perhaps one of the oldest and still unresolved problems concerning the pathophysiology of migraine is the origin of the pain. During his introductory lecture Professor Lance covered both the historical and current data implicating blood vessels in the pathophysiology of migraine. The question of arterial hypertension and its relationship to headache arose in discussion. The point was made that rapid changes in pressure can induce headache, such as may be seen with pheochromocytoma, but that slowly evolving changes in blood pressure, such as is seen in primary hypertension, generally speaking do not cause headache. The interesting question of sex headache arose, and while it is clear that some patients with migraine have headache after orgasm, it remains unclear as to why so many patients with migraine, who may have orgasm, do not have headache. Certainly vasodilator agents, such as nitrates or ethanol, may induce headache. It is yet to be determined why sudden expansion of blood vessels is not necessarily a robust cause of headache in migraineurs.

A model for the pathophysiology of migraine is presented in Professor Lance's chapter. One of the problems identified with current models of migraine is the difficulty such a model may present in explaining the time cause of the evolution of the attack. Whereas most neurogenic phenomena occur soon after the stimuli, migraine can often take hours to develop after some biochemical challenge. It is certainly plausible that there are brain stem mechanisms that take some time to develop; in view of the clinical observations, there must be some plausible explanation for the delay. It is accepted that the basis for such a delay and the basis for the slowly developing aspects of the disease are not known at the moment.

There was discussion concerning the biological effects of endothelial-derived nitric oxide synthase (eNOS). Current directions include culturing human tissue, in particular lung tissue from patients with pulmonary hypertension, to examine the mechanisms by which the plexiform lesion and other structural changes in the affected lung may relate to the pathophysiology of the disease. Techniques such as oligonucleotide antisense probes are being used to inhibit synthesis of proteins selectively to determine their function in culture. Some remarks were directed to the genetic components of hypertension and recent data suggesting polymorphisms in the eNOS gene in arteriosclerotic patients. After heart/lung transplantation, with the removal of the affected lung, systemic hypertension apparently settles. This implies some local pathology or some local pathophysiological process particularly related to the lung. Whether this involves such mechanisms as the balance between endothelin and eNOS is uncertain. In patients with pulmonary hypertension it appears that eNOS is reduced whereas endothelin in the lung is increased. There are currently no data concerning endothelin receptors in the lung in these patients.

Some discussion concerned the methodology for measurement of neuropeptides. Some exiting new mass spectroscopy methods, including matrix-assisted laser desorption time-of-flight (MALD-TOF) mass spectroscopy were explored. The ability to differentiate structures on the basis of their charge and mass was emphasized and the utility of this as a research tool considered. The highly refined method of capillary electrophoresis, which offers the prospect of measuring small amounts of chemicals in the cerebrospinal fluid, was reviewed. It is important in the measurement of the neuropeptides to have not only radioimmunoassay determinations but also high-performance liquid chromatography characterization of the peptides. Mass spectroscopy then provides a further characterization of what is being measured. Such careful methodologies are important to avoid the problem of not measuring fragments of peptides that may have biological activity. Conversely, it is important that fragments determined by measurement techniques be tested in biological assays for their ability to have biological effects.

SECTION II

Messenger Molecules in Cranial Blood Vessels

Headache Pathogenesis: Monoamines, Neuropeptides, Purines, and Nitric Oxide, edited by J. Olesen and L. Edvinsson.
Lippincott–Raven Publishers, Philadelphia © 1997.

4

Messenger Molecules in the Cranial Sympathetic Nervous System

Lars Edvinsson

Department of Internal Medicine, Lund University Hospital, S-221 85 Lund, Sweden

Vascular resistance in regional circulatory beds is regulated by metabolic factors, chemical stimuli, perfusion pressure, and nerves. There always has been general agreement among investigators that the first three factors are important in regulation of the cerebral circulation (1). However, the contribution of neural stimuli to cerebrovascular control has been controversial, and it has only been in the last decade and a half that the importance of this mode of control has been fully appreciated, even though it is more than 300 years since Thomas Willis (1664) described nerve fiber profiles on the anterior and the posterior cerebral arteries. This was confirmed at the end of the 19th century by others, who noted that part of the perivascular fibers around the major vessels were sympathetic and originated in the superior cervical ganglion. Later observations amply supported this view using silver impregnation techniques (for review, see ref. 2). The development of the histofluorescence method made it possible to define in detail the origin, distribution, and identity of the sympathetic adrenergic innervation in cerebral vessels from various animals and the human. This was later extended by using immunocytochemistry with specific antibodies directed against either enzymes involved in the catecholamine synthesis (tyrosine hydroxylase or dopamine-β-hydroxylase) or neuropeptides. Studies of innervation pattern *in humans* clearly shows that the sympathetic innervation dominates markedly over the parasympathetic and the sensory innervation (3). A neural influence in the control of the cerebral circulation was suggested six decades ago, and now we know part of the role of the sympathetic nerves in the brain circulation; much still awaits to be elucidated, however, largely due to the many co-transmitters involved (4).

ANATOMY

Adrenergic Innervation

In general the sympathetic nerve fibers in the cerebral circulation consist of those neurons that innervate brain vessels and whose cell bodies are located mainly in the superior cervical ganglion, but to some degree also lower sympathetic ganglia such as the stellate ganglion. These postganglionic fibers form a well-developed plexus in cerebral arteries and arterioles in the adventia, and the nerve fiber seen at the adventia-medial border (5,6). The sympathetic nervous system arises in hypothalamic neurons and passes to the intermediolateral cell column of the spinal cord and synapse before proceeding out to the superior cervical ganglion.

Nielsen and Owman (5) were the first to give a comprehensive description of noradrenaline in perivascular nerve fibers of brain vessels. This was supported by a string of papers on different species using histochemistry and biochemistry (2). Arteries as well as veins receive a dense supply of adrenergic fibers. Small arterioles are sometimes accompanied by only one fiber; sympathetic nerve fibers have also been seen in the walls of intracerebral arteries with diameters down to 15 µm. In some species, cerebral vessels in caudal areas of the brain are supplied to a limited extent by fibers originating from sympathetic ganglia other than the superior cervical ganglia (7). In addition, innervation is highly heterogeneous. Innervation of arteries arising from the internal carotid system is denser than in vessels of the vertebral system. Approximately 60% to 90% of the arterioles in the medial geniculate body, parietal and temporal cortices, caudate nucleus, inferior colliculus, thalamus, and hypothalamus are innervated, in contrast to 10% to 30% of arterioles in the medulla, occipital cortex, and cerebellum (8). Variation in the density of innervation is suggestive of preferential sympathetic effects in certain areas of the brain. The general picture is that the nerve fibers may follow blood vessels for a short distance when they enter the cerebral tissue, and thus many intracerebral vessels appear to lack perivascular adrenergic nerves.

Removal of the superior cervical ganglion eliminates, mainly unilaterally, the sympathetic nerve fibers, as demonstrated by histochemistry and quantitative biochemistry. Labeled noradrenaline is taken up into the perivascular nerve terminals via a specific uptake mechanism that is absent after sympathetic denervation. Sympathetic stimulation, on the other hand, results in the release of noradrenaline from the perivascular nerves. This release can be modified by interaction with presynaptic α- and β-adrenoceptors, as well as by many other neurotransmitters, controlling the amount of released catecholamine (1).

Neuropeptide Y

An interesting finding is that neuropeptide Y (NPY) is co-localized with noradrenaline in sympathetic nerve endings in the cerebral as well as other parts of the

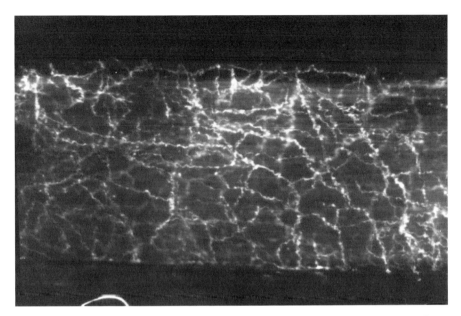

FIG. 1. Whole-mount preparation of rat cerebral artery demonstrating a ground plexus of neuropeptide Y-immunoreactive nerve fibers surrounding the blood vessel.

circulation (9–15). NPY, a 36-amino acid peptide with tyrosine at the N and C terminals, was first isolated from porcine brain by Tatemoto (16). This peptide has a wide distribution in the central and peripheral nervous system. NPY-containing perivascular nerves in the cerebral circulation were first observed in 1983 by immunocytochemistry and quantitative radioimmunoassay (10). The NPY fibers are particularly abundant around the major arteries at the base of the brain (Fig 1). The fibers show a dense network around cerebral cortical arteries, arterioles, and veins. NPY co-localizes with noradrenaline in the perivascular ground plexus.

Sympathectomy or treatment with 6-hydroxydopamine causes a marked decrease in the number of NPY-immunoreactive fibers and in the levels of NPY in cerebral blood vessels. Retrograde tracing using application of True Blue on the middle cerebral artery has resulted in the appearance of the tracer in ganglion cells of the superior cervical ganglion. Here NPY and True Blue co-localize with the noradrenaline-synthesizing enzymes: dopamine β-hydroxylase and tyrosine hydroxylase (17,18). This finding clearly demonstrates co-localization of the two neurotransmitters, noradrenaline and NPY, in the sympathetic nervous system innervating the cerebral circulation. Co-release of NPY could be involved in presynaptic or postsynaptic activities, such as control of neurotransmitter release or modulation of degree of constriction.

Neuropeptide Y expression has been found to be plastic, and environmental factors may trigger or suppress expression of specific genes (19). Both during development and in culture, neonatal sympathetic neurons start making acetylcholine and reduce synthesis of noradrenaline in response to target-derived signals (20). Sympathetic neurons that undergo such a cholinergic switch modify their neuropeptide expression; for example, sympathetic neurons innervating the sweat glands of neonatal rats acquire immunoreactivity for vasoactive intestinal peptide (VIP) and calcitonin gene-related peptide (CGRP) (20). In culture, superior cervical ganglion neurons increase their immunoreactivity for substance P, VIP, and somatostatin.

Postganglionic sympathectomy produces dramatic changes in innervation of target tissues, including a depletion of NPY and an increase in innervation by neuropeptide-containing sensory fibers. Thus, superior cervical ganglionectomy produces an increase of substance P and CGRP in the iris and ciliary body (21), and an increase of CGRP in rat cerebral vessels (22). In addition, sympathectomy may increase expression of "sympathetic" neuropeptides in parasympathetic ganglia; sympathetic ganglionectomy in the rat produces increased NPY expression in parasympathetic ganglia and in fibers innervating cerebral blood vessels (23). In addition, there are age- and disease-dependent changes in autonomic and sensory neuropeptides (13).

Ultrastructure

Electron microscopy early complemented these observations and extended our knowledge to include the organization of the nerve terminal region. Thus, varicosities containing electron-dense, granular vesicles, indicating adrenergic nerves, have been demonstrated in the walls of cerebral arteries (6,24,25). In addition, electron-lucent vesicles have been found, suggestive of nonadrenergic nerves. The terminals containing the electron-dense vesicles degenerate and disappear after surgical removal of the superior cervical ganglia, whereas terminals with electron-lucent vesicles remain. In feline cerebral arteries a thorough ultrastructural study observed the proportion of granular and agranular vesicles to be 40% and 60%, respectively. In the rabbit basilar artery the corresponding ratios were 98% and 2% (26,27). Both types of nerve terminals are separated from the smooth muscle cells by a distance of 80 to 90 nm, which is comparable with the terminal organization observed in peripheral blood vessels and fulfills accepted criteria for a functional innervation. The difference noted in nerve terminal organization and distribution of vesicles suggests a difference in the physiological role of the cerebrovascular autonomic nerves in various species as noted during transmural nerve stimulation. Furthermore, the two types of varicosities approach each other intimately to within 25 nm—thus the vasomotor nerves may interact at the terminal level (6).

Ultramorphological studies using immunoelectron microscopy demonstrated populations of vesicles in sympathetic nerves in blood vessel walls, one smaller, putatively noradrenergic, and one larger, showing immunoreactivity toward NPY. Thus, this morphological observation fits very well with the study by Fried and colleagues (28) separating on a biochemical mode the two vesicle populations and this was later illustrated by ultramorphology (29).

The choroid plexus is a specialized part of the brain circulation involved in the formation of cerebrospinal fluid (CSF). Both electron-dense and electron-lucent vesicles have been demonstrated in the choroid plexus (7). These nerve terminals closely approach the smooth muscle cells of both blood vessels and epithelial cells, suggesting a neural influence on CSF formation also.

Pharmacological Characterization of Cerebrovascular Adrenoceptors

A clear-cut demonstration and characterization of α- and β-adrenoceptors in cerebral blood vessels appeared in 1974 (30) for the cat and 2 years later for the human (31). The classical sympathomimetic agents (noradrenaline, adrenaline, and phenylephrine) contracted feline and human cerebral arterial segments with intact endothelium in a concentration-dependent manner. The response was blocked by phentolamine, piperoxane, dibenamine, and phenoxybenzamine, indicating the presence of an α-adrenoceptor. Subsequent studies have shown that oxymetazoline and clonidine (α_2-agonists) are potent agonists and that noradrenaline-induced contractions in feline cerebral arteries can be blocked by yohimbine and rauwolscine (α_2-blockers) but to a lesser extent than by prazosin (α_1-antagonist) (32). These investigations and other comparable studies have demonstrated the presence of α_2-adrenoceptor sites in feline and canine cerebral arteries. Interspecies variation appears to exist; the human, guinea pig, and rat have α_1-adrenoceptors, whereas the cat, dog, and rabbit have α_2-adrenoceptors (for review, see ref. 1). It has been suggested that vascular α_1-adrenoceptors are located at the neuron-effector junction while postsynaptic α_2-adrenoceptors are located extrajunctionally. This suggestion partly explains the dilatory responses obtained in cat and dog cerebral arteries during electrical field stimulation, since the α_2-adrenoceptors are considered to respond primarily to exogenously applied catecholamines. Furthermore, the rabbit basilar artery has a low degree of sensitivity to noradrenaline, whereas the rat basilar artery does not react when exposed to noradrenaline. Noradrenaline may also interact with β-adrenoceptor sites in cerebral vessels and thus dilation may be induced by sympathomimetic agents. This response can be shifted toward higher concentrations by propranolol and practolol, indicating the presence of a β-adrenoceptor of the β_1 type (30). Later studies have proposed that there is a mixture of β_1- and β_2-adrenoceptors in other species, e.g., in the human.

Peptidergic Receptors

Neuropeptide Y results in strong and potent constriction of cerebral arteries and veins in vitro and in vivo (Fig. 2). The responses are mediated via the NPY Y_1 subtype of receptors, as shown by agonist potency (NPY, Pro^{34}-NPY, NPY$_{13-36}$) and antagonist (α-trinositol and BIBP 3226) experiments as well as by reverse transcriptase polymerase chain reaction demonstration of the cloned human NPY Y_1-receptor

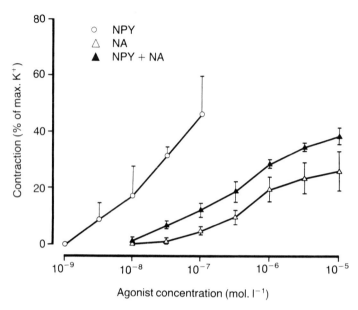

FIG. 2. Concentration-dependent contractions of human cerebral arteries with neuropeptide Y (NPY), noradrenaline alone (NA), and noradrenaline in the presence of 10^{-8} M neuropeptide Y. Mean value ± SEM.

(11,13,33,34). The responses to noradrenaline and NPY are mediated via influx of intracellular calcium, increase in inositol phosphate turnover, reduction in adenylyl cyclase activity, and increase in intracellular calcium, which all result in binding of actin and myosin filaments, and subsequent constriction (Fig. 3). In addition, NPY in cerebral vessels can antagonize the effects of substance P and acetylcholine, possibly via an NPY Y_1-receptor (35,36).

It has frequently been shown in many mammals, including humans, that cerebral arteries are more sensitive to depletion of extracellular calcium and to "calcium antagonists" than peripheral arteries during activation with a depolarizing solution (e.g., potassium ions). In studies comparing rabbit basilar and ear arteries, it was found that the basilar artery primarily utilizes extracellular calcium ions during activation with noradrenaline, while the ear artery uses an additional tightly bound intracellular pool of calcium (37). Therefore, when extracellular calcium is removed from the tissue bath, the rate of decline in both the rapid transient contraction and the slower contractile component of the arterial response to noradrenaline is faster in the basilar artery than in the ear artery. Administration of a "calcium antagonist" leads to complete relaxation of constricted cerebral arteries (38,39). These observations would indicate that only small calcium pools exist in cerebral arteries. The vessels are thus extremely dependent on an adequate supply of extracellular calcium for their activation, a fact worthy of contemplation when designing treatments of disorders in which there is supposedly an intense constriction of cranial arteries.

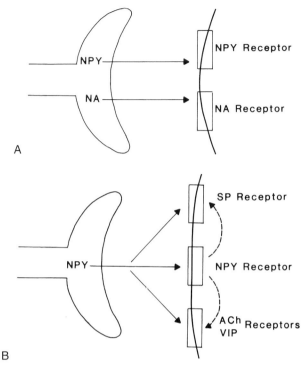

FIG. 3. Modes of interaction between noradrenaline (NA) and neuropeptide Y (NPY) shown for the cerebral circulation: a direct effect on the NPY Y_1-receptors (**A**) and inhibition of relaxant responser to substance P (SP) and acetylcholine (ACh) (**B**). VIP, vasoactive intestinal peptide.

Responses of the Cerebral Microcirculation

In Situ

Upon sympathetic nerve stimulation, arteries and veins constrict in a frequency-dependent manner (40,41). The response is more pronounced and appears to last longer in veins than in arteries. The microapplication of noradrenaline around an individual pial vessel results in a dose-dependent constriction of both arteries and veins. Similarly, the effect is more pronounced in veins than in arteries—with regard to maximum contraction and to sensitivity (42). The responses of cerebral arteries and veins to sympathetic nerve stimulation or microapplication of noradrenaline are markedly attenuated by α-adrenoceptor antagonists such as phentolamine, phenoxybenzamine, and yohimbine. These investigations in vivo support the existence of an α-adrenoceptor of a character similar to that found in studies of isolated cerebral vessel segments. The constriction obtained in situ after sympathetic nerve stimulation is in contrast to the data in vitro during electrical field stimulation. This can, however, be explained by the selectivity of the stimulation. Thus, stimulation of the superior cervical ganglion causes release of noradrenaline and NPY, whereas field stimulation in vitro may release several other transmitters from parasympathetic and sensory nerves. Isoproterenol has been found to induce a slight dilation, indicative of the presence of β-adrenoceptors. Taken together, ample evidence demonstrates the presence of a contractile α-adrenoceptor and a dilatatory β-adrenoceptor in situ.

Is there any physiological evidence for the existence of a transmitter role for NPY? Stimulation of the superior cervical ganglion in situ results in constriction of cerebral arteries and veins, which can only in part be blocked by α-adrenoceptor antagonists (43). Thus, these indirect data give support for an additional signal substance in the sympathetic nerve fibers, but the final conclusion awaits the experiments with selective NPY blockers (e.g., BIBP 3226).

PHYSIOLOGICAL EFFECTS

As outlined in the volume by Edvinsson et al. (1), experiments to unravel the influence of the sympathetic perivascular nerves in the cerebral circulation have been extensive, but only after critical analysis of the methodology has a clear picture emerged. Administration of sympathetic agonists or antagonists, and stimulation or denervation of the sympathetic nerves have (at normotension and normocapnia) mainly resulted in weak (5% to 15%) or no effects at all on resting cerebral blood flow. Even though stimulation or denervation of the sympathetic nerves only marginally changes resting cerebral blood flow, these nerves have marked effects on cerebral blood volume, i.e., cerebral capacitance, intracranial pressure, and cerebral spinal fluid formation.

Amines may, under some conditions, increase the cerebral perfusion. Thus, when noradrenaline or adrenaline is given systemically in sufficient amounts, an increase in cerebral blood flow is observed concomitantly with an enhanced cerebral metabolism. The effect is probably due to an action of the sympathomimetics on cerebral neurons, resulting in an enhanced metabolism and increase in flow (44). This effect is, however, achieved only when the amines increase the arterial blood pressure to such a degree that the integrity of the blood-brain barrier is changed. Thus, this response to the catecholamines is not found when the hypertensive action is abolished. Similarly, cerebral blood flow increases are obtained when noradrenaline is administered in a way that circumvents the blood-brain barrier, e.g., given intraventricularly or after disruption of the blood-brain barrier by a hypertonic solution.

Stimulation In Vitro

Despite the dense innervation by sympathetic nerves, considerable confusion has existed as to the detailed responses to transmural nerve stimulation, which differs greatly from those seen in peripheral vessels; considerable species variation also exists (1). Rabbit basilar arteries constrict in response to transmural nerve stimulation, but the response is resistant to α-adrenergic antagonists. However, the constrictor response is abolished by chronic reserpinization, bilateral superior cervical gangliectomy, or cold storage. The data imply a response mediated via sympathetic adrenergic neurons but not by noradrenalin. Both adenosine triphosphate and NPY have been suggested as candidate mediator molecules. Studies have revealed a somewhat wider synaptic cleft in cerebral vessels compared with other vessels. On the other hand, transmural nerve stimulation in the cat causes dilation. This seems to be mediated via perivascular peptides that mainly mediate relaxation.

In Vivo

Topical application of noradrenaline and electrical stimulation of sympathetic nerves have been used to simulate reflex activation; these interventions presumably produce near-maximal effects on cerebral vessels. During baseline conditions in anesthetized animals, topical application of noradrenaline is a constrictor agent of arteries and veins; these effects are blocked with typical α-adrenoceptor antagonists (41,42). The stimulation of the superior cervical trunk in the cat results in constriction of cerebral arterioles with a diameter >100 μm, but there is no change in vessels of smaller diameter. This effect can be attenuated by α-adrenergic antagonism. It is quite interesting that cerebral veins appear to constrict more than arterioles on sympathetic stimulation (40). This is supported by microapplication of noradrenaline, which constricts cerebral veins more potently than arterioles (42). This finding correlates with the effects on intracranial capacitance.

Cerebral blood volume has received little attention in the past. However, sympathetic nerve stimulation or the systemic administration of either noradrenaline or tyramine may reduce cerebral blood volume by about 20% (45,46). This response is attenuated by the α-adrenoceptor antagonists phentolamine and phenoxybenzamine. Cerebral blood volume and intracranial pressure are enhanced after sympathectomy. Furthermore, sympathetic nerve stimulation may concomitantly reduce intracranial pressure (46) and constrict cerebral arteries and veins, indicating a role in the regulation of cerebral capacitance (40,43).

During normotension, electrical stimulation of sympathetic pathways causes constriction of cerebral arterioles and reduces cerebral blood flow in some species (40,47–51). Thus, species differences exist in cerebrovascular responsiveness to sympathetic nerve stimulation. In the cat, sympathetic stimulation constricts pial arterioles, but cerebral blood flow fails to fall because of compensatory downstream dilation (52). To understand better how sympathetic nerves may influence the cerebral circulation, stimulation or denervation of the superior cervical ganglion has been performed in conjunction with manipulation of other regulatory principles. A larger decrease in cerebral blood flow is seen during hypercapnic dilation, since the vessels are markedly dilated, and a larger response is unravelled. The converse is seen during hypocapnia.

Autoregulation

Marked hypertension, beyond the upper limits of autoregulation, results in a flow increase that varies passively with the arterial blood pressure. This "breakthrough" leads to the formation of edema and, rarely, intracerebral hemorrhage. Sympathetic nerve stimulation may extend the upper limit of the autoregulation and thus protect the brain against such damage. The confines of the lower limit of autoregulation—when tested by hemorrhagic hypotension—may be extended toward lower levels by acute sympathectomy or by administration of α-adrenoceptor blockers (53,54). Whereas acute denervation may shift the lower limit of the autoregulation toward lower blood pressure levels (55–57), chronic sympathetic denervation does not shift the limits of autoregulation (1). The shift of the upper limit of cerebral autoregulation toward higher pressure during the sympathetic activation is probably a physiological mechanism protecting the brain against the damage that may occur when the blood pressure is increased due to a general sympathetic activation (Fig. 4). In con-

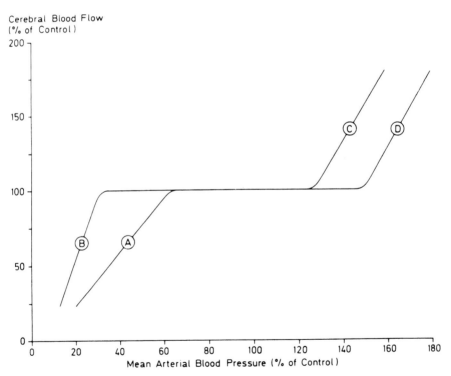

FIG. 4. Effect of stimulation of the sympathetic nerves on autoregulation of cerebral blood flow. Lines A and C, control; line D, during sympathetic stimulation; line B, during sympathetic blockade. In the autoregulatory range, and sympathetic constriction extends the upper limit of autoregulation. At a lower end sympathetic constriction may counterbalance the autoregulatory dilation, hence blockade may extend it further toward the left.

scious animals the upper limit of autoregulation is considerably more difficult to reach because of a concomitant sympathetic activation.

Thus, the sympathetic nerves may have a protective effect that acts to defend the brain from damage in acute hypertension. The transmitters and receptors involved have been verified by studies using specific adrenoceptor antagonists and an NPY blocker (58), which can in part block the response. The studies thus show that noradrenaline and NPY are both active as mediators for vasoconstriction in acute hypertension. Furthermore, this is supported by neuropathology studies showing that sympathetic denervation may enhance the damage to the brain in situations of experimentally raised perfusion pressure.

Reductions in blood pressure within the physiological range are often associated with a low sympathetic tone. Consequently, a tendency to a shift toward lower pressure of the autoregulation curve affords some protection to the brain against hypertension-induced ischemia. In another setting, the sympathetic tone is not low at low blood pressures but may in some instances be high, for example, during hemorrhagic hypotension. Here a resulting upper shift of the lower limit of autoregulation is not advantageous for the brain but is rather related to general regulatory mechanisms of the body in response to shock. In experimental hemorrhage hypotension, blockade of sympathetic adrenergic receptors or acute denervation can result in a shift of the lower limits of autoregulation toward lower levels of blood pressure (53,54).

A marked cerebrovascular hypertrophy, which is attenuated by sympathetic denervation, has been found in stroke-prone, spontaneously hypertensive rats (59). This vascular hypertrophy may protect cerebral vessels by reducing the wall stress. It has been speculated that the sympathetic nerves not only have a trophic influence on cerebrovascular smooth muscle in chronic hypertension but also serve to protect against stroke in the presence of severe hypertension (60).

Sympathetic Influence on Choroid Plexus Function

Studies of intracranial pressure, cerebral blood volume, and CSF production have all revealed that the sympathetic nerves can indeed have a significant role in intracranial pressure regulation. This has been interpreted as due to the positive effects on cerebral capacitance (cerebral blood volume) and CSF production.

The observation of adrenergic nerve fibers in the choroid plexus suggests a neurogenic influence on the vascular bed and the secretory epithelium (61). Since blood flow through the choroid plexus may be a rate-limiting factor influencing CSF formation, the reactivity to catecholamines in isolated choroidal arteries has been examined. These vessels were found to be supplied with both α- and β-adrenoceptors. However, as choroid plexus blood flow appears not to change during electrical stimulation of the superior cervical ganglion, the vasomotor influence in situ of the sympathetic nerves does not seem to be of major significance.

Direct evidence for a physiological effect of the sympathetic nerves on the secretory epithelium of the choroid plexus has been obtained by quantitative determina-

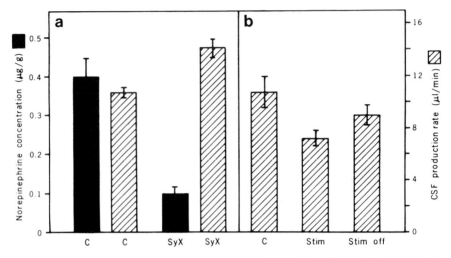

FIG. 5. a: At 1 week following sympathetic denervation (SyX) of rabbit choroid plexus, marked reductions in norepinephrine concentration concomitant with highly significant increase in rate of CSF production compared with unoperated controls (C) were observed. Differences between mean values (± SEM) according to Student's t-test: $p < 0.001$ in both groups. **b:** CSF production rate before (C) and during bilateral electrical stimulation of superior cervical ganglia (Stim), which markedly reduces rate of production (difference, based on paired observations, was highly significant: ($p < 0.001$). After stimulation was stopped (Stim off), production rate tended to normalize (Stim vs. Stim off: $p = 0.01$). Vertical brackets denote means ± SEM.

tions of carbonic anhydrase activity, which is an enzyme considered to be of importance for the production of CSF; it increases by 25% to 50% after either superior cervical sympathectomy or injection of reserpine. These findings were the first to indicate that sympathetic innervation has an inhibitory role on carbonic anhydrase activity and probably on CSF production (7).

The ventriculocisternal perfusion technique of Pappenheimer is a dynamic method for studying the influence of the sympathetic nerves on the rate of CSF production. The mean production rate of CSF is decreased by about 30% following intermittent electrical stimulation of the sympathetic trunks in the neck (62). After the stimulation has been discontinued, the production rate of CSF returns toward baseline conditions (Fig. 5).

Bilateral excision of the superior cervical ganglia, which produces extensive sympathetic denervation of the choroid plexus, results in an increase by about 30% of the bulk CSF production when compared with a control group. These results are in agreement with the enhanced carbonic anhydrase activity in the choroid plexus noted after sympathectomy and with direct measurement of the intracranial pressure (46,63).

Intraventricular perfusion with noradrenaline in increasing concentrations results in a dose-related reduction of CSF production. This reduction is attenuated both by the α-adrenoceptor antagonist phentolamine and by the β-adrenoceptor inhibitor

TABLE 1. *Effects of sympathetic nerves on the cerebrovascular bed in situ*

Constriction of pial arteries and veins
Decrease of cerebral blood flow and cerebral blood volume
Decrease of cerebrospinal fluid formation
Decrease of intracranial pressure
Protection against "breakthrough" of autoregulation in acute hypertension
Trophic influence on cerebrovascular smooth muscle in chronic hypertension

propranolol. The results suggest that both α- and β-adrenoceptors are involved in regulation of CSF production (62).

CONCLUSIONS

Cerebral vessels are innervated by sympathetic, parasympathetic, and sensory fibers. The sympathetic nerves constitute the richest innervation of the cerebral circulation, in arteries, arterioles, and veins. Activation of these nerves elicits a number of effects, summarized in Table 1. The most important effects seem to be those of modulation of autoregulation and control of intracranial pressure, blood volume, and CSF production.

REFERENCES

1. Edvinsson L, MacKenzie ET, McCulloch J. *Cerebral blood flow and metabolism.* Lippincott–Raven, Philadelphia, 1993;1–683.
2. Edvinsson L. Neurogenic mechanisms in the cerebral circulation. Autonomic nerves, amine receptors and their effects on cerebral blood flow. *Acta Physiol Scand Suppl* 1975;427:1–35.
3. Edvinsson L, Jansen I, Cunha e Sa M, Gulbenkian S. Demonstration of neuropeptide containing nerves and vasomotor responses to perivascular peptides in human cerebral arteries. *Cephalalgia* 1994;14:88–96.
4. Benarroch EE. Neuropeptides in the sympathetic system: presence, plasticity, modulation, and implications. *Ann Neurol* 1994;36:6–13.
5. Nielsen KC, Owman C. Adrenergic innervation of pial arteries related to the circle of Willis in the cat. *Brain Res* 1967;6:773–776.
6. Edvinsson L, Nielsen KC, Owman C, Sporrong B. Cholinergic mechanisms in pial vessels. *Z Zellforsch* 1972;134:311–325.
7. Edvinsson L, Håkanson M, Lindvall, M, Owman C, Svensson KG. Ultrastructural and biochemical evidence for a sympathetic neural influence on the choroid plexus. *Exp Neurol* 1975;48:241–251.
8. Edvinsson L, Owman C. Sympathetic innervations and adrenergic receptors in intraparenchymal cerebral arteries of baboon. In: Ingvar DH, Lassen, NA, eds. *Proceedings of the 8th International Symposium on Cerebral Function, Metabolism and Circulation.* Copenhagen: Munksgard, 1977; 403–405.
9. Allen JM, Schon F, Todd N, Yeats JC, Crockard HA, Bloom SR. Presence of neuropeptide Y in human circle of Willis and its possible role in cerebral vasospasm. *Lancet* 1984;1:550–552.
10. Edvinsson L, Emson P, McCulloch J, Tatemoto K, Uddman R. Neuropeptide Y: cerebrovascular innervation and vasomotor effects in the cat. *Neurosci Lett* 1983;43:79–84.
11. Edvinsson L, Emson P, McCulloch J, Tatemoto K, Uddman R. Neuropeptide Y: immunocytochemical localization to and effect upon feline pial arteries and veins *in vitro* and *in situ*. *Acta Physiol Scand* 1984;122:155–163.

12. Edvinsson L, Copeland JR, Emson PC, McCulloch J, Uddman R. Nerve fibers containing neuropeptide Y in the cerebrovascular bed: immunocytochemistry, radioimmunoassay and vasomotor effects. *J Cereb Blood Flow Metab* 1987;7:45–57.
13. Edvinsson L, Ekman R, Jansen I, Ottosson A, Uddman R. Peptide-containing nerve fibers in human cerebral arteries: immunocytochemistry, radioimmunoassay and *in vitro* pharmacology. *Ann Neurol* 1987;21:432–437.
14. Nakakita K. Peptidergic innervation in the cerebral blood vessels of the guinea pig: an immunohistochemical study. *J Cereb Blood Flow Metab* 1990;10:819–826.
15. Uddman R, Ekbland R, Edvinsson L, Håkanson R, Sundler F. Neuropeptide Y-like immunoreactivity in perivascular nerve fibers of guinea-pig. *Regul Pept* 1985;10:243–257.
16. Tatemoto K. Neuropeptide Y. Complete amino acid sequence of the brain peptide. *Proc Natl Acad Sci USA* 1982;79:5485–5489.
17. Edvinsson L, Hara H, Uddman R. Retrograde tracing of nerve fibers to the rat middle cerebral artery with true blue: colocalization with different peptides. *J Cereb Blood Flow Metab* 1989;9:212–218.
18. Suzuki N, Hardebo JE, Kåhrström J, Owman C. Neuropeptide Y coexists with vasoactive intestinal polypeptide in parasympathetic cerebrovascular nerves originating in the sphenopalatine, otic and internal carotid ganglia of the rat. *Neuroscience* 1990;36:507–519.
19. Zigmond RE, Hyatt-Sachs H, Baldwin C, et al. Phenotypic plasticity in adult sympathetic neurons: changes in neuropeptide expression in organ culture. *Proc Natl Acad Sci (USA)* 1992;89:1507–1511.
20. Landis SC. Neurotransmitter plasticity in sympathetic neurons. In: *Handbook of chemical neuroanatomy: the peripheral nervous system*, vol 6. Amsterdam: Elsevier, 1988;65–115.
21. Cole DF, Bloom SR, Burnstock G, et al. Increase in SP-like immunoreactivity in nerve fibres of rabbit iris and ciliary body one to four months following sympathetic denervation. *Exp Eye Res* 1983; 37:191–197.
22. Schon F, Ghatei M, Allen JM, et al. The effect of sympathectomy on calcitonin gene-related peptide levels in the rat trigeminovascular system. *Brain Res* 1985;348:197–200.
23. Björklund H, Hökfelt T, Goldstein M, et al. Appearance of the noradrenergic markers tyrosine hydroxylase and neuropeptide Y in cholinergic nerves of the iris following sympathectomy. *J Neurosci* 1985;5:1633–1640.
24. Nielsen KC, Owman C, Sporrong B. Ultrastructure and the autonomic innervation apparatus in the main pial arteries of rats and cats. *Brain Res* 1971;27:25–32.
25. Nelson E, Rennels M. Neuromuscular contacts in intracranial arteries of the cat. *Science* 1970; 167:301–302.
26. Lee TJ-F, Saito A. Vasoactive intestinal polypeptide-like substance: the potential transmitter for cerebral vasodilatation. *Science* 1981;224:898–901.
27. Lee TJ-F, Sarwinski S. Nitric oxidergic neurogenic vasodilatation in porcine basilar artery. *Blood Vessels* 1991;28:407–412.
28. Fried G, Terenius L, Hökfelt T, Goldstein M. Evidence for differential localization of noradrenaline and neuropeptide Y (NPY) in neuronal storage vesicles isolated from rat vas deference. *J Neurosci* 1985;5:450–458.
29. Jansen Olesen I, Edvinsson L, et al. The peptidergic innervation of the human superficial temporal artery: immunohistochemistry, ultrastructure and vasomotility. *Peptides* 1995;16:275–287.
30. Edvinsson L, Owman C. Pharmacological characterization of adrenergic alpha and beta receptors mediating the vasomotor responses of cerebral arteries in vitro. *Circ Res* 1974;35:835–849.
31. Edvinsson L, Owman C, Sjöberg N. O. Autonomic nerves, mast cells, and amine receptors in human brain vessels. A histochemical and pharmacological study. *Brain Res* 1976;15:377–393.
32. Skärby TVC, Andersson K-E, Edvinsson L. Pharmacological characterization of postjunctional α-adrenoceptors in isolated feline cerebral and peripheral arteries. *Acta Physiol Scand* 1983;117:63–73.
33. Nilsson T, Cantera L, Edvinsson L. Presence of neuropeptide Y Y_1 receptor mediating vasoconstriction in human cerebral arteris. *Neurosci Lett* 1996;204:145–148.
34. Abounader R, Villemure JG, Hamel E. Characterization of neuropeptide Y (NPY) receptors in human cerebral arteries with selective agonists and the new Y_1 antagonist BIBP 3226. *Br J Pharm* 1995;116:2245–2250.
35. Fallgren B, Ekblad E, Edvinsson L. Co-existence of neuropeptide and differential inhibition of vasodilator responses by neuropeptide Y in guinea-pig uterine arteries. *Neurosci Lett* 1989;1900:71–76.
36. Nilsson T, You J, Sun X, et al. Characterization of neuropeptide Y receptors mediating contraction, potentiation and inhibition of relaxation. *Blood Pressure* 1996;5:164–169.
37. McCalden TA, Bevan JA. Sources of activator calcium in rabbit basilar artery. *Am J Physiol* 1981;241:H129–H133.

38. Brandt L, Andersson KE, Edvinsson L, Ljunggren B. Effect of extracellular calcium and of calcium antagonists on the contractile responses of isolated human pial and mesenteric arteries. *J Cereb Blood Flow Metab* 1981;1:339–347.
39. Edvinsson L. Characterization of the contractile effect of neuropeptide Y in feline cerebral arteries. *Acta Physiol Scand* 1985;125:33–41.
40. Auer L, Johansson BB, Lund S. Reaction of pial arteries and veins to sympathetic stimulation in the cat. *Stroke* 1981;12:528–531.
41. Kuschinsky W, Wahl M. α-Receptor stimulation by endogenous and exogenous noradrenaline and blockade by phentolamine in pial arteries in cats. A microapplication study. *Circ Res* 1975;37:168–174.
42. Edvinsson L, McCulloch J, Uddman R. Feline cerebral veins and arteries: comparison of autonomic innervation and vasomotor responses. *J Physiol (Lond)* 1982;325:161–173.
43. Auer L, Edvinsson L, Johansson BB. Effect of sympathetic nerve stimulation and adrenoceptor blockade on pial arterial and venous calibre and on intracranial pressure in the cat. *Acta Physiol Scand* 1983;119:213–217.
44. MacKenzie ET, McCulloch J, O'Keane M, Pickard JD, Harper AM. Cerebral circulation and norepinephrine: Relevance of the blood-brain barrier. *Am J Physiol* 1976;231:483–488.
45. Edvinsson L, Nielsen KC, Owman C, West KA. Sympathetic adrenergic influence on brain vessels as studied by changes in cerebral blood volume of mice. *Eur Neurol* 1971/72;6:193–202.
46. Edvinsson L, Lindvall M, Owman C, West KA. Autonomic nervous control of cerebrospinal fluid production and intracranial pressure. In: Wood JH, ed. *Neurobiology of cerebrospinal fluid*, vol 2. New York: Plenum, 1983;661–676.
47. Wei EP, Raper AJ, Kontos HA, Patterson JL Jr. Determinants of response of pial arteries to norepinephrine and sympathetic nerve stimulation. *Stroke* 1975;6:654–658.
48. Sercombe R, Lacombe P, Aubineau P, et al. Is there an active mechanism limiting the influence of the sympathetic system on the cerebral vascular bed? Evidence for vasomotor escape from sympathetic stimulation in the rabbit. *Brain Res* 1979;164:81–102.
49. Busija DW, Heistad DD, Marcus ML. Effects of sympathetic nerves on cerebral vessels during acute, moderate increases in arterial pressure in dogs and cats. *Circ Res* 1980;46:696–702.
50. Heistad DD, Marcus ML. Effects of sympathetic nerves on cerebral vessels in dog, cat, and monkey. *Am J Physiol* 1978;235:H544–H552.
51. Gross PM, Heistad DD, Strait MR, et al. Cerebral vascular responses to physiological stimulation of sympathetic pathways in cats. *Circ Res* 1979;44:288–294.
52. Baumbach BL, Heistad DD. Effects of sympathetic stimulation and changes in arterial pressure on segmental resistance of cerebral vessels in rabbits and cats. *Circ Res* 1983;52:527–533.
53. Edvinsson L, MacKenzie ET, Robert J-P, et al. Cerebrovascular responses to haemorrhagic hypotension in anaesthetized cats. Effects of α-adrenoceptor anatagonists. *Acta Physiol Scand* 1985;123:317–323.
54. Fitch W, MacKenzie ET, Harper AM. Effects of decreasing arterial blood pressure on cerebral blood flow in the baboon. Influence of the sympathetic nervous system. *Circ Res* 1975;37:550–557.
55. Edvinnson L, Owman C, Siesjö BK. Physiological role of cerebrovascular sympathetic nerves in the autoregulation of cerebral blood flow. *Brain Res* 1976;117:519–523.
56. Bill A, Linder J. Sympathetic control of cerebral blood flow in acute arterial hypertension. *Acta Physiol Scand* 1976;96:114–121.
57. MacKenzie ET, McGeorge AP, Graham DI, Fitch W, Edvinsson L, Harper AM. Effects of increasing arterial pressure of cerebral blood flow in the baboon: influence of the sympathetic nervous system. *Pflugers Arch* 1979;378:189–195.
58. Goadsby PJ, Edvinsson L. Examination of the involvement of neuropeptide Y (NPY) in cerebral autoregulation using the novel NPY antagonist PP56. *Neuropeptides* 1993;24:27–33.
59. Hart MN, Heistad DD, Broby MJ. Effect of chronic hypertension and sympathetic denervation on wall-lumen ratio of cerebral arteries. *Hypertension* 1980;2:419–423.
60. Sadoshima S, Busija DW, Heistad DD. Mechanisms of protection against stroke in stroke-prone spontaneously hypertensive rats. *Am J Physiol* 1983;244:H406–H412.
61. Edvinsson L, Nielsen KC, Owman C, West KA. Adrenergic innervation of the mammalian choroid plexus. *Am J Anat* 1974;139:299–308.
62. Lindvall M, Edvinsson L, Owman C. Sympathetic nervous control of cerebrospinal fluid production from the choroid plexus. *Science* 1978;201:176–178.
63. Lindvall M, Edvinsson L, Owman C. Effect of sympathomimetic drugs and corresponding receptor antagonists on the rate of cerebrospinal fluid production. *Exp Neurol* 1979;64:132–145.

5

Messenger Molecules in the Cranial Parasympathetic Nervous System

Rolf Uddman and *Anders Luts

*Department of Otorhinolaryngology, Malmö University Hospital, S-205 02 Malmö, Sweden; and *Departments of Physiology and Neuroscience, and Psychiatry, University of Lund, S-221 85 Lund, Sweden*

The autonomic nervous system plays an important role in the regulation of regional blood flow to cranial structures as evidenced by the rich supply of nerve fibers around most blood vessels. The classical neurotransmitter in the sympathetic component, norepinephrine, has been mapped in several species by catecholamine histofluorescence. The classical transmitter in the parasympathetic component, acetylcholine (ACh), has been more difficult to map due to shortcomings in the methods available. In recent years, an increasing number of neurotransmitter candidates have been discovered in the autonomic nervous system and, in particular, the parasympathetic component. Many of these transmitters are small peptides. Immunocytochemical studies have revealed that cranial blood vessels are surrounded by numerous nerve fibers containing different neurotransmitters that derive from parasympathetic ganglia.

The parasympathetic fibers arise from the superior salivatory nucleus and travel in the facial (seventh cranial) nerve through the otic and sphenopalatine ganglia. The origin of nerve fibers surrounding cranial blood vessels has been assessed in the rat by tracing studies and denervations. Such studies have revealed that most parasympathetic fibers to cranial arteries derive from the sphenopalatine and otic ganglia (1–3). In addition, it has been suggested that at least some of the fibers derive from local microganglia in, for example, the cavernous plexus and external rete.

ACETYLCHOLINE

The classical postganglionic neurotransmitter in the parasympathetic nervous system is ACh, and for several years parasympathetic innervation of cranial structures was defined as cholinergic. Acetylcholinesterase (AChE) staining has been used to delineate cholinergic fibers, and histological studies have shown a rich supply of

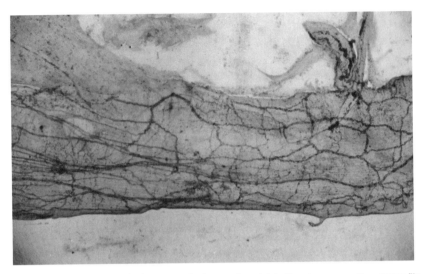

FIG. 1. Cat cerebral artery, whole mount. A plexus of acetylcholinesterase-positive nerve fibers surrounds the artery.

AChE-positive nerve fibers around large cerebral blood vessels in both animals (Fig. 1) and humans (4–6). Immunochemical studies have revealed ACh, acetylcholine transferase, and AChE in cerebral blood vessels from laboratory animals (7–10). In addition, cerebral blood vessels possess a temperature- and time-dependent uptake mechanism for [^{3}H]choline (8). Transmural nerve stimulation or application of potassium release [^{3}H]choline from cerebral arteries (11,12). Cholinomimetic agents, such as ACh and carbacholine, dilate most cerebral blood vessels by an atropine-sensitive mechanism (13). This effect is mediated via the release of an endothelium-derived relaxing factor now thought to be nitric oxide.

VASOACTIVE INTESTINAL PEPTIDE

Vasoactive intestinal peptide (VIP) is a 28-amino acid peptide belonging to a family of regulatory peptides that includes hormones such as secretin and glucagon. VIP is encoded by a large precursor molecule that, in addition, encodes peptide histidine isoleucine (PHI). In humans, the corresponding peptide is peptide histidine methionine, differing from PHI by having methionine in the C-terminal position instead of isoleucine. The distribution of PHI is identical to that of VIP, and double immunostaining has shown that VIP and PHI are co-localized in nerve cell bodies in parasympathetic ganglia. Neurons in these ganglia contain, in addition, AChE and choline acetyltransferase and are thus considered cholinergic (14). Further, a moderate supply of nerve cell bodies in parasympathetic ganglia contain neuropeptide Y (NPY), which is co-localized with VIP. Immunocytochemistry has revealed varying amounts of nerve fibers containing VIP in the cardiovascular system. Generally, arteries have a rich supply whereas veins have a scarcer supply (15,16). Cerebral blood vessels are richly invested by VIP-containing fibers (17–19). High concentrations of VIP are found in feline and porcine pial vessels. Also, a population of the NPY-containing fibers that surround pial arteries is co-localized with VIP (20). The functional significance of this co-localization remains to be investigated.

Pharmacological studies with peptide analogs suggest the existence of several classes of VIP receptors. Two types of receptors capable of specific binding of VIP have been described. One of these, also known as the PACAP II receptor, recognizes VIP and pituitary adenylate cyclase-activating peptide (PACAP) with similar affinity. This receptor is present in a variety of peripheral tissues. A second VIP receptor, for which helodermin is a potent ligand, has been described in lung carcinoma cells. Recently, cDNAs encoding rat and human forms of the VIP receptors have been cloned (21–23). VIP and PHI cause relaxation of isolated cerebral arteries (17,24,25). The relaxation occurs in parallel with activation of adenylate cyclase (25,26). In several tissues, low-frequency nerve stimulation gives rise to responses that are atropine sensitive, whereas high-frequency stimulation, when applied in bursts, gives rise to atropine-resistant responses. The release of VIP is greatly enhanced during high-frequency stimulation. Microapplication of VIP or PHI elicits a concentration-dependent dilation of pial arterioles and veins in situ (27,28).

PITUITARY ADENYLATE CYCLASE-ACTIVATING PEPTIDE

PACAP is a VIP-like peptide originally isolated from ovine hypothalami (29). PACAP occurs in two forms, one with 38 residues (PACAP-38) and the other with 27 residues (PACAP-27); they both derive from a 176-amino acid precursor molecule (30). The N-terminal sequence (1–28) exhibits 68% sequence identity with VIP whereas the sequence 29–38 does not seem to have any homologues. The PACAP gene has been cloned in several species and its transcript identified in different tissues. In situ hybridization and immunocytochemistry have revealed the expression of PACAP in both parasympathetic (otic and sphenopalatine) and sensory ganglia (cervical dorsal root and trigeminal) (31,32). In the trigeminal ganglion PACAP is synthesized in a population of small to medium-sized neurons. In dorsal root ganglia, cells expressing PACAP constituted about 10% and those expressing calcitonin gene-related peptide 46% of the total number of nerve cell bodies. In the otic and sphenopalatine ganglia, most of the nerve cell bodies contain immunoreactive PACAP and PACAP mRNA (32). In these ganglia PACAP is, as a rule, co-expressed with VIP.

Transection of the efferent output from the sphenopalatine ganglion in the rat gives rise to a marked loss of neurons in the ganglion. In the remaining neurons a twofold increase in PACAP mRNA can be seen, as judged by determination of the optical density of in situ hybridization labeling of the ganglia. Around cerebral blood vessels there is a moderate supply of nerve fibers containing PACAP (Fig. 2). The effects of PACAP seem to be mediated through at least three different receptors, all G-protein coupled and seven-transmembrane spanning (33–36). One (the PACAP

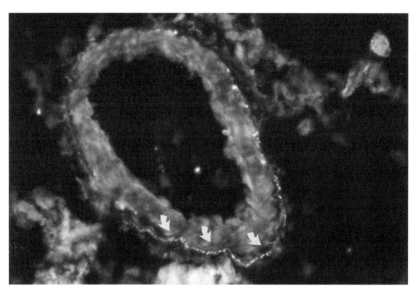

FIG. 2. A small blood vessel from the circle of Willis of the cat. Section shows PACAP-containing nerve fibers (*arrows*) in the adventitia-media border.

type I receptor) recognizes VIP and secretin poorly, a second (the PACAP type II or VIP 1 receptor) recognizes both VIP and secretin, and a third (the PACAP type III or VIP 2 receptor) recognizes VIP but not secretin (37). Of the PACAP type I receptor, several splice variants have been identified. The addition of PACAP-27, PACAP-38, and VIP on isolated large cerebral blood vessels of laboratory animals results in identical concentration-dependent dilations (38,39). Intracisternal injections of PACAP-27, PACAP-38, and VIP dilate canine cerebral arteries (40). Intracerebral microinjections of PACAP effect a moderate increase in cerebral blood flow (38).

HELOSPECTIN-LIKE PEPTIDES

Helospectin I and helospectin II are two closely related peptides consisting of 38 and 37 amino acid residues, respectively. Helospectin II is identical to helospectin I except for the lack of serine in position 38. The peptides belong to the family of VIP-related peptides. There is evidence that helospectin-like peptides occur in endocrine-like cells and in neurons in the central and peripheral nervous system (41–43). In the sphenopalatine and otic ganglia, a subpopulation of VIP-immunoreactive nerve cell bodies seems to contain helospectin. A moderate supply of nerve fibers containing helospectin-like immunoreactivity can be seen in the adventitia and adventitia-media order of cat cerebral arteries (44). Double immunostaining has shown that most of these fibers contain VIP. Helospectin I and helospectin II produce concentration-dependent relaxations of feline cerebral arteries amounting to 50% to 80% of the precontraction induced by the prostaglandin analog U 46619. The maximum effects are similar to those of VIP, whereas the potency is lower. Cortical injections of helospectins reveal a moderate increase in local cerebral blood flow (44).

NITRIC OXIDE

The identification of nitric oxide (NO) as a neuronal messenger has raised particular interest because of its chemical identity, its wide distribution, and its broad spectrum of effects. NO is formed from L-arginine during its conversion to L-citrulline; this reaction is facilitated by the enzyme nitric oxide synthase (NOS). There are at least three types of NOS: neuronal-, endothelial- and macrophage-type enzyme (45). The neuronal and endothelial enzymes are constitutive, whereas the macrophage type is induceable. The formation of neuronal NO is Ca^{2+} calmodulin dependent and requires nicotinamide adenine dinucleotide phosphate and O_2. Since NO is a highly labile molecule, information on its cellular localization has largely been attained by immunocytochemistry and in situ hybridization for NOS or by the histochemical technique for demonstration of NADPH-diaphorase, which stains neurons containing NOS. In the sphenopalatine ganglion virtually all nerve cell bodies express NOS. In the trigeminal ganglion and in cervical dorsal root ganglia, a few small- to medium-sized cell bodies express NOS (46,47).

Double immunostaining in rats has revealed that a major population of VIP-containing nerve cell bodies in the otic and sphenopalatine ganglia contains NOS (47) (Fig.3). Around cerebral blood vessels a rich supply of NOS-immunoreactive nerve fibers can be seen, and bilateral sectioning of parasympathetic fibers from the sphenopalatine ganglia eliminates NOS-immunoreactive nerve fibers in the cerebral circulation (46,48,49). Several experiments have indicated that NO is a likely candidate for mediating nonadrenergic, noncholinergic relaxation of smooth muscle. A similar mediator role has also been proposed for VIP. The combined action of VIP and VIP-like peptides with NO and their mediation via multiple pathways may well ensure a more effective smooth muscle relaxation (50). The physiological role of NO on cerebral blood vessels has been investigated in a number of studies. Transmural nerve stimulation of cerebral blood vessels causes a dilation that is abolished by NO synthase inhibition and is restored by L-arginine, a substrate of NOS (51). The NOS inhibitor 7-nitroindazole, which is supposed to be relatively specific for the neuronal isoform of the enzyme, reduces cerebral blood flow on injection (52), whereas L-arginine, a precursor of NO, dilates pial arterioles, increases regional cerebral blood flow, and decreases infarction size in rats (53,54).

Numerous neurotransmitters have been discovered within the parasympathetic nervous system. Most of these transmitters have strong and distinct effects on cranial blood vessels. So far, a clear physiological role for these transmitters, has not been found. They do not seem to be directly involved in several basic cerebrovascular responses such as hypoxic or hypercapnic vasodilation or in autoregulation. Their effects may be to increase cerebral blood flow in times of threat when ordinary metabolic factors are impaired. The physiological significance of these multiple

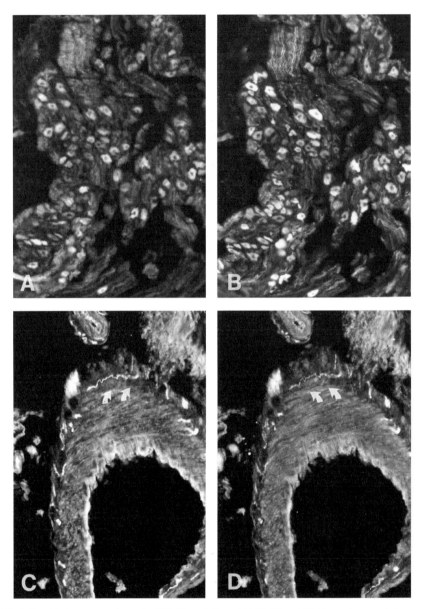

FIG. 3. Double immunostaining for VIP (**A** and **C**) and NOS (**B** and **D**). Rat sphenopalatine ganglion (**A** and **B**). Virtually all VIP-containing nerve cell bodies also contain NOS. Rat cerebral arteries (**C** and **D**). VIP and NOS co-exist in the same nerve fibers around the blood vessel (*arrows*).

transmitters may be fully revealed only after the development of specific receptor blocking agents.

REFERENCES

1. Walters BB, Gillespie SA, MA. Cerebrovascular projections from the sphenopalatine and otic ganglia to the middle cerebral artery of the cat. *Stroke* 1986;17:488–494.
2. Edvinsson L, Hara H, Uddman R. Retrograde tracing of nerve fibers to the rat middle cerebral artery with True Blue: colocalization with different peptides. *J Cereb Blood Flow Metab* 1989;9:212–228.
3. Suzuki N, Hardebo J-E, Owman C. Origins and pathways of cerebrovascular vasoactive intestinal polypeptide-positive nerves in rat. *J Cereb Blood Flow Metab* 1988;8:697–712.
4. Edvinsson L, Nielsen K, Owman C, Sporrong B. Cholinergic mechanisms in pial vessels. Histochemistry, electron microscopy and pharmacology. *Z Zellforsch* 1972;134:311–325.
5. Burnstock G. Cholinergic and purinergic regulation of blood vessels. In: Bohr DF, Somlyo AD, Sparks HW, Geiger SR, eds. *Handbook of physiology Sect. 2. The cardiovascular system*, vol. II. *Vascular smooth muscle*. American Physiological Society. Baltimore: Waverly Press, 1980;567–612.
6. Hara H, Hamill GS, Jacobowitz DM. Origin of cholinergic nerves to the rat major cerebral arteries: coexistence with vasoactive intestinal polypeptide. *Brain Res* 1985;14:179–188.
7. Hardebo J-E, Edvinsson L, Emson PC, Owman C. Isolated brain microvessels: enzymes related to adrenergic and cholinergic functions. In: Owman C, Edvinsson L, eds. *Neurogenic control of the brain circulation*. London: Pergamon, 1977;105–113.
8. Florence VM, Bevan JA. Biochemical determination of cholinergic innervation in cerebral arteries. *Circ Res* 1979;45:212–218.
9. Duckles SP. Evidence for a functional cholinergic innervation of cerebral arteries. *J Pharmacol Exp Ther* 1981;217:544–548.
10. Estrada C, Hamel E, Krause DN. Biochemical evidence for cholinergic innervation of intracerebral blood vessels. *Brain Res* 1983;266:261–270.
11. Hamel E, Assumel-Lurdin C, Edvinsson L, MacKenzie ET. Cholinergic innervation of small pial vessels: specific uptake and release processes. *Acta Physiol Scand* 1986;127[Suppl 552]:13–16.
12. Hamel E, Assumel-Lurdin C, Edvinsson L, Fage D, MacKenzie ET. Neuronal versus endothelial origin of vasoactive acetylcholine in pial vessels. *Brain Res* 1987;420:391–396.
13. Edvinsson L, Falck B, Owman C. Possibilities for a cholinergic action on smooth musculature and on sympathetic axons in brain vessels mediated by muscarinic and nicotinic receptors. *J Pharmacol Exp Ther* 1977;200:117–126.
14. Lundberg JM, Hökfelt T, Schultzberg M, Uvnäs-Wallensten K, Köhler C, Said SI. Occurrence of vasoactive intestinal polypeptide (VIP)-like immunoreactivity in certain cholinergic neurons in the rat: evidence from combined immunohistochemical and acetylcholinesterase staining. *Neuroscience* 1979;4:1539–1559.
15. Uddman R, Ekblad E, Edvinsson L, Håkanson R, Sundler F. VIP nerve fibres around peripheral blood vessels. *Acta Physiol Scand* 1981;112:65–70.
16. Della NG, Papka RG, Furness JB, Costa M. Vasoactive intestinal peptide-like immunoreactivity in nerves associated with the cardiovascular system of guinea-pigs. *Neuroscience* 1983;9:605–619.
17. Larsson LI, Edvinsson L, Fahrenkrug J, et al. Immunohistochemical localization of a vasodilatory peptide (VIP) in cerebrovascular nerves. *Brain Res* 1976;113:400–404.
18. Edvinsson L, Fahrenkrug J, Hanko J, Owman C, Sundler F, Uddman R. VIP (vasoactive intestinal polypeptide)-containing nerves of intracranial arteries in mammals. *Cell Tissue Res* 1980;208:135–142.
19. Kobayashi S, Kyoshima K, Olschowka JA, Jacobowitz DM. Vasoactive intestinal polypeptide immunoreactive and cholinergic nerves in whole mount preparation of the major cerebral arteries of the rat. *Histochemistry* 1983;79:377–381.
20. Gibbins IL, Morris JL. Co-existence of immunoreactivity to neuropeptide Y and vasoactive intestinal peptide in non-adrenergic axons innervating guinea pig cerebral arteries after sympathectomy. *Brain Res* 1988;44:402–406.
21. Ishihara T, Shigemoto R, Mori K, Takahashi K, Nagata S. Functional expression and tissue distribution of a novel receptor for vasoactive intestinal polypeptide. *Neuron* 1992;8:811–819.

22. Lutz EM, Sheward WJ, West KM, Morrow JA, Fink G, Harmar AJ. The VIP2 receptor: molecular characterization of a cDNA encoding a novel receptor for vasoactive intestinal peptide. *FEBS Lett* 1993;334:3–8.
23. Sreedharan SP, Patel DR, Huang J-X, Goetzl EJ. Cloning and functional expression of a human neuroendocrine vasoactive intestinal peptide receptor. *Biochem Biophys Res Commun* 1993;193:546–553.
24. Toda N. Relaxant responses to transmural stimulation and nicotine of dog and monkey cerebral arteries. *Am J Physiol* 1982;243:H145–H153.
25. Suzuki Y, McMaster D, Lederis K, Rorstad OP. Characterization of the relaxant effect of vasoactive intestinal peptide (VIP) and PHI on isolated brain arteries. *Brain Res* 1984;322:9–16.
26. Lee TJ-F, Saito A, Berezin I. Vasoactive intestinal polypeptide-like substance: the potential transmitter for cerebral vasodilatation. *Science* 1984;224:898–901.
27. McCulloch J, Edvinsson L. Cerebral circulatory and metabolic effects of vasoactive intestinal polypeptide. *Am J Physiol* 1980;238:H449–H456.
28. Edvinsson L, McCulloch J. Distribution and vasomotor effects of peptide HI (PHI) in feline cerebral blood vessels in vitro and in situ. *Regul Pept* 1985;10:345–356.
29. Miyata A, Arimura A, Dahl RR, Minomino N, Uehara A. Isolation of a novel 38 residue hypothalamic polypeptide which stimulates adenylate cyclase in pituitary cells. *Biochem Biophys Res Commun* 1989;164:567–574.
30. Kimura C, Ohkubo S, Ogi K, et al. A novel peptide which stimulates adenylate cyclase: molecular cloning and characterization of the ovine and human cDNAs. *Biochem Biophys Res Commun* 1990;166:81–89.
31. Mulder H, Uddman R, Moller K, et al. Pituitary adenylate cyclase activating polypeptide expression in sensory neurons. *Neuroscience* 1994;63:307–312.
32. Mulder H, Uddman R, Moller K, et al. Pituitary adenylate cyclase activating polypeptide is expressed in autonomic neurons. *Regul Pept* 1995;59:121–128.
33. Shivers BD, Görcs TJ, Gottschall PE, Arimura A. Two high affinity binding sites for pituitary adenylate cyclase-activating polypeptide have different tissue distributions. *Endocrinology* 1991;128:3055–3065.
34. Morrow JA, Lutz EM, West KM, Fink G, Harmar AJ. Molecular cloning and expression of a cDNA encoding a receptor for pituitary adenylate cyclase-activating polypeptide (PACAP). *FEBS Lett* 1993;329:99–105.
35. Pisegna JR, Wank SA. Molecular cloning and functional expression of the human pituitary adenylate cyclase-activating polypeptide type I receptor. *Proc Natl Acad Sci USA* 1993;90:6345–6349.
36. Inagaki N, Yoshida H, Mizuta M, et al. Cloning and functional characterization of a third pituitary adenylate cyclase-activating polypeptide receptor subtype expressed in insulin-secreting cells. *Proc Natl Acad Sci USA* 1994;91:2679–2683.
37. Usdin TB, Bonner TI, Mezey E. Two receptors for vasoactive intestinal polypeptide with similar specificity and complementary distributions. *Endocrinology* 1994;135:2662–2678.
38. Udman R, Goadsby P, Jansen I, Edvinsson L. PACAP, a VIP-like peptide: immunohistochemical localization and effect upon cat pial arteries and cerebral blod flow. *J Cereb Blood Flow Metab* 1993;13:291–297.
39. Anzai M, Suzuki Y, Takayasu M, et al. Vasorelaxant effect of PACAP-27 on canine cerebral arteries and rat intracerebral arterioles. *Eur J Pharmacol* 1995;285:173–179.
40. Seki Y, Suzuki Y, Baskaya MK, et al. The effects of pituitary adenylate cyclase-activating polypeptide on cerebral arteries and vertebral artery blood flow in anesthetized dogs. *Eur J Pharmacol* 1995;275:259–266.
41. Bjartell A, Persson P, Absood A, Sundler F, Håkanson R. Helodermin-like peptides in noradrenaline cells of the adrenal medulla. *Regul Pept* 1989;26:27–34.
42. Luts A, Uddman R, Håkanson R, Absood A, Sundler F. Chemical coding of endocrine cells of the airways. Presence of helodermin-like peptides. *Cell Tissue Res* 1991;265:425–433.
43. Kivipelto L, Absood A, Håkanson R, Sundler F, Panula P. Helodermin- and helospectin-like immunoreactivity in the rat brain. An immunochemical and immunohistochemical study. *Neuroscience* 1992;47:135–153.
44. Jansen-Olesen I, Goadsby PJ, Uddman R, Edvinsson L. Vasoactive intestinal peptide (VIP) like peptides in the cerebral circulation of the cat. *J Auton Nerv Syst* 1994;49:97–103.
45. Förstermann U, Schmidt HH, Pollock JS, et al. Isoforms of nitric oxide synthase. Characterization and purification from different cell types. *Biochem Pharmacol* 1991;42:1849–1857.

46. Nozaki K, Moskowitz MA, Maynard KI, et al. Possible origins and distribution of immunoreactive nitric oxide synthase-containing nerve fibers in cerebral arteries. *J Cereb Blood Flow Metab* 1993; 13:70–79.
47. Uddman R, Mulder H, Sundelin J, Elsås T, Sundler F. Nitric oxide synthase expression in cervical autonomic and sensory ganglia in rat: relationship to neuropeptides. *Cell Vision* 1994;1:306–312.
48. Bredt DS, Hwang PM, Snyder SH. Localization of nitric oxide synthase indicating a neural role for nitric oxide. *Nature* 1994;347:768–770.
49. Yoshida K, Okamura T, Kimura H, Bredt DS, Snyder SH, Toda N. Nitric oxide synthase-immunoreactive nerve fibers in dog cerebral and peripheral arteries. *Brain Res* 1993;629:67–72.
50. Said SI. Nitric oxide and vasoactive intestinal peptide: cotransmitters of smooth muscle relaxation. *NIPS* 1992;7:181–183.
51. Toda N, Okamura T. Neurogenic nitric oxide (NO) in the regulation of cerebroarterial tone. *J Chem Neuroanat* 1996;10:259–265.
52. Kelly PAT, Ritchie IM, Arbuthnott GW. Inhibition of neuronal nitric oxide synthase by 7-nitroindazole: effects upon local cerebral blood flow and glucose use in the rat. *J Cereb Blood Flow Metab* 1995;15:766–773.
53. Morikawa E, Huang Z, Moskowitz MA. L-arginine decreases infarct size caused by middle cerebral arterial occlusion in SHR. *Am J Physiol* 1992;263:H1632–H1635.
54. Morikawa E, Rosenblatt S, Moskowitz MA. L-arginine dilates rat pial arterioles by nitric oxide-dependent mechanisms and increases blood flow during focal cerebral ischaemia. *Br J Pharmacol* 1992;107:905–907.

6

Messenger Molecules in the Cranial Sensory Nervous System

Norihiro Suzuki

Department of Neurology, Keio University, Tokyo 160, Japan

The assumption that cranial blood vessels cause headache pain is quite feasible since they possess the densest sensory innervation in the cranium, and mechanical stimulation of the dural or main cerebral arteries elicits pain as vascular headache (1). Both vascular and neurogenic mechanisms for the generation of pain from cranial blood vessels in migraine have been suggested (2). Several lines of evidence suggest that activation of perivascular sensory afferent nerves rather than vasodilation per se causes headache pain in migraine. The hypothesis that neurotransmitter release from trigeminal sensory afferent nerve fibers is crucial for the development of the headache phase of migraine was postulated by Moskowitz et al. in 1979 (3). Accordingly, analysis of transmitter molecules in the cranial sensory nervous system is one of the critical issues in research on the mechanisms of vascular headache.

The cranial blood vessels have been demonstrated to be equipped with ample sensory nerve fibers that store tachykinins (neurokinins), i.e., substance P (SP), neurokinin A (NKA), calcitonin gene-related peptide (CGRP), dynorphin B (dyn B), and nitric oxide (NO).

SENSORY NERVE FIBERS AROUND CEREBRAL VESSELS

Substance P

Substance P (SP) was detected in the equine brain and intestine by von Euler and Gaddum in 1931 (4) and was suggested to be a transmitter in both the central and peripheral nervous systems, particularly in primary sensory neurons (5). Since SP was observed in the blood vessel wall and shows strong vasodilatory activity, it has been regarded as one of the putative physiological neurovasodilator substances.

Substance P-containing cerebrovascular nerve fibers have been observed in many species. Like other perivascular nerve fibers, they are located in the adventitia-medial border. Evidence from retrograde axonal tracing, immunohistochemistry, and capsaicin treatment is consistent with the concept that SP is synthesized in sensory ganglia and transported to the nerve terminals by fast transport. Capsaicin treatment also causes loss of SP immunoreactivity from the cerebral vessels, as shown in cats and rabbits (6). Trigeminal ganglionectomy reduces SP levels in the feline circle of Willis by less than half. This implies the existence of other sources of cerebrovascular SP nerve fibers. Release of SP can be elicited by antidromic stimulation of the sensory neurons, which is associated with vasodilation (7). SP has been shown to be a potent vasodilator in vivo and in vitro through activation of specific vascular receptors (8,9), although tachyphylaxis to the effect of exogenous SP has been observed (10). It is notable that SP has a vasoconstrictor action (11).

The vasodilatory effect of SP on the artery is characteristically endothelium dependent (10,12), while that on the veins does not seem to require an intact endothelium (13,14).

Several studies on the relation between the trigeminal ganglion and the intracranial vasculature suggested that SP is involved in the pathophysiology of vascular headache (15–17). SP release upon antidromic stimulation appears to be associated with extravasation due to disruption of the blood-brain barrier (18).

Neurokinin A

Neurokinin A(NKA) has been isolated from the mammalian central nervous system and demonstrated in the primary sensory neurons of unmyelinated C-types. NKA has also been demonstrated to co-exist with SP in the nerve fibers of the cerebral blood vessels as well as in the trigeminal ganglion cell bodies (19). NKA is also sensitive to capsaicin. Both tachykinins are noted to co-exist with CGRP in certain populations of nerve fibers. Although no evidence shows that these neuropeptides may potentiate the vessel relaxant effects of one another in vitro, NKA potently relaxes vascular smooth muscle in an endothelium-dependent manner (12).

Calcitonin Gene-Related Peptide

Alternative processing of RNA transcribed from the calcitonin gene gives rise to a 37-amino acid peptide in nonthyroid tissues (20). The localization of nerves containing calcitonin gene-related peptide (CGRP) shows a marked overlap with the distribution of SP-containing fibers, which are capsaicin-sensitive. Capsaicin directly activates a subclass of sensory neurons to produce release, and ultimately depletion, of SP and CGRP and can also produce long-lasting blockade of transmission along the axon (21). CGRP is also observed in nerve fibers associated with pial arteries where it is also stored together with SP. Accordingly, CGRP co-localizes with SP in a population of trigeminal ganglion cells (22,23) and disappears after section of the ipsilateral trigeminal nerve (24). This peptide is a more potent vasodilator than SP, but, in contrast to the latter, its effect is endothelium independent (22,24). Indeed, the vessel dilation elicited by CGRP was not affected by the nitric oxide synthase (NOS) inhibitor L-nitroarginine (25). Furthermore, CGRP inhibits vasoconstriction mediated by activation of the adrenergic nerves (22,24) and increases the duration of the vasoconstrictor response to noradrenalin (24).

Calcitonin gene-related peptide has mainly been found in the sensory system co-localizing with SP. Several parasympathetic ganglia, however, also reveal a small population of CGRP-containing cell body and perisomatic axons, as well as the motor end plate of the striate muscles, cerebral meninges, chemosensitive nasal and oral epithelia, dermal papillae, and hair follicles (26). This finding may imply that CGRP contributes not only to evocation of nociceptive response to irritants, but also to maintenance or renewal of tissue under physiological or pathological conditions.

Recent studies have shown a functional coupling of CGRP and NO in mechanisms of the neurogenic vasodilation (27–30). Part of the CGRP-induced dilation of the cerebral vessels is mediated by NO through ATP-sensitive K^+ channels (27). Thus, concepts on the functional aspects of CGRP are expanding from the primary sensory system to more comprehensive systems.

Dynorphin B

In the rat, guinea pig, and monkey, dynorphin B (dyn B) has been demonstrated in the trigeminal ganglion cells and the perivascular nerve fibers in the pial arteries by immunohistochemistry (31–33). Although dyn B has been shown to co-exist with SP and CGRP in the nerve fibers of the pial vessels of the guinea pig, neither vasomotor function nor relevance to sensory transduction could be detected in vitro (33).

Nitric Oxide

Recent experiments have implied that at least some sensory neurons, such as those in the dorsal root ganglia, are likely to contain NOS (34,35). Some studies suggest that NO released from capsaicin-sensitive sensory nerve terminals contributes to vasodilatory response by activation of the nerves. It is not yet known, however, whether peptides contained in the sensory neurons contribute to this vascular response remaining after inhibition of NOS.

In cat cerebral arteries, nicotine can produce a component of the vasodilator response that is blocked by capsaicin and seems to be due to release of a vasodilator from sensory nerve terminals (36). This vasodilation is blocked by CGRP desensitization, but is not affected by NOS inhibitors (37). Thus, so far, few studies have demonstrated a vasodilatory role for NO after release from the peripheral ends of sensory neurons.

ORIGINS AND DISTRIBUTION OF AGENTS STORED IN THE SENSORY NERVES IN ANIMALS AND HUMANS

SP-containing nerve fibers supplying cerebral blood vessels have been demonstrated by immunohistochemistry in the human, pig, cat, rabbit, guinea pig, and cat (23,38–43). Utilizing horseradish peroxidase tracing and nerve transection in the cat, it has been shown that these fibers originate in the ophthalmic division of the trigeminal ganglion (15,41,44,45). CGRP has also been shown to be stored in the cerebrovascular nerve fibers in the human, cat, rabbit, guinea pig, rat, and mouse (22,24,46–50). These two peptides co-exist in the same neurons in the trigeminal ganglion (23,51,52). Accordingly, the number of cerebrovascular nerves storing CGRP decreases after trigeminal ganglionectomy (46,47) or ganglion lesioning (49). In the monkey, denervation experiments have shown that the maxillary and ophthalmic divisions are the sources of unmyelinated and myelinated sensory fibers in pial vessels (53,54). Trigeminal innervation to the perforators of the circle of Willis also has been demonstrated by horseradish peroxidase anterograde tracing technique in the rabbit (55).

Rat Fibers

In the rat, SP- and CGRP-containing nerve fibers were observed in all regions of pial vessels (56). The nerve density was higher in the rostral portion of the circle of Willis and its branches compared with the caudal portion and the vertebrobasilar system. The two peptides appeared in the same position in the vessel wall, an indication that they co-existed. However, CGRP-containing nerve fibers were more abundant than those of SP-containing fibers.

After bilateral transection of the nasociliary nerve (a branch of the first division of the trigeminal ganglion), SP/CGRP-containing nerve fibers in the rostral half of the circle of Willis and its branches were eliminated, whereas the number only decreased in the caudal half, in the proximal segment of the middle cerebral artery, and in the rostral two-thirds of the basilar artery. Fibers in the internal carotid arteries, the caudal third of the basilar artery, and the vertebral arteries were not affected by nerve section.

The retrograde axonal tracer study in which True Blue was applied to the proximal segment of the middle cerebral artery demonstrated accumulation of tracer in several SP/CGRP-containing cells in the ophthalmic division of the ipsilateral trigeminal ganglion as well as in a few cells in the maxillary division and the internal carotid ganglion (56,57). No accumulation of tracer was demonstrated in SP/CGRP-positive cells of the other cranial ganglia. The rostral part and some of the caudal part of the pial arteries at the base of the brain are innervated by SP/CGRP-containing nerve fibers originated from the trigeminal and the internal carotid ganglion. The great majority of trigeminal nerve fibers reach the vessels via the nasociliary nerve of the ophthalmic division, which enters the cranial cavity through the ethmoidal

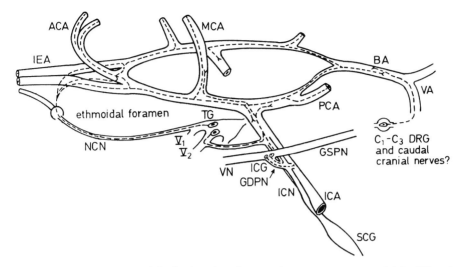

FIG. 1. Origins, pathways, and distribution of cerebrovascular sensory nerves containing SP and CGRP in the rat. The sensory nerves in the pial vessels originate in the following cranial ganglia: (a) the ophthalmic division of the trigeminal ganglion (TG, V_1)—the nerve fibers originating in TG (V_1) innervate, via the nasociliary nerve (NCN), the circle of Willis, and its branches from rostral to caudal; (b) the maxillary division of the trigeminal ganglion (TG, V_2)—those originating in TG (V_2) innervate, via an extradural branch on the skull base, the internal carotid artery (ICA), and its intracranial ramifications; (c) the internal carotid (mini-)ganglion (ICG)—the nerve fibers, originating mainly in the caudal part of ICG, innervate the ICA and its intracranial ramifications via a short direct branch to the artery; and (d) upper cervical dorsal root ganglia (DRG, C_1–C_5)—those originating in DRG innervate the caudal third of the basilar and vertebral artery. ACA, anterior cerebral artery; BA, basilar artery; GDPN, greater deep petrosal nerve; GSPN, greater superficial petrosal nerve; ICN, internal carotid nerve; IEA, internal ethmoidal artery (olfactory artery); MCA, middle cerebral artery; PCA, posterior cerebral artery; SCG, superior cervical ganglion; VA, vertebral artery; VN, vidian nerve (nerve of pterygoid canal). From Suzuki et al. (56).

foramen, whereas fibers from the internal carotid ganglion project directly to the internal carotid artery.

The origin and pathways of SP/CGRP nerve fibers in the pial arteries are summarized in Fig. 1. The pathway between the trigeminal ganglion and the cerebral vessels has not been previously known, with the exception of branches to the cavernous sinus segment of the internal carotid artery in the monkey (53,54,58). In these monkey studies, the ophthalmic trigeminal division was shown to innervate (via short branches within the cavernous sinus) this portion of the internal carotid artery, whereas the maxillary division was shown to project to the artery via branches, called the recurrent branches of the orbitociliary nerve, leaving the nerve deep in the orbital fossa. In contrast to the monkey and human, the cavernous sinus portion of the internal carotid artery in the rat is extremely short in length and is located just medial to the radix of the trigeminal ganglion where the ganglion is not yet divided into its three branches. Instead, in the rat, the nasociliary nerve was shown to be a cerebrovascular pathway of the ophthalmic division of the trigeminal ganglion (56). This nerve enters into the cranial cavity from the orbital fossa through the ethmoidal foramen together with the intracranial branches of the pterygopalatine ganglion. It is notable that most of the two vasodilatory peptidergic vasodilatory systems (the sensory system with SP/CGRP and the parasympathetic system with VIP) reaches the pial vessels through the same foramen and thus innervates the vessels from a rostral to caudal direction.

No clear-cut evidence has yet been obtained for a similar sensory nerve pathway to the cerebral vessels in the human. Interestingly, ganglion cells and nerve fibers were found in the falx cerebri of the anterior cranial fossa in a study on an infant of 4 months (59,60). They were suggested to be connected with the anterior ethmoidal branch of the trigeminal nerve (which is a continuation of the nasociliary nerve), to supply the vascular plexus of the falx and the territory of the anterior cerebral artery.

A flow increase upon electrical stimulation of the nasociliary nerve in the rat, i.e., the intracranial or cerebrovascular branch of the trigeminal ganglion, was reported (61). There have been several studies on cerebral blood flow changes during trigeminal stimulation (62–65). However, criticism of stimulation of the trigeminal ganglion itself is unavoidable in these studies. One study was able to show stimulation of the trigeminal nerves projecting to the cerebrovascular beds selectively, without activation of other branches or central connection (61) (Fig. 2). A maximal increase in blood flow was obtained with continuous stimulation at 10 Hz and a considerable increase induced in the ipsilateral parietal registration site (Fig. 3). For comparison, an enhanced level of SP is found in the aqueous humor of albino rabbits upon electrical stimulation of the trigeminal nerve at 15 Hz, 10 V, and 5 msec impulse duration (66). Increased flow in the anterior facial vein has been reported in the rat upon electrical stimulation of the mental nerve at 15 Hz, 11 V, and 5 msec impulse duration (67). Taken together, it is possible that optimal frequencies for the antidromic trigeminal sensory stimulation range around 10 to 15 Hz. The results demonstrated that the trigeminal cerebrovascular nerves, apart from transferring sensory information, may also contribute to flow regulation.

Monkey Fibers

The source of innervation of the middle cerebral artery with SP- and CGRP-containing nerve fibers appears to be threefold (68). The major contribution comes from the ophthalmic division of the ipsilateral trigeminal ganglion. The pathway for these fibers was demonstrated in cynomolgus monkeys using the electron microscope; denervation was shown with nerve sections (53,54). The fibers bridge to the cavernous plexus from the ophthalmic nerve shortly rostral to the ganglion, and an additional bridge exists between the plexus and the rostral segment of the internal carotid artery just before the artery bends upward in the sinus (Fig. 4). A few early reports in humans have identified fine branches connecting the internal carotid artery with the medial surface of the ophthalmic nerve shortly rostral to the ganglion (69,70). However, it was not clarified whether such fibers were sensory or sympa-

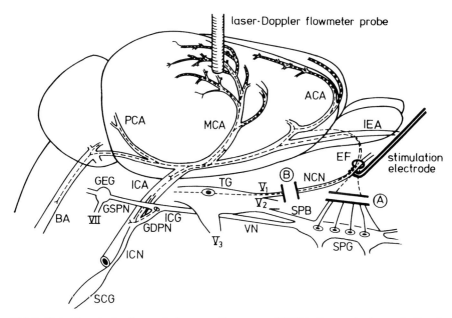

FIG. 2. Main trigeminal pathway via the nasociliary nerve (NCN) to the cerebral vessels, the site of nerve stimulation and the laser-Doppler flow probe. The nerve is stimulated just outside the ethmoidal foramen (EF). The postganglionic nerve fibers from the sphenopalatine ganglion (SPG), which carry cerebrovascular parasympathetic nerves, were transected (A) 2 weeks before nerve stimulation to avoid concomitant activation of the parasympathetic and sensory nerves. The proximal part of the NCN was also transected (B) just before nerve stimulation to exclude involvement of activation of the trigeminal ganglion cells, which may activate central sensory pathways in the brain stem. GEG, geniculate ganglion; SPB, sphenopalatine branch of the maxillary trigeminal nerve; V_3, mandibular nerve; VII, facial nerve. Other abbreviations are the same as in Fig. 1 legend. From Suzuki et al. (61).

thetic in nature. In contrast to the case of the rat, no evidence in the monkey shows that there are pathways via the nasociliary nerve from the ophthalmic division of the trigeminal ganglion through the ethmoidal foramen and the basal frontal dura mater to the circle of Willis.

The fibers from the maxillary division of the trigeminal ganglion apparently travel in the orbitociliary nerve branch to run through the cavernous nerve plexus and bridge to the internal carotid artery together with fibers from the ophthalmic division (53,68). Some SP-containing fibers from the ophthalmic and maxillary divisions join the recurrent nerve of the plexus to run along the abducent nerve to innervate the basilar artery and its branches (53,68). Occasionally there are a few SP- or CGRP-containing neurons in the abducent nerve, which may represent aberrant trigeminal neurons in this pathway. Furthermore, in the monkey, some SP-containing fibers from the ophthalmic division leave the plexus to join the tentorial nerve, which follows the trochlear nerve to the rostral origin of the tentorium cerebri and innervates the tentorium, dura mater of the occipital region, and falx cerebri and their sinuses (71).

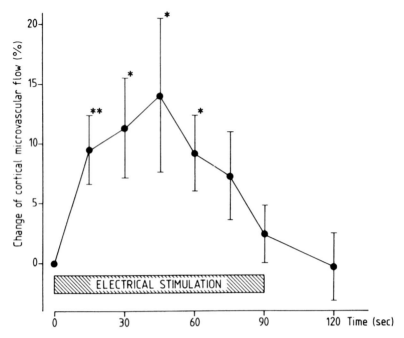

FIG. 3. Change of cortical blood flow relative to resting flow values upon electrical stimulation of the nasociliary nerve (5 V, 10 Hz, 0.5 msec impulse duration). Values are expressed as means ± SEM of ten observations. Modified t-test: *, $p < 0.05$; **, $p < 0.01$ in comparison with resting flow values. From Suzuki et al. (61).

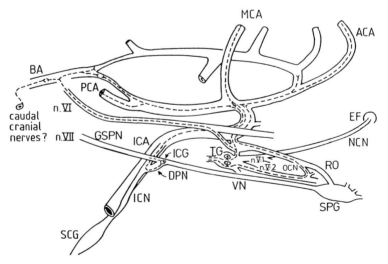

FIG. 4. Origins and pathways of sensory nerve fibers to the internal carotid artery and pial arteries in the monkey. (The figure represents those on the right side.) DPN, deep petrosal nerve; OCN, orbitociliary nerve; RO, rami orbitales of sphenopalatine ganglion. Other abbreviations are the same as those in Figs. 1 and 2 legends. From Hardebo et al. (68).

The third source of the sensory nerve fibers to the middle cerebral artery is a subdivision of the ipsilateral internal carotid ganglion. The fibers reach the internal carotid artery via the deep petrosal nerve and run in bundles along the artery to reach the pial vessels or form a terminal network on the artery.

The upper cervical dorsal root ganglia may contribute to sensory innervation of the infratentorial vessels.

Human Fibers

The intracranial portion of the internal carotid artery and its pial branches as well as some veins on the brain surface are known to be pain sensitive for applied stimuli at single locations along their courses (72). SP, CGRP, and NKA have been demonstrated in human cerebral arteries by immunohistochemistry and biochemical measurements, which made it possible to map out cerebrovascular sensory nerve fibers. The probable origins and pathways of sensory nerve fibers in the cerebral vessels in humans, based on the findings in humans and monkeys, are outlined in Figure 5 (73).

Substance P- and CGRP-containing sensory nerve fibers to the internal carotid artery and its branches in humans are mainly derived from the ophthalmic division of the trigeminal ganglion. The fibers leave the ophthalmic trunk shortly distal to the ganglion and run a short course through the nerve plexus in the cavernous sinus wall. Some of these fibers join and follow the abducent nerve backward to innervate the basilar artery and its branches.

Recently, two ganglionic cell groups, located close together, were demonstrated

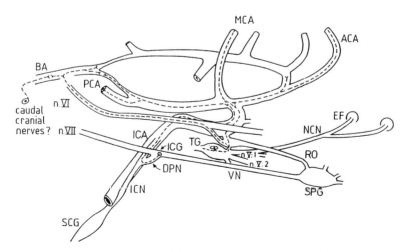

FIG. 5. Probable origins and pathways of the sensory nerve fibers to the intracranial segment of the internal carotid artery and the cerebral arteries in humans. Abbreviations are the same as those in Fig. 4 legend. From Suzuki and Hardebo (73).

on the ventrolateral surface of the human internal carotid artery, where the greater superficial petrosal nerve is joined by the greater deep petrosal nerve to form the vidian nerve (nerve of the pterygoid canal). One of the two ganglionic cell groups was shown by immunohistochemistry to contain SP and CGRP. The nerve fibers containing SP and CGRP from this ganglion may innervate the internal carotid arterial tree in humans.

The proximal portion of the basilar artery may receive sensory nerve fibers from caudal cranial nerves and upper cervical dorsal root ganglia.

REFERENCES

1. Ray BS, Wolff HG. Experimental studies on headache: pain sensitive structures of the head and their significance in headache. *Arch Surg* 1940;41:813–856.
2. Moskowitz MA, Macfarlane R. Neurovascular and molecular mechanisms in migraine headache. *Cerbrovasc Brain Metab Rev* 1993;5:159–177.
3. Moskowitz MA, Reinhard JF, Romero J, Melamed E, Pettibone DJ. Neurotransmitters and the fifth cranial nerve: is there a relation to the headache phase of migraine? *Lancet* 1979;2:883–885.
4. von Euler US, Gaddum JH. An unidentified depressor substance in certain tissue extracts. *J Physiol (Lond)* 1931;72:74–87.
5. Lembeck F. Zur Frage der zentralen Uebertragung afferenter Impulse. III. Mitteilung. Das Vorkommen und die Bedeugung der Substanz P in den dorsalen Wurzeln des Rueckenmarks. *Naunyn Schmiedbergs Arch Exp Pathol Pharmacol* 1953;219:197–213.
6. Duckles SP, Buck SH. Substance P in the cerebral vasculature: depletion by capsaicin suggested a sensory role. *Brain Res* 1982;245:171–174.
7. Lembeck F, Holzer P. Substance P as neurogenic mediator of antidromic vasodilation and neurogenic plasma extravasation. *Naunyn-Schmiedbergs Arch Pharmacol* 1979;310:175–183.
8. Edvinsson L, McCulloch J, Uddman R. Substance P: immunohistochemical localization and effect upon cat pial arteries in vitro and in situ. *J Physiol (Lond)* 1981;318:251–258.
9. Edvinsson L, Uddman R. Immunohistochemical localization and dilatory effect of substance P on human cerebral vessels. *Brain Res* 1982;232:466–471.
10. Furchgott RF. Role of endothelium in the vascular smooth muscle. *Circ Res* 1983;53:557–573.
11. Regoli D, D'Orlean-Juste P, Escher E, Mizrahi J. Receptors for substance P. I. The pharmacological preparations. *Eur J Pharmacol* 1984;97:161–170.
12. Jansen I, Alafaci C, McCulloch J, Uddman R, Edvinsson L. Tachykinins (substance P, neurokinin A, neuropeptide K, and neurokinin B) in the cerebral circulation: vasomotor responses in vitro and in situ. *J Cereb Blood Flow Metab* 1991;11:567–575.
13. Regoli D, Mizrahi J, D'Orlean-Juste P, Escher E. Receptors for substance P. II. Classification by agonist fragments and homologues. *Eur J Pharmacol* 1984;97:171–177.
14. Regoli D, Escher E, Drapeau G, D'Orlean-Juste P, Mizrahi J. Receptors for substance P. *Eur J Pharmacol* 1984;97:179–189.
15. Mayberg M, Langer RS, Zervas NT, Moskowitz MA. Perivascular meningeal projections from cat trigeminal ganglia: possible pathway for vascular headache in man. *Science* 1981;213:228–230.
16. Moskowitz MA. The neurobiology of vascular head pain. *Ann Neurol* 1984;16:157–168.
17. Hardebo JE. The involvement of trigeminal substance P neurons in cluster headache. An hypothesis. *Headache* 1984;24:294–304.
18. Markowitz S, Saito K, Buzzi MG, Moskowitz MA. The development of neurogenic plasma extravasation in the rat dura mater does not depend upon the degranulation of mast cells. *Brain Res* 1989; 477:157–165.
19. Edvinsson L, Brodin E, Jansen I, Uddman R. Neurokinin A in cerebral vessels: characterization, localization and effects in vitro. *Regul Pept* 1988;20:191–197.
20. Amara SG, Jonas V, Rosenfeld MG, Ong ES, Evans RM. Alternative RNA processing in calcitonin gene expression generates mRNAs encoding different polypeptide products. *Nature* 1982; 298:171–174.

21. Buck SH, Burks TF. The neuropharmacology of capsaicin: review of some recent observations. *Pharmacol Rev* 1986;38:179–226.
22. Hanko J, Hardebo JE, Kahrstrom J, Owman C, Sundler F. Calcitonin gene-related peptide is present in mammalian cerebrovascular nerve fibers and dilates pial and peripheral arteries. *Neurosci Lett* 1985;57:91–95.
23. Hanko J, Hardebo JE, Kahrstrom J, Owman C, Sundler F. Existence and coexistence of calcitonin gene-related peptide (CGRP) and substance P in cerebrovascular nerves and trigeminal ganglion cells. *Acta Physiol Scand* 1986;suppl 552:29–32.
24. McCulloch J, Uddman R, Kingman T, Edvinsson L. Calcitonin gene-related peptide: functional role in cerebrovascular regulation. *Proc Natl Acad Sci USA* 1986;83:5731–5735.
25. Claing A, Telemaque S, Cadieux A, Fournier A, Regoli D, D'Orleans-Juste P. Nonadrenergic and noncholinergic arterial dilation and vasoconstriction are mediated by calcitonin gene-related peptide and neurokinin-1 receptors, respectively, in the mesenteric vasculature of the rat after perivascular stimulation. *J Pharmacol Exp Ther* 1992;263:1226–1232.
26. Silverman JD, Kruger L. Calcitonin gene-related peptide immunoreactive innervation of rat head with emphasis on specialized sensory structures. *J Comp Neurol* 1989;280:303–330.
27. Kitazono T, Heistad DD, Faraci FM. Role of ATP-sensitive K^+ channels in CGRP-induced dilatation of basilar artery in vivo. *Am J Physiol* 1993;265:H581–H585.
28. Hughes SR, Brain, SD. Nitric oxide-dependent release of vasodilator quantities of calcitonin gene-related peptide from capsaicin-sensitive nerves in rabbit skin. *Br J Pharmacol* 1994;111:425–430.
29. Wahl M, Scilling L, Parsons AA, Kaumann A. Involvement of calcitonin gene-related peptide (CGRP) and nitric oxide (NO) in the pial artery dilatation elicited by cortical spread depression. *Brain Res* 1994;637:204–210.
30. Brian JE Jr, Heistad DD, Faraci FM. Mechanisms of endotoxin-induced dilatation of cerebral arterioles. *Am J Physiol* 1995;269:H783–H788.
31. Maskowitz MA, Brezina LR, Kuo C. Dynorphin B-containing perivascular axons and sensory neurotransmitter mechanisms in brain blood vessels. *Cephalalgia* 1986;6:81–86.
32. Moskowitz MA, Saito K, Brezina L, Dickson J. Nerve fibers surrounding intracranial and extracranial vessels from human and other species contain dynorphin B-like immunoreactivity. *Neuroscience* 1987;23:731–737.
33. Hardebo JE, Suzuki N. Dynorphin B is present in sensory and parasympathetic nerves innervating pial arteries. *J Auton Nerve Syst* 1994;47:171–176.
34. Aimi Y, Fujimura M, Vincent SR, Kimura H. Localization of NADPH-diaphorase-containing neurons in sensory ganglia of the rat. *J Comp Neurol* 1991;306:382–392.
35. Terenghi G, Riverosmoreno V, Hudson JD, Ibrahim NBN, Polak JM. Immunohistochemistry of nitric oxide synthase demonstrates immunoreactive neurons in spinal cord and dorsal root ganglia of man and rat. *J Neurol Sci* 1993;118:34–37.
36. Toda N. Mediation by nitric oxide of neurally induced human cerebral artery relaxation. *Experientia* 1993;49:51–53.
37. Toda N, Okamura T. Nitroxidergic innervation in cerebral arteries. *Can J Physiol Pharmacol* 1994; 72[suppl 4]:20.
38. Chan-Palay V. Innervation of cerebral blood vessels by norepinephrine, indoleamine, substance P and neurotensin fibers and the leptomeningeal indoleamine axons: their roles in vasomotor activity and local alterations of brain blood composition. In: Owman C, Edvinsson L, eds. *Neurogenic control of brain circulation*. Oxford: Pergamon Press, 1977;39–57.
39. Uddman R, Edvinsson L, Owman C, Sundler F. Perivascular substance P: occurrence and distribution in mammalian pial vessels. *J Cereb Blood Flow Metab* 1981;1:227–232.
40. Edvinsson L, Uddman R. Immunohistochemical localization and dilatory effect of substance P on human cerebral vessels. *Brain Res* 1982;232:466–471.
41. Liu-Chen L-Y, Mayberg MR, Moskowitz MA. Immunohistochemical evidence for a substance P-containing trigeminovascular pathway to pial arteries in cats. *Brain Res* 1983;268:162–166.
42. Yamamoto K, Matsuyama T, Shiosaka S, et al. Overall distribution of substance P-containing nerves in the wall of the cerebral arteries of the guinea pig and its origins. *J Comp Neurol* 1983;215:421–426.
43. Hara H, Weir B. Different distribution of substance P and vasoactive intestinal polypeptide in the cerebral arterial innervation in rat and guinea pig. *Anat Anz* 1987;163:19–23.
44. Mayberg MR, Zervas NT, Moskowitz MA. Trigeminal projections to supratentorial pial and dural blood vessels in cat demonstrated by horse radish peroxidase histochemistry. *J Comp Neurol* 1984;223:46–56.

45. Saito K, Liu-Chen L-Y, Moskowitz MA. Substance P-like immunoreactivity in rat forebrain leptomeninges and cerebral vessels originate from the trigeminal but not sympathetic ganglia. *Brain Res* 1987;403:66–71.
46. Uddman R, Edvinsson L, Ekman R, Kingman T, McCulloch J. Innervation of the feline cerebral vasculature by nerve fibers containing calcitonin gene-related peptide: trigeminal origin and co-existence with substance P. *Neurosci Lett* 1985;362:131–136.
47. Wanaka A, Matusyama T, Yoneda S, et al. Origins and distribution of calcitonin gene-related peptide containing nerves in the wall of the cerebral arteries of the guinea pig with special reference to coexistence with substance P. *Brain Res* 1986;362:185–192.
48. Edvinsson L, Ekman R, Jansen I, McCulloch J, Uddman R. Calcitonin gene-related peptide and cerebral blood vessels: distribution and vasomotor effects. *J Cereb Blood Flow Metab* 1987;7:720–728.
49. Tsai S-H, Tew JM, McLean JH, Shipley MT. Cerebral arterial innervation by nerve fibers containing calcitonin gene-related peptide (CGRP). I. Distribution and origin of CGRP perivascular innervation in the rat. *J Comp Neurol* 1988;271:435–444.
50. Tsai S-H, Tew JM, Shipley MT. Cerebral arterial innervation. II. Development of calcitonin gene-related peptide and norepinephrine in the rat. *J Comp Neurol* 1989;279:1–12.
51. Gulbenkian S, Merighi A, Wharton J, Varndell IM, Polak JM. Ultrastructural evidence for the coexistence of calcitonin gene-related peptide and substance P in sensory vesicles of peripheral nerves in the guinea pig. *J Neurocytol* 1986;15:535–542.
52. O'Connor TP, van der Kooy D. Enrichment of a vasoactive neuropeptide (calcitonin gene related peptide) in the trigeminal sensory projection to the intracranial arteries. *J Neurosci* 1988;8:2468–2476.
53. Ruskell GL, Simons T. Trigeminal nerve pathways to the cerebral arteries in monkeys. *J Anat* 1987;155:67–77.
54. Simons T, Ruskell GL. Distribution and termination of trigeminal nerves to the cerebral arteries in monkeys. *J Anat* 1988;159:57–71.
55. Zhang Q-J, Kobayashi S, Hongo K. Trigeminal sensory innervation on perforators of the circle of Wilis in rabbits by wheat germ agglutinin-conjugated horse radish peroxidase anterograde tracing. *J Auton Nerv Syst* 1993;48:199–205.
56. Suzuki N, Hardebo JE, Owman C. Origins and pathways of cerebrovascular nerves storing substance P and calcitonin gene-related peptide in rat. *Neuroscience* 1989;31:427–438.
57. Hardebo JE, Suzuki N, Owman C. Origins of substance P and calcitonin gene-related peptide-containing nerves in the internal carotid artery of rat. *Neurosci Lett* 1989;101:39–45.
58. Ruskell GL. Ocular fibers of the maxillary nerve in monkeys. *J Anat* 1974;118:195–203.
59. Sinclair JG. A ganglionic plexus in human falx cerebri. *Texas Rep Biol Med* 1951;9:348–352.
60. Sinclair JG. Development of the anterior cerebral nerve plexus. *Texas Rep Biol Med* 1951;9:805–810.
61. Suzuki N, Hardebo JE, Kahrstrom J, Owman C. Effects on cortical blood flow of electrical stimulation of trigeminal cerebrovascular nerve fibers in the rat. *Acta Physiol Scand* 1990;138:307–315.
62. Lambert GA, Bogduk N, Goadsby PJ, Duckworth JW, Lance JW. Decreased carotid arterial resistance in cats in response to trigeminal stimulation. *J Neurol Surg* 1984;61:307–315.
63. Goadsby PJ, Lambert GA, Lance JW. Stimulation of the trigeminal ganglion increases flow in the extracerebral but not the cerebral circulation in the monkey. *Brain Res* 1986;381:63–67.
64. Goadsby PJ, Duckworth JW. Effects of stimulation of trigeminal ganglion on regional cerebral blood flow in cats. *Am J Physiol* 1987;253:R270–R274.
65. Lambert GA, Goadsby PJ, Zagami AS, Duckworth JW. Comparative effects of stimulation of the trigeminal ganglion and the superior sagittal sinus on cerebral blood flow and evoked potentials in the cat. *Brain Res* 1988;453:142–149.
66. Bill A, Stjernschantz J, Mandahl A, Brodin E, Nilsson G. Substance P: release on trigeminal stimulation, effects in the eye. *Acta Physiol Scand* 1979;106:371–373.
67. Couture R, Cuello AC. Studies on the trigeminal antidromic vasodilatation and plasma extravasation in the rat. *J Physiol (Lond)* 1984;346:273–285.
68. Hardebo JE, Arbab M, Suzuki N, Svengaard NA. Pathways of parasympathetic and sensory cerebrovascular nerves in monkeys. *Stroke* 1991;22:331–342.
69. McNaughton FL. The innervation of the intracranial blood vessels and dural sinuses. *Assoc Res Nerv Ment Dis* 1938;18:178–200.
70. Northfield DWC. Some observations on headache. *Brain* 1938;61:133–162.
71. Ruskell GL. The tentorial nerve in monkeys is a branch of the cavernous plexus. *J Anat* 1988;157:67–77.

72. Dalessio DJ. *Wolff's headache and other head pain*, 6th ed. New York: Oxford University Press, 1993.
73. Suzuki N, Hardebo JE. Anatomical basis for a parasympathetic and sensory innervation of the intracranial segment of the internal carotid artery in man. Possible implication for vascular headache. *J Neurol Sci* 1991;104:19–31.

7

Endothelial Messengers and Cerebral Vascular Tone Regulation

Tony J-F. Lee

Department of Pharmacology, Southern Illinois University School of Medicine, Springfield, Illinois 62794-1222

Acetylcholine (ACh) was thought to be the transmitter mediating cerebral neurogenic vasodilation when the "cholinergic" nerves innervating cerebral blood vessels were reported (1). This assumption of the role of ACh was logical based on the findings that ACh dilated cerebral and peripheral arteries and decreased systemic blood pressures (1), but was questioned half a century later based on the finding that the neurogenic vasodilation in isolated cerebral arteries was not blocked by atropine (2). It was later discovered that the ACh-induced dilation in isolated large cerebral arterial rings of the cat, like that found in the aorta (3), was endothelium dependent (4). Thus, ACh induced only constriction of cerebral arteries after the endothelium was mechanically removed. In this denuded preparation, however, neurogenic vasodilation persists (Fig. 1). This finding provides direct evidence indicating that ACh is not the transmitter mediating vasodilation, at least in the large arteries at the base of the brain, and points out the significance of cerebral vascular endothelial cells via release of vasodilating factors in regulating cerebral vascular tone and circulation. Since then, similar findings have been observed in cerebral arteries in different species, including human (5). Based on similar pharmacological characteristics of dilator substances released from the endothelial cells and perivascular nerves, Lee et al. (6) proposed for the first time that the noncholinergic, nonadrenergic vasodilator transmitter was similar to the relaxing substance released from the endothelium. The endothelium-derived relaxing factor (EDRF) (7) is now identified as nitric oxide (NO) or a NO-releasing substance (8–10). Likewise, the transmitter mediating cerebral neurogenic vasodilation is also found to be NO (11 13). It is now evident that cerebral vascular endothelial cells release not only dilator factors but also constricting factors (5,14). This chapter reports the currently described endothelium-derived relaxing and contracting factors (Fig. 2) and their mechanisms of action. The potential interaction between perivascular nerves and endothelium in regulating cerebrovascular tone is also discussed.

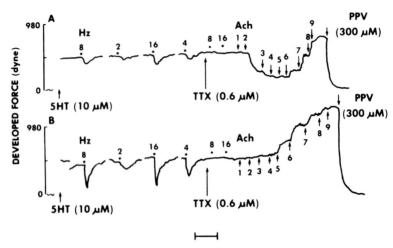

FIG. 1. Response of a segment of middle cerebral artery from a control (**A**) and a segment of the artery in which the endothelium was rubbed (**B**) to acetylcholine (ACh) and transmural nerve stimulation (TNS). Trains of 200 biphasic square wave pulses of 0.3 msec duration at different frequencies (2, 4, 8, and 16 Hz) were delivered at supramaximal voltage. The active muscle tone was produced by serotonin (5-HT), 10 µM. TNS induced a frequency-dependent relaxation in both control and endothelium rubbed arteries. The TNS-induced dilator response was abolished by tetrodotoxin (TTX), 0.6 µM. ACh induced relaxation in control artery. In contrast, ACh induced constriction exclusively in the artery with the endothelium rubbed. At the end of each experiment, papaverine (PPV) was given to induce maximum relaxation. Numbers with arrow indicate the final concentration (M) of ACh in the bath: 1, 10^{-8}; 2, 10^{-7}; 3, 3×10^{-7}; 4, $3, \times 10^{-6}$; 5, 10^{-5}; 6, 3×10^{-5}; 7, 10^{-4}; 8, 3×10^{-4}; 9, 10^{-3}. Scale bar = 5 min. (4)

PROSTACYCLIN AND OTHER CYCLOOXYGENASE PRODUCTS

Prostaglandin I_2 (PGI_2; prostacyclin), a metabolite of arachidonic acid, was first described by Moncada et al. (15) to be released from the endothelial cells. PGI_2 induces potent vasodilation in most vasculatures, by activating adenylate cyclase and the resulting increased production of cyclic adenosine monophosphate (16). The endothelial synthesis of PGI_2 in large cerebral arteries and cultured microvessels has been demonstrated (5,14,17,18). Bradykinin (via stimulation of B_2 receptors on the endothelial cells), thrombin, and A23187 are potent stimuli for PGI_2 production (17,19–21).

PGI_2 induces relaxation of isolated large cerebral arteries (22–25) and pial arterioles in vivo (26). In isolated goat middle cerebral arterial rings, serotonin-induced, concentration-dependent contraction was enhanced in mechanically denuded arteries and in endothelium-intact arteries pretreated with indomethacin (27). In the rabbit middle cerebral arteries, histamine-induced relaxation was inhibited by inhibitor of PGI_2 (5). Dilation of pial arterioles in response to angiotensin II and A23187 was also shown to be blocked by indomethacin (28). These results suggest that products of cyclooxygenase such as PGI_2 released from endothelium play an active role in

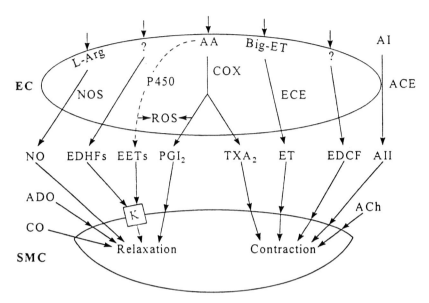

FIG. 2. Illustration of endothelium-derived relaxing and contracting factors. EC, endothelial cell; SMC, smooth muscle cell; L-Arg, L-arginine; NOS, nitric oxide synthase; NO, nitric oxide; EDHF, endothelium-derived hyperpolarizing factor; K, potassium channel; AA, arachidonic acid; P450, cytochrome P450; ROS, reactive oxygen species; EETs, epoxyeicosatrienoic acids; COX, cyclooxygenase; TXA_2, thromboxane A_2; ET, endothelin; ECE, endothelin converting enzyme; EDCF, endothelium-derived contracting factor; AI, angiotensin I; ACE, angiotensin converting enzyme; AII, angiotensin II; ACh, acetylcholine; ADO, adenosine; CO, carbon monoxide. Adenosine, acetylcholine, and carbon monoxide have been shown to be formed in the endothelial cells.

regulating cerebral vascular tone of large and small arteries. PGD_2, another product of cyclooxygenase and a potential vasodilator, has been shown to be released from human brain endothelial cells (18). Arginine-vasopressin, catecholamine, thrombin, protein kinase C-activated phorbol ester, and A23187 greatly stimulated the secretion of endothelial PGD_2.

ENDOTHELIUM-DERIVED RELAXING FACTORS

Numerous vasoactive substances, such as bradykinin, substance P, serotonin, adenosine triphosphate (ATP), adenosine diphosphate (ADP), histamine, thrombin, arginine vasopressin, endothelin, and lipid peroxidation products such as 4-hydroxynonenal have been shown to induce endothelium-dependent relaxation in large cerebral arteries and pial arterioles from a number of species including human (5,29). EDRF in cerebral endothelial cells is identified as NO or its derivatives (10,11–13,30). NO is produced by not only endothelial cells but also by perivascular

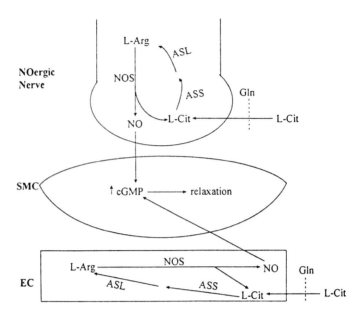

FIG. 3. Conversion of L-citrulline (L-Cit) to form L-arginine (L-Arg) in endothelial cell (EC) and perivascular nerve in cerebral blood vessel. The conversion is catalyzed by argininosuccinate synthase (ASS) and argininosuccinate lyase (ASL) in both cells. L-citrulline uptake into both cells is blocked by glutamine (Gln). NO, nitric oxide; NOS, nitric oxide synthase; cGMP, cyclic guanosine monophosphate; SMC, smooth muscle cell.

neurons and smooth muscle cells in cerebral blood vessels (11,12,13,31,32). NO is produced from L-arginine by NO synthase (NOS) with citrulline as a byproduct (8,9,33). The constitutive form of NOS and its marker, reduced nicotinamide adenine dinucleotide phosphate (NADPH)-diaphorase, are localized in the endothelium of large and small pial vessels, in parenchymal vessels as small as 3 μm in diameter (34–36), and in perivascular neurons (12,37). Biochemical measurement of cyclic guanosine monophosphate (cGMP) content and physiological and pharmacological examinations of changes in vascular tone or vessel diameter consistently support the role of the arginine-NO-cGMP pathway in mediating endothelium-dependent vasodilation (5,6). Furthermore, endothelial cells and cerebral perivascular neurons recycle L-citrulline, the byproduct of NOS, to form L-arginine, the substrate of NOS (37,38) (Fig. 3). This is indicated by the findings that increased arterial tone induced by nitro-L-arginine is reversed by L-citrulline and L-arginine (38). Our morphologic results also indicate that endothelial cells in cerebral arteries contain argininosuccinate synthase (ASS) and argininosuccinate lyase (ASL) immunoreactivities. Both ASS and ASL are necessary enzymes for conversion of L-citrulline to L-arginine as is found in cerebral perivascular nerves (37). This finding of L-citrulline recycling to form L-arginine in the endothelium and perivascular nerves verifies the origins of

NO in endothelium and perivascular neurons and provides the first direct evidence that NO can be released from cerebral perivascular nerves. This recycling mechanism also provides a means for an "unlimited" supply of NO in mediating both endothelium-dependent and neurogenic vasodilation (39).

The receptor subtypes on endothelial cells mediating NO release in response to numerous agonists are not fully characterized. Species variation is significant. The endothelium-mediated relaxation of large cerebral arteries and microvessels in response to ACh has been shown pharmacologically to be mediated by M_3 muscarinic receptors (40–42). The similar receptor subtype has also been shown to mediate endothelium-dependent relaxation in the aorta of the spontaneously hypertensive rat (43). This receptor subtype, however, was not expressed in the cultured human cerebral microvessel endothelial cells, which strongly expressed the M_2 and M_5 muscarinic receptors (44).

Serotonin (5-HT)-induced contraction of large cerebral arteries in most species (4,27,45–47) is enhanced after inhibition of NO synthesis or de-endothelization, suggesting that 5-HT can also act on the endothelium to release NO and modulate its contractile effect. The 5-HT receptors on the endothelial cells mediating NO release have been suggested to be 5-HT2B/2C (46).

The histamine-induced cerebral arterial constriction is also limited by its effect on releasing dilator factor from the endothelium (25,48). Thus, endothelial damage or lesion will result in an increase in histamine-induced contraction. The dilator factors, both NO and PGI_2, released from endothelial cells in response to histamine have been shown to be mediated by H_1 receptors in the primate (48) and H_3 receptors in the rabbit (25). In clinical studies, histamine-induced, probably NO-mediated, migraine headache has been suggested to involve H_1 receptors (49,50). Regional variation in cerebral vasomotor control by endothelium-derived NO is also apparent. NO has been shown to play a greater role in pial vessels of the posterior than the anterior circulation (51), in large arteries than in small ones (5), and in arteries than in veins (52).

The regional heterogeneity in endothelium-mediated response also occurs to many other agonists. Arginine-vasopressin-induced, endothelium-dependent relaxation, mediated by the V_1-vasopressinergic receptor coupled to NOS, was found in the circle of Willis and brain stem arteries, but not in the middle cerebral arteries of the dog (53,54). Furthermore, the EDRFs mediating bradykinin-induced, endothelium-dependent relaxation are different between large cerebral arteries and arterioles. The relaxation mediated by B_2 receptors on the endothelium (17,20) appears to be due to endothelium-derived NO in the large arteries and hydroxyl radical and hydrogen peroxide in the arterioles (30,55–57).

Consistent with findings from in vitro studies, endothelium-dependent dilation in response to agonists has also been observed in the cerebral circulation in vivo. Topical application of ACh, substance P, and bradykinin dilates pial arterioles and the basilar arteries (5). Intravascular administration of ACh and substance P produces increase in cerebral blood flow (5). Synthesis of NO or EDRF in cerebral vessels in vitro and in vivo appears to occur under basal conditions (5,11). Based on NOS knock-out experiments, it has been shown that endothelial NOS plays a role in regulating the basal cerebral blood flow (58). NO also appears to mediate vasodilation and increased cerebral blood flow during hypercapnia (59). Removal or injury of the endothelium did not abolish the hypercapnia-induced dilation (60,61). The neuronal but not endothelial source of NO may contribute to blood flow augmentation during moderate hypercapnia (58). In a recent report, hypercapnia-induced cerebral arteriolar dilation is shown to be associated with activation by CO_2 of ATP-sensitive potassium channels (62). It is, however, not clear if different levels of hypercapnia may have different effects on different sources of NO.

Whether or not NO participates in autoregulation of cerebral blood flow remains unsettled. Wang et al. (61) reported that autoregulation of cerebral blood flow during decreases in arterial pressure was not altered by inhibition of NO synthesis, suggesting that endothelium-derived NO does not contribute to decreases in cerebral vascular resistance that occur during decreases in perfusion pressure. This is different from the finding by Kobari et al. (63) that in anesthetized cats cerebral blood flow remained constant with blood pressure changes.

ENDOTHELIUM-DERIVED HYPERPOLARIZING FACTOR

Along with the production of NO, ACh and several agonists such as bradykinin, 5-HT, and histamine can induce vasodilation via hyperpolarization of smooth muscle cells in cerebral arteries and arterioles that is not mediated by NO (64). Using a sandwich preparation (65) and a perfusion-superfusion cascade method in the presence of inhibitors of NO synthase and cyclooxygenase (66), endothelial cells in guinea pig carotid arteries and canine carotid arteries were shown to release, in response to ACh and bradykinin, respectively, a substance that hyperpolarized and relaxed the vascular smooth muscle. The effects were blocked by tetraethylammonium (TEA), an inhibitor of Ca^{2+}-activated K^+ channels, suggesting that endothelial cells released a diffusible endothelium-derived hyperpolarizing factor (EDHF) that activated Ca-dependent K^+ channels in vascular smooth muscle. EDHF may also produce hyperpolarization and relaxation of vascular smooth muscle through stimulation of Na-K-ATPase (65,67). In cerebral circulation, ample evidence indicates that activation of potassium channels produces hyperpolarization of smooth muscle and relaxation of cerebral arteries in vitro and in vivo (5). Since activation of potassium channels is a major mechanism of cerebral vasodilation (68), identification of the nature of EDHF has been intensively pursued.

Campbell et al. (69) recently reported that the cytochrome P450 inhibitors such as SKF525A and miconazole significantly attenuated relaxation and completely inhibited hyperpolarization of isolated bovine coronary arteries with intact endothelium induced by methacholine. The relaxation was inhibited by TEA. Furthermore, in vessels prelabeled with [^{3}H]arachidonic acid, methacholine stimulated the release of epoxyeicosatrienoic acids (EETs). Arachidonic acid relaxed precontracted coronary arteries, which were blocked by TEA. The EETs indeed hyperpolarized and relaxed coronary smooth muscles. These effects were attenuated by TEA. The EETs also increased the open-state probability of Ca^{2+}-activated K^+ channel in the coronary smooth muscle (69). These results suggest that EETs, metabolites of arachidonic acid by the P450 epoxygenase pathway, are EDHF in bovine coronary arteries. This is consistent with the finding in carotid arteries of the rabbit (70). But findings in guinea pig carotid arteries indicated that metabolites of arachidonic acids through cyclooxygenase, lipoxygenase, or cytochrome P450 monooxygenase were not involved in ACh-induced, endothelium-dependent hyperpolarization (71). In this latter study, miconazole, a specific inhibitor of P450 epoxygenase, was not used. In cerebral circulation, miconazole was shown to decrease baseline cerebral blood flow by 30% with inhibition of conversion of arachidonic acids to EETs (72). These results support the notion that endogenous P450 epoxides of arachidonic acids play a role via activation of potassium channels in the regulation of basal blood flow in cerebral microcirculation.

In large cerebral arteries, superoxide anion is considered a vasoconstrictor because it is a potent inactivator of NO and it selectively inhibits PGI_2 synthesis (73). The endothelium-dependent contraction of the canine basilar artery in response to ACh is in part mediated by superoxide anion and is the balance between superoxide and NO. In contrast, oxygen-derived radicals including superoxide anion, hydroxyl radical, hydrogen peroxide, and peroxynitrite, which are released on application of bradykinin, are shown to be strong dilators in the cerebral microcirculation of the cat and mice (74–76). In anesthetized cats equipped with a cranial window, exogenous hydrogen peroxide and peroxynitrite induced dilation of cerebral arterioles, which was inhibited by glyburide, an inhibitor of ATP-sensitive potassium channels. In the same preparations, dilation induced by superoxide, generated by xanthine oxidase acting on xanthine in the presence of catalase, was not affected by glyburide but was inhibited completely by TEA. The vasodilations induced by these three reactive oxygen species were not affected by inhibition of soluble guanylate cyclase with LY83583.

These results suggest that hydrogen peroxide, peroxynitrite, and superoxide induce cerebral arteriolar dilation by activating ATP-sensitive potassium channels and Ca-dependent potassium channels, respectively, and that activation of soluble guanylate cyclase is not involved in the dilator action of these oxygen radicals (74). Evidence that potassium channels are involved in cerebral vasodilation during hypercapnia has also been presented (62). These authors reported that hypercapnia-induced dilation in cat cerebral arterioles was blocked by nitro-L-arginine (L-NNA) and glyburide but not by LY83583. L-NNA also blocked dilation induced by ATP-sensitive potassium channel openers. These data suggest that arginine analogs inhibit hypercapnic vasodilation by blocking ATP-sensitive K^+ channels, independently of activation of guanylate cyclase. Furthermore, cerebral arterial dilations during hypoxia (77,78) and changes in intravascular pressure (79) have also been shown to be due to activation of potassium channels. Wellman and Bevan (80) have also reported that flow-induced shear stress activates inward rectifier potassium channels in endothelial cells, leading to increased synthesis/release of NO in the endothelium.

ENDOTHELIUM-DERIVED CONTRACTING FACTOR

The major endothelium-derived contracting factors (EDCFs) shown in cerebral circulation are endothelin-1 (ET-1) and cyclooxygenase products of arachidonic acid. Lypoxygenase products and cytochrome P450 monooxygenase products are also potential candidates (5,14,81). ET produces potent contraction of large cerebral arteries, pial arteries, and parenchymal arterioles via activation of ET_A receptors on smooth muscle from a variety of species including human in vitro (5). In vivo, topical application of low concentrations of ET produced dilation of pial arterioles, probably by acting on ET_B receptors on the endothelium to release NO. Formation of ET in cultured cerebral endothelial cells has been shown to be stimulated by angiotensin II, vasopressin, thrombin, and 5-HT (5).

ACh induces endothelium-dependent dilation in cerebral arteries of most species; it induced endothelium-dependent constriction in the dog, and possibly porcine, basilar arteries (82–85). Thromboxane A_2, the primary cyclooxygenase product of arachidonic acid, has been shown to mediate endothelium-dependent contraction in the canine basilar arteries (82–84). Endothelium-dependent contractions in canine basilar arteries have been shown in response to a large number of other agonists including A23187, ADP, ATP, norepinephrine, hydrogen peroxide, prostaglandin H_2, angiotensin, serotonin, histamine, nicotine, somatostatin, and tetrahydrobiopterin (84,86).

NEURAL-ENDOTHELIAL MODULATION

Several reports have indicated that endothelium can modulate perivascular nerve-elicited responses. In isolated cerebral arterial rings of the cat and pig, transmural nerve stimulation (TNS) elicits tetrodotoxin-sensitive, NO-mediated relaxation (85,87). The relaxation is significantly enhanced in arteries without endothelial cells (85,87) (Fig. 1). In porcine basilar arteries with endothelial cells, the TNS-induced relaxation is increased by glutamate, suggesting that N-methyl-D-aspartate receptors on the endothelium may modulate neurogenic vasodilation (38). These results suggest the presence of potential functional interactions between endothelium and perivascular nerves in regulating cerebral vascular tone. Due to the large distance between nerve and endothelium, particularly in large arteries, direct modulation through activation of receptors on endothelial cells by mediators from the nerves or vice versa is questionable (87). The nature of nerve-endothelial modulation remains to be determined.

CONCLUSIONS

Since the discovery of EDRF, investigation of endothelial regulation of vascular tone has been intensified. Several relaxing and contracting factors have been identified, and the numbers are increasing. The identification of several EDHFs and demonstrations of ACh (88), adenosine (5), and heme oxygenase (89) in cerebral arterial endothelium further emphasize the significant role of endothelial cells in regulating cerebral vascular functions in health and disease.

ACKNOWLEDGMENTS

This work was supported by NIH HL 27763 and HL47574. We thank Ms. Dawn Melcher for preparing the manuscript.

REFERENCES

1. Chorobski J, Penfield W. Cerebral vasodilator nerves and their pathway from the medulla oblongata. *Arch Neurol Psychiatry* 1932;28:1257–1289.
2. Lee TJF, Su C, Bevan JA. Nonsympathetic dilator innervation of cat cerebral arteries. *Experientia* 1975;31:1424–1425.
3. Furchgott RF, Zawadzki JV. Acetylcholine relaxes arterial smooth muscle by releasing a relaxing substance from endothelial cells. *Fed Proc* 1980;39:581.
4. Lee TJF. Direct evidence against acetylcholine as the dilator transmitter in the cat cerebral artery. *Eur J Pharmacol* 1980;68:393–394.
5. Faraci FM. Regulation of the cerebral circulation by endothelium. *Pharmacol Ther* 1992;56:1–22.
6. Lee TJF, Fang YX, Nickols GA. Cyclic nucleotides and cerebral vasodilation. In: Seylaz J, MacKenzie ET, eds. *Neurotransmission and cerebrovascular function*. Amsterdam: Elsevier, 1989; 277–280.
7. Furchgott RF, Zawadzki JV. The obligatory role of endothelial cells in the relaxation of arterial smooth muscle by acetylcholine. *Nature* 1980;288:373–376.
8. Palmer RMJ, Ferrige AG, Moncada S. Nitric oxide release accounts for the biological activity of endothelium-derived relaxing factor. *Nature* 1987;327:524–526.
9. Ignarro LJ. Biological action and properties of endothelium-derived nitric oxide formed and released from artery and vein. *Circ Res* 1989;65:1–21.
10. Kukreja RC, Wei EP, Kontos HA, Bates JN. Nitric oxide and S-nitroso-L-cysteine as endothelium-derived relaxing factors from acetylcholine in cerebral vessels in cats. *Stroke* 1993;24:2010–2014.
11. Lee TJF, Sarwinski SJ. Nitric oxidergic neurogenic vasodilation in the porcine basilar artery. *Blood Vessels* 1991;28:407–412.
12. Chen FY, Lee TJF. Role of nitric oxide in neurogenic vasodilation of porcine cerebral artery. *J Pharmacol Exp Ther* 1993;265:339–345.
13. Toda N, Okamura T. Mechanism underlying the response to vasodilator nerve stimulation in isolated dog and monkey cerebral arteries. *Am J Physiol* 1990;259:H1511–1517.
14. Akopov S, Sercombe R, Seylaz J. Cerebral vascular reactivity: role of endothelium/platelet/leukocyte interactions. *Cerebrovasc Brain Metab Rev* 1996;8:11–94.
15. Moncada S, Gryglewski RJ, Bunting S, Vane JR. An enzyme isolated from arteries transforms prostaglandin endoperoxide to an unstable substance that inhibits platelet aggregation. *Nature* 1976; 263:663–665.
16. Gorman RR, Bunting S, Miller OV. Modulation of human platelet adenylate cyclase by prostacyclin. *Prostaglandins* 1977;13:377–338.
17. Wiemer G, Popp R, Scholkens BA, Gogelein H. Enhancement of cytosolic calcium, prostacyclin and

nitric oxide by bradykinin and ACE inhibitor ramiprilat in porcine brain capillary endothelial cells. *Brain Res* 1994;638:261–266.
18. Spatz M, Stanimirovic D, Bacic F, Uematsu S, McCarron RM.Vasoconstrictive peptides induce endothelin-1 and prostanoids in human cerebromicrovascular endothelium. *Am J Physiol* 1994;266: C654–C660.
19. Okumura R, Hatake K, Wakabayashi I, Suehiro A, Hishida S, Kakishita E. Vasorelaxant effect of trapidil on human basilar artery. *J Pharm Pharmacol* 1992;44:425–428.
20. Wahl M, Schilling L. Effects of bradykinin in the cerebral microcirculation. In: Phillis JE, ed. *The regulation of cerebral blood flow*. Boca Raton: CRC Press, 1993;315–328.
21. Moore SA, Spector AA, Hart MN. Eicosanoid metabolism in cerebromicrovascular endothelium. *Am J Physiol* 1988;254:C37–C44.
22. Uski T, Andersson KE, Brant L, Edvinsson L, Ljunggren B. Responses of isolated feline and human cerebral arteries to prostacyclin and some of its metabolites. *J Cereb Blood Flow Metab* 1983;3: 238–245.
23. Parsons AA, Whalley ET. Effects of prostanoids on human and rabbit basilar arteries precontracted *in vitro*. *Cephalalgia* 1989;9:165–171.
24. Shirahase H, Usui H, Manabe K, Kurahashi K, Fujiwara M. Vasorelaxing effects of prostaglandin I_2 on the canine basilar artery and coronary arteries. *J Pharmacol Exp Ther* 1989;248:769–773.
25. Ea Kim L, Javellaud J, Oudart N. Endothelium-dependent relaxation of rabbit middle cerebral artery to a histamine H_3-agonist is reduced by inhibitors of nitric oxide and prostacyclin. *Br J Pharmacol* 1992;105:103–106.
26. Ellis EF, Wei EP, Kontos HA. Vasodilation of cat cerebral arterioles by prostaglandins D_2, E_2, G_2, and I_2. *Am J Physiol* 1979;237:H381–385.
27. Miranda FJ, Torregrosa G, Salom JB, et al. Endothelial modulation of 5-hydroxytryptamine-induced contraction in goat cerebral arteries. *Gen Pharmacol* 1993;24:649–653.
28. Haberl RL, Anneser F, Villringer A, Einhaupl KM. Angiotensin II induces endothelium-dependent vasodilation of rat cerebral arterioles. *Am J Physiol* 1990;258:H1840–1846.
29. Martinez MC, Bosch-Morrell F, Raya A, et al. 4-Hydroxynonenal, a lipid peroxidation product, induces relaxation of human cerebral arteries. *J Cereb Blood Flow Metab* 1994;14:693–696.
30. Rosenblum WI. Hydroxyl radical mediates the endothelium-dependent relaxation produced by bradykinin in mouse cerebral arterioles. *Circ Res* 1987;61:601–603.
31. Ueno M, Lee TJF. Endotoxin decreases the contractile responses of the porcine basilar artery to vasoactive substances. *J Cereb Blood Flow Metab* 1993;13:712–719.
32. Gonzalez C, Estrada C. Nitric oxide mediates the neurogenic vasodilation of bovine cerebral arteries. *J Cereb Blood Flow Metab* 1991;11:366–370.
33. Moncada S, Palmer RMJ, Higgs EA. Nitric oxide: physiology, pathophysiology and pharmacology. *Pharmacol Rev* 1991;43:109–142.
34. Bredt DS, Hwang PM, Snyder SH. Localization of nitric oxide synthase indicating a neural role for nitric oxide. *Nature* 1990;347:768–770.
35. Lovick TA, Key BJ. Distribution of nicotinamide adenine dinucleotide phosphate (NADPH)-dependent diaphorase staining in intraparenchymal blood vessels of the rat brain. *Neurosci Lett* 1995; 196:113–115.
36. Gabbott PL, Bacon SJ. Histochemical localization of NADPH-dependent diaphorase (nitric oxide synthase) activity in vascular endothelial cells in the rat brain. *Neuroscience* 1993;57:79–95.
37. Yu JG, O'Brien WE, Lee TJF. Morphological evidence for L-citrulline conversion to L-arginine via the argininosuccinate pathwway in porcine cerebral perivascular nerves. *J Cereb Blood Flow Metab* (in press).
38. Lee TJF, Sarwinski S, Ishine T, Lai CC, Chen FY. Inhibition of cerebral neurogenic vasodilation by L-glutamine and nitric oxide synthase inhibitors and its reversal by L-citrulline. *J Pharmacol Exp Ther* 1996;276:353–358.
39. Chen FY, Lee TJF. Arginine synthesis from citrulline in perivascular nerves of cerebral artery. *J Pharmacol Exp Ther* 1995;273:895–901.
40. Dauphin F, Hamel E. Muscarinic receptor subtype mediating vasodilation in feline middle cerebral artery exhibits M3 pharmacology. *Eur J Pharmacol* 1990;178:203–213.
41. Garcia-Villalon AL, Krause DN, Ehlert FJ, Duckles SP. Heterogeneity of muscarinic receptor subtypes in cerebral blood vessels. *J Pharmacol Exp* 1991;258:304–310.
42. Alonso MJ, Arribas S, Marin J, Balfagon G, Salaices M. Presynaptic M_2-muscarinic receptors on noradrenergic nerve endings and endothelium-derived M_3 receptors in cat cerebral arteries. *Brain Res* 1991;567:76–82.
43. Boulanger CM, Morrison KJ, Vanhoutte PM. Mediation by M3-muscarinic receptors of both en-

dothelium-dependent contraction and relaxation to acetylcholine in the aorta of the spontaneously hypertensive rat. *Br J Pharmacol* 1994;112:519–524.
44. Elhusseiny A, Cohen Z, Olivier A, Yong W, Stanimirovic D, Hamel E. Expression of muscarinic receptor mRNAs in human brain microvascular fractions, cultured vascular cells and astrocytes. *Soc Neurosci Abst* 1996;22:692.8.
45. Faraci FM, Heistad DD. Endothelium-derived relaxing factor inhibits constrictor responses of large cerebral arteries to serotonin. *J Cereb Blood Flow Metab* 1992;12:500–506.
46. Fozard JR. The 5-hydroxytryptamine-nitric oxide connection: the key link in the initiation of migraine. *Arch Int Pharmacodyn Ther* 1995;329:111–119.
47. Brian JE Jr, Kennedy RH. Modulation of cerebral arterial tone by endothelium-derived relaxing factor. *Am J Physiol* 1993;264(4 Pt 2):H1245–1250.
48. Ayajiki K, Okamura T, Toda N. Involvement of nitric oxide in endothelium-dependent, phasic relaxation caused by histamine in monkey cerebral arteries. *Jpn J Pharmacol* 1992;60:357–362.
49. Olesen J, Iversen HK, Thomsen LL. Nitric oxide supersensitivity: a possible molecular mechanism of migraine pain. *Neuroreport* 1993;4:1027–1030.
50. Lassen LH, Thomsen LL, Olesen J. Histamine induced migraine via the H1-receptor. Support for the NO hypothesis of migraine. *Neuroreport* 1994;6:1475–1479.
51. Kijita Y, Takayasu M, Suzuki Y, et al. Regional differences in cerebral vasomotor control by nitric oxide. *Brain Res Bull* 1995;38:365–369.
52. Lee TJF, Ueno M, Sunagane N, Sun MH. Serotonin relaxes porcine pial veins. *Am J Physiol* 1994;266:H1000–H1006.
53. Katusic ZS. Endothelial L-arginine pathway and regional cerebral arterial reactivity to vasopressin. *Am J Physiol* 1992;262(5 Pt 2):H1557–1562.
54. Suzuki Y, Satoh S, Oyama H, Takayasu M, Shibuya M, Sugita K. Vasopressin mediated vasodilation of cerebral arteries. *J Auton Nervous Syst* 1994;49:S129–132.
55. Kontos HA, Wei EP, Kukreja RC, Ellis EF, Hess ML. Differences in endothelium-dependent cerebral dilation by bradykinin and acetylcholine. *Am J Physiol* 1990;258:H1261–1266.
56. Mayhan WG. Impairment of endothelium-dependent dilation of basilar artery during chronic hypertension. *Am J Physiol* 1990;259:H1455–1462.
57. Copeland JR, Willoughby KA, Tynan TM, Moore SF, Ellis EF. Endothelial and nonendothelial cyclooxygenase mediate rabbit pial arteriole dilation by bradykinin. *Am J Physiol* 1995;268(1 Pt 2):H458–466.
58. Ma J, Meng W, Ayata C, Huang PL, Fishman MC, Moskowitz MA. L-NNA-sensitive regional cerebral blood flow augmentation during hypercapnia in type III NOS mutant mice. *Am Physiol Soc* 1996;271:H1717–H1719.
59. Iadecola C, Pelligrino DA, Moskowitz MA, Lassen NA. Nitric oxide synthase inhibition and cerebrovascular regulation. *J Cereb Blood Flow Metab* 1994;14:175–192.
60. Gotoh F, Fukuuchi Y, Amano T, et al. Role of endothelium in responses of pial vessels to changes in blood pressure and to carbon dioxide in cats. *J Cereb Blood Flow Metab* 1987;7:S275.
61. Wang Q, Paulson OB, Lassen NA. Is autoregulation of cerebral blood flow in rats influenced by nitro-L-arginine, a blocker of the synthesis of nitric oxide? *Acta Physiol Scand* 1992;145:297–298.
62. Kontos HA, Wei EP. Arginine analogues inhibit responses mediated by ATP-sensitive K^+ channels. *Am J Physiol* 1996;271:H1498–H1506.
63. Kobari M, Fukuuchi Y, Tomita M, Tanahashi N, Takeda H. Role of nitric oxide in regulation of cerebral microvascular tone and autoregulation of cerebral blood flow in cats. *Brain Res* 1994;667:255–262.
64. Brayden JE. Membrane hyperpolarization is a mechanism of endothelium-dependent cerebral vasodilation. *Am J Physiol* 1990;69:1415–1420.
65. Chen G, Yamamoto Y, Miwa K, Suzuki H. Hyperpolarization of arterial smooth muscle induced by endothelial humoral substances. *Am J Physiol* 1991;260:H1888–1892.
66. Mombouli JV, Bissiriou I, Agboton VD, Vanhoutte PM. Bioassay of endothelium-derived hyperpolarizing factor. *Biochem Biophys Res Commun* 1996;221:484–488.
67. Feletou M, Vanhoutte PM. Endothelium-dependent hyperpolarization of canine coronary smooth muscle. *Br J Pharmacol* 1988;93:515–524.
68. Kitazono T, Faraci FM, Taguchi H, Heistad DD. Role of potassium channels in cerebral blood vessels. *Stroke* 1995;26:1713–1723.
69. Campbell WB, Gebremedhin D, Pratt PF, Harder DR. Identification of epoxyeicosatrienoic acids as endothelium-derived hyperpolarizing factors. *Circ Res* 1996;78:415–423.

70. Lischke V, Busse R, Hecker M. Inhalation anesthetics inhibit the release of endothelium-derived hyperpolarizing factor in the rabbit carotid artery. *Anesthesiology* 1995;83:574–582.
71. Corriu C, Feletou M, Canet E, Vanhoutte PM. Inhibitors of the cytochrome P450-mono-oxygenase and endothelium-dependent hyperpolarizations in the guinea-pig isolated carotid artery. *Br J Pharmacol* 1996;17:601–610.
72. Alkayed NJ, Birks EK, Hudetz AG, Roman RJ, Henderson L, Harder DR. Inhibition of brain *P*-450 arachidonic acid epoxygenase decreases baseline cerebral blood flow. *Am J Physiol* 1996;271: H1541–1546.
73. Katusic ZS. Superoxide anion and endothelial regulation of arterial tone. *Free Radic Biol Med* 1996; 20:443–448.
74. Wei EP, Kontos HA, Beckman JS. Mechanisms of cerebral vasodilation by superoxide hydrogen peroxide, and peroxynitrite. *Am J Physiol* 1996;271:H1262–1996.
75. Wei EP, Kontos HA. H_2O_2 and endothelium-dependent cerebral arteriolar dilation: implications for the identity of endothelium-derived relaxing factor generated by acetylcholine. *Hypertension* 1990; 16:162–169.
76. Taguchi H, Heistad D, Kitazono T, Faraci F. Dilatation of cerebral arterioles in response to activation of adenylate cyclase is dependent on activation of Ca^{2+}-dependent K^+ channels. *Circ Res* 1995;76: 1057–1062.
77. Gebremedhin D, Bonnet P, Green AS, et al. Hypoxia increases the activity of Ca(2+)-sensitive K+ channels in cat cerebral arterial muscle cell membranes. *Pflugers Arch* 1994;428:621–630.
78. Fredricks KT, Liu Y, Rusch NJ, Lombard JH. Role of endothelium and arterial K+ channels in mediating hypoxic dilation of middle cerebral arteries. *Am J Physiol* 1994;267:H580–586.
79. Knot HJ, Nelson MT. Regulation of membrane potential and diameter by voltage-dependent K+ channels in rabbit myogenic cerebral arteries. *Am J Physiol* 1995;269:H348–355.
80. Wellman GC, Bevan JA. Barium inhibits the endothelium-dependent component of flow but not acetylcholine-induced relaxation in isolated rabbit cerebral arteries. *JPET* 1995;274:47–53.
81. Harder DR, Campbell WB, Roman RJ. Role of cytochrome P-450 enzymes and metabolites of arachidonic acid in the control of vascular tone. *J Vasc Res* 1995;32:79–92.
82. Shirahase H, Fujiwara M, Usui H, Kurahashi K. A possible role of thromboxane A2 in endothelium in maintaining resting tone and producing contractile response to acetylcholine and arachidonic acid in canine cerebral arteries. *Blood Vessels* 1987;24:117–119.
83. Katusic ZS, Shepherd JT, Vanhoutte PM. Endothelium-dependent contractions to calcium ionophore A23187, arachidonic acid and acetylcholine in canine basilar arteries. *Stroke* 1988;19:476–479.
84. Shirahase H, Kanda M, Shimaji H, Usui H, Rorstad OP, Kurahashi K. Somatostatin-induced contraction mediated by endothelial TXA2 production in canine cerebral arteries. *Life Sci* 1993;53:1539–1544.
85. Lee TJF, Kinkead L, Sarwinski S. Norepinephrine and acetylcholine transmitter mechanism in pig cerebral blood vessels. *J Cereb Blood Flow Metab* 1982;2:439–450.
86. Kinoshita H, Katusic ZS. Exogenous tetrahydrobiopterin causes endothelium-dependent contractions in isolated canine basilar artery. *Am J Physiol* 1996;271:H738–H743.
87. Lee TJF. Cholinergic mechanisms in the large cat cerebral arteries. *Circ Res* 1982;50:870–879.
88. Yu JG, Lee TJF. Choline acetyltransferase-immunoreactivities in cerebral blood vessels. *Chin J Pharmacol Toxicol* 1992;6:28–35.
89. Zakhary R, Gaine SP, Dinerman JL, Ruat M, Flavahan NA, Snyder SH. Heme oxygenase 2: endothelial and neuronal localization and role in endothelium-dependent relaxation. *Proc Natl Acad Sci USA* 1996;93:795–798.

8
Discussion Summary: Messenger Molecules in Cranial Blood Vessels

Patrick P. A. Humphrey

Glaxo Institute of Applied Pharmacology, University of Cambridge, Cambridge CB2 1QJ, United Kingdom

There was much discussion about the role of the sympathetic nervous system and the enigma of its modest vasoconstrictor effect in controlling cerebral blood flow, despite its relatively dense innervation. The experimental observation that sympathetic stimulation has little effect on basal cerebral blood flow is consistent with in vitro data showing that noradrenaline is weak in contracting isolated cerebral arteries. However, noradrenaline is more potent in stimulating large arteries rather than small arteries, consistent with it not having a profound effect on resistance vessels. Furthermore, it was said that noradrenaline is potent in contracting cerebral veins. This was of particular interest in relation to the effect of the sympathetic nervous system in the control of cerebrovascular capacitance.

Apparently dihydroergotamine is being used experimentally in the treatment of cerebral edema associated with severe head trauma. The basis for this could be the potent α-adrenoceptor agonist activity of dihydroergotamine. The sympathetic innervation to the large cerebral arteries appears to be important in supporting autoregulation within the brain, such that during sympathetic stimulation blood flow is maintained, despite markedly increased pressures that would otherwise lead to excessive increases in flow. This would seem to provide an important protective mechanism in various hypertensive conditions. It was speculated that α-adrenoceptor agonists might be used clinically in benign intracranial hypertension. Stimulation of the sympathetic nervous system will also reduce cerebrospinal fluid (CSF) pressure by inhibition of its secretion within the choroid plexus, and again this may be an important mechanism in controlling cerebral edema. Consideration was also given to the role of neuropeptide Y (NPY), which is co-released with noradrenaline, although stored in separate vesicles within sympathetic nerve terminals. It appears to provide supporting actions complimentary to those of noradrenaline, causing a modest vasoconstriction and potentiating other vasoconstrictors. Interestingly, in terms of the arterial to venous selectivity, NPY is more potent on arteries than on veins, which is the opposite of the case for noradrenaline.

The puzzling multiplicity of neurotransmitters in the parasympathetic nervous system was discussed. They include not only acetylcholine but also vasoactive intestinal peptide (VIP), pituitary adenylate cyclase-activating peptide (PACAP), and heliospectin. The role of PACAP is unclear, but it is also found in sensory nerves, and one may speculate that it has an antinociceptive function. Heliospectin and similar peptides are also present and cause modest vasorelaxation, but their precise role is unknown. Obviously acetylcholine and VIP have profound vasodilator actions, and nitric oxide (neuronal) may also be important in this respect. The co-existence of these multiple transmitters raises the question of the importance and relevance of co-transmission; what role do they all play? One wonders too whether they have a homogeneous role throughout the parasympathetic nervous system or whether indeed they might have differential roles at different locations within the system. It is clear that the parasympathetic nervous system is involved in the control of cerebral blood flow causing vasodilation and increases in cerebral blood flow, but the exact mediators involved remain unclear. Acetylcholine acts through activation of endothelial nitric oxide synthase (NOS) to release nitric oxide (NO), and this will be highly dependent on the integrity of the endothelium and the presence of muscarinic receptors. Other mediators like VIP and heliospectin cause vascular smooth relaxation directly, but the exact roles of NPY (present in small quantities in the parasympathetic system) and PACAP remain to be determined.

It would seem that the parasympathetic nervous system does not have a profound controlling influence on basal cerebral blood flow, but under pathophysiological conditions is important in maintaining an adequate cerebral blood flow. This seems to be particularly evident in animal models of stroke. However, it is not entirely clear how important the additional vasodilator actions of NO are under pathological conditions such as ischemia and the relative contributions from perivascular nerves and the endothelium. As regards any cross-talk between the various nervous systems (sympathetic, parasympathetic, and sensory), it seems likely that when mediators are released in large amounts due to excessive stimulation, they may feed back on the nerve terminals of the other systems and modify presynaptic release of relevant transmitters.

In the sensory nervous system, redundancy of neurotransmitters seems to be less apparent, with the major mediators being substance P and calcitonin gene-related peptide (CGRP). Substance P was first isolated from dorsal root ganglia and the spinal cord and is more potent than glutamate as a depolarizing agent. It also has a vasodilator action (physiologically beneficial?) within the cerebrovasculature, and these effects appear to be mediated through NK_1 receptors on endothelial cells. CGRP is co-stored with substance P, but the ratio of the concentrations of the two transmitters seems to vary quite markedly according to the location, with CGRP being seen in general in much higher concentrations than substance P. This seems to be in keeping with the work of Edvinsson and Goadsby, who showed that during a migraine attack CGRP, but not substance P, is measurable in the external jugular venous blood. Discussions led to the view that there is no reason to believe that substance P is more metabolically labile under the experimental conditions employed. This suggests that CGRP is the predominant mediator released and that the blood vessels involved in the pathophysiology of migraine are those that are innervated by predominantly CGRP-containing sensory nerves. The role of neuronally released NO was also discussed, but the relative distribution of nNOS within the sensory nervous system was not known. There is, however, evidence that extraneuronal NO will activate sensory nerves and release CGRP.

The question was raised as to whether glutamate is released from trigeminal sensory nerve terminals. There is apparently no evidence for this but it seems surprising if it is not, since glutamate is believed to be the main transmitter at the rostral end, where nerves terminate in the nucleus caudalis. As regards the precise role of the two major known transmitters (substance P and CGRP) at the peripheral level of sensory nerve terminals, there was general agreement that substance P is probably involved in extravasation and to some degree vasodilation, while CGRP causes profound and prolonged vasodilation, which may be an important component of the migraine pathophysiology. However, an additional contribution of other vasodilator mediators such as prostaglandins and NO to the pathophysiology of headache must also be seriously considered.

The role of the endothelium is apparently complex and paradoxical in that it is capable of secreting both vasoconstrictor agents and vasodilator agents. The vasoconstrictor agents include endothelin in particular, but the powerful vasodilator mediators it and other stimuli can release were the focus of discussion. They obviously include adenosine, prostacyclin, and endothelium-derived relaxing factor (now known to be NO). The latter appears to be the most obvious substance of interest in relation to migraine pathophysiology. There was extensive debate about whether endogenous NO might be involved in vascular headache and what the mechanism might be. It is certainly a potent vasodilator, and this could arguably explain the lowering of thresholds for perivascular sensory nerve activation; in addition, NO is able to activate nerves in its own right. NO may also initiate other inflammatory sequelae, which makes it a potential candidate for the initiation of the pathophysiology of headache. However, the question of what the most likely source is was raised; is it likely to be produced by endothelial NOS or neuronal NOS, or perhaps more likely by inducible NOS? The consensus was that low levels of NO might be released from endothelial cells, causing modest physiological degrees of vasodilation, not making it an obvious candidate in a pathophysiological scenario. It was agreed that neuronal NOS might be important in terms of release of NO from excessively activated nerves, causing further activation of sensory nerves and a cascade of further release of CGRP and substance P. However, the most likely sources for the pathological release of NO might be the action of inducible NOS enzyme such that events might be initiated several hours before the headache pain; certainly the levels of NO would be anticipated to be higher than those produced by constitutive NOS activity.

Other vasodilator mediators considered were the metabolites of P450 enzyme activity on arachidonic acid, such as the epoxyeicosatrienoic acids species. Inhibition of cytochrome P450 enzyme with miconazole is associated with vasoconstriction and a decrease in cerebral blood flow. How specific the mechanism of this agent is remains to be determined, and it is not known what subtype of P450 enzyme it might inhibit. There was also some discussion about the roles of endothelium-derived hyperpolarizing factor (EDHF) and reactive oxygen species, both of which activate potassium channels. The former may have a physiologically relevant role, but reactive oxygen species are more likely to be linked to neuronal injury and subsequent pathological events. The nature of EDHF remains elusive, but it seems not to be related to NO in any way, as was first thought. It was not known whether the recently available endothelial NOS "knock-out" mouse makes EDHF or not, but it will clearly be an interesting animal in which to study potential pathophysiology mechanisms. In the light of questions about whether eNOS is differentially located within cerebral blood vessels vis-à-vis those in the periphery, it would be interesting to examine the role of endothelial NO in cerebral blood flow control mechanisms.

A final conclusion was that it was problematic that what one finds in one species does not necessarily occur in another, as for example thromboxane A_2 release from dog basilar artery in response to neurogenic stimulation. Therefore it is important to study mechanisms across a number of species, before concluding about any clinical relevance. Arguably it is best to carry out studies on man, both in vitro and in vivo; although opportunities are obviously limited they should be actively sought. It was also concluded that if NO is critical in migraine pathophysiology, it would be interesting to determine how the NOS genes might differ in various individuals with migraine. It would also be important to know how age and gender, which greatly affect the prevalence of migraine, might influence NOS activity.

SECTION III

Role of Messenger Molecules in Pain Processing

9

Messenger Molecules Involved in Sensitization of Peripheral Nerve Endings

Stephen B. McMahon

Department of Physiology, St. Thomas' Hospital Medical School, London, SE1 7EH, United Kingdom

The pain of vascular headache depends critically on sensory inflow via trigeminal afferent neurons, as illustrated by the pain relief offered by peripheral interventions, such as pressure on extracranial vessels when these are involved in pain, and the presumed peripheral sites of action of sumatriptan, assumed not to cross the blood-brain barrier. Moreover, the neuropeptide calcitonin gene-related peptide (CGRP) is known to be released during vascular headaches into the cerebral circulation. Since this peptide is found almost exclusively in small-diameter primary sensory neurons, this finding strongly suggests that nociceptive trigeminal afferents are active during migraine and other vascular headaches. Cerebral perivascular afferents appear to be the relevant ones, on the basis of the referred pain patterns seen in migraine, the ability of cerebral artery distension to mimic migraine pain, and the pulsatile nature (with cardiac cycle) of these pains (1).

What is less clear are the factors responsible for the activation of nociceptive afferents under these conditions. Nociceptors in general are known to be responsive to a variety of forms of stimulation. Several chemical mediators are known to sensitize nociceptors, and these are considered in some detail below. Many nociceptors are also excited by extremes of temperature, but it seems unlikely that perivascular sensory neurons are exposed to such temperatures during migraine attacks, or indeed during almost any disease state (2).

A third form of sensitivity of nociceptors is to strong mechanical stimuli. In the case of cutaneous nociceptors, excitation usually requires tissue-damaging or tissue-threatening levels of mechanical stimuli (2,3). In the case of innervation of the viscera, the issue is less clear-cut, with much evidence in support of the so-called intensity-encoding mechanism, that is, sensory neurons in some systems fire at low levels of activity to physiological, innocuous levels of stimulation and at higher levels when exposed to supraphysiological, presumed noxious levels (see ref. 4 for full discussion). In this context one must assume that the central nervous system sets the threshold level above which activity is recognized as painful. In the case of migraine, many sufferers report pulsatile pain, modulated by the cardiac cycle. In these cases, the mechanical activation of cerebral perivascular afferents is strongly suggested. There is now overwhelming evidence that during the painful phase of migraine attacks, cerebral vessels dilate moderately. One presumptive final pathway for migraine pain, therefore, is the increased level of trigeminal afferent activity, arising because of dilation. In support of this hypothesis, it is true that many stimuli producing cerebral vasodilation (e.g., infusions of histamine or glyceryl trinitrate) also produce pain.

The fundamental question, to which we currently have no precise answer, is whether dilation of cerebral vessels alone is a sufficient stimulus for the production of migraine pain. The problem is that several maneuvers that increase blood pressure (e.g., physical exercise), and are therefore likely to increase transmural pressure, do not normally produce headache. Another potential problem is that the temporal relationship between headache and dilation is sometimes complex. For instance, when glyceryl trinitrate is infused into human subjects, it induces an initial pain that rises during the infusion and then rapidly subsides. However, in migraineurs (and only migraineurs) it usually precipitates a second painful episode, a genuine migraine attack, after several hours of delay. It is not known whether the second painful phase is associated with vasodilation. If dilation alone is not sufficient to explain the pain of migraine, one must propose an additional process of sensitization of primary afferent nociceptors (or possibly a secondary sensitization of central processing mechanisms, as discussed by Woolf in Chapter 10, *this volume*) as a critical event in the generation of headache. This one issue is critical for theories of migraine, since in the former case (i.e., dilation alone sufficient) the challenge is to understand how multiple precipitating factors can lead to dilation, whereas in the latter case (nociceptor sensitization required), the challenge is one of identifying the mediators and processes that lead to nociceptor sensitization of perivascular afferents.

Given that it is relatively straightforward to study electrophysiological trigeminal perivascular afferents in experimental animals, and to monitor directly the sensitivity of these afferents to vascular dilation, it is surprising how limited the information is on this subject. In one recent report, nociceptors innervating rat dural sinuses were shown to be activated and mechanically sensitized by a variety of putative inflammatory mediators (6).

For the purposes of this chapter, I will assume that nociceptors are sensitized in migraineurs during attacks and will therefore briefly review the factors that have been proposed as mediators of sensitization in a variety of nociceptive systems.

CHEMICAL MEDIATORS OF NOCICEPTOR SENSITIZATION

Injury and inflammation have been shown to produce direct sensitization of nociceptors innervating a variety of tissues (2). Most of the evidence we have relates to cutaneous nociceptors in experimental animals. However, in comparing nociceptors

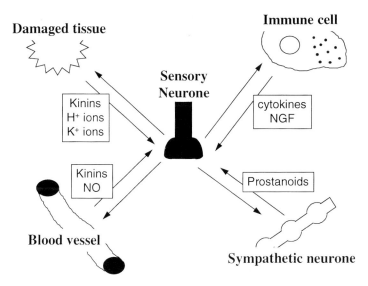

FIG. 1. Nature and source of mediators of inflammatory pain. Modified from Dray et al. (10). NGF, nerve growth factor.

from diverse origins, one is struck by the overwhelming similarities in chemical sensitivities. Figure 1 shows schematically the principal mediators that have been identified as sensitizers of nociceptors following tissue injury or inflammation. It shows that endogenous molecules from a variety of tissue elements can participate, as follows: First, tissue-damaging stimuli disrupt cellular elements and liberate potassium ions and these may directly excite nociceptors (5). Kinins, particularly kallidin, is produced in seconds within damaged tissue and may then both activate and sensitize nociceptors (6). The pH of inflamed tissue falls, in some cases to quite extreme levels, and hydrogen ions can themselves activate and sensitize nociceptors (7). Indeed, there is some suggestion that protons may be the natural ligand for the capsaicin receptor.

Bradykinin is produced from blood products at levels that are capable of powerfully exciting many nociceptors. There has recently been a resurgence of interest in the role of bradykinin, and there is convincing evidence that this kinin may be an important endogenous mediator in a variety of animal models of inflammation (6). Given the keen interest in the migraine field regarding the possibility that nitric oxide (NO) may be the principal mediator of cerebral dilation, its role as a nociceptor sensitizer is considered in more detail below.

There is a long history of interest in products of arachidonic acid metabolism as powerful modulators of pain sensitivity. More recently a body of opinion has emerged postulating that prostanoids may be released from sympathetic postganglionic neurons in a number of experimental inflammatory conditions (8).

There has been a growing interest in the role of immune-competent cells in the generation of abnormal pain states. Of course, the role of these cells in the inflammatory response in general has been much studied, but the possibility that they liberate mediators impacting on primary sensory nociceptors directly is a newer concept. With the cloning of the relevant receptors, it is now becoming apparent that many nociceptors express receptors for several cytokines such as some of the interleukins, tumor necrosis factor-α and leukocyte inhibitory factor (9). Immune cells are also a source of nerve growth factor (NGF), a molecule only recently promoted to the position of inflammatory mediator of pain (see below).

Figure 1 also attempts to illustrate that many of these mediators may interact with one another. In part, this is likely to result from the peripheral release by nociceptors of sensory neuropeptides such as substance P and CGRP, but there are potentially important interactions not shown in the figure. For instance, in addition to direct actions on nociceptors, bradykinin can release several of the other mediators shown, such as prostanoids from sympathetic neurons (8) and NO (see below).

The role of many of these mediators has been the focus of several excellent reviews (8,10,11). Therefore, here I will elaborate further on only two molecules. First, I will discuss the evidence relating to NO as a mediator, because of the central role ascribed by some to this molecule in the pathogenesis of migraine. Second, I will discuss NGF as a mediator, since much of this information is new, and most is unlikely to have reached the headache community as yet.

NITRIC OXIDE

Nitric oxide (NO) is a diffusible gas, identified as an endothelium-derived relaxing factor (12). There is growing evidence that it may be the factor responsible for the vasodilation of cerebral blood vessels, a cardinal event in the generation of vascular headache (see Chapter 44, *this volume*). Additional evidence now suggests that this molecule may be important in the generation of abnormal pain states. First, there have been repeated reports that NO contributes to the process of central sensitization (13). This process has an increasingly well-understood physiology and pharmacology and is recognized as a clinically important mechanism explaining in part the hyperalgesia associated with inflammatory pain (as discussed by Woolf in Chapter 10, *this volume*). However, in this case the NO is produced by neurons in the dorsal horn of the spinal cord (and trigeminal equivalent) as a result of nociceptive inputs. Thus, peripheral changes in NO synthesis, suggested to occur in vascular headache, almost certainly have little relevance to this phenomenon.

Additionally, a smaller body of experimental data suggests that the peripheral processes of nociceptors might be directly or indirectly affected by NO. Unfortunately, the literature is somewhat conflicting, but some findings are relatively consistent. Thus, one effect of bradykinin is to liberate NO in peripheral tissues (14). Moreover, the hyperalgesic effects of bradykinin injections in rodents are blocked by peripheral administration of NO synthase inhibitors (15). Similarly, NO synthase inhibitors can markedly reduce responses in another animal model of persistent pain—the second phase of the formalin response—as measured both electrophysiologically and behaviorally (16,17). However, in this latter study, an opposite effect of a NO donor (that is, antinociception) was seen at high doses (17). Since NO regulates local blood flow and is critical for the production of inflammatory edema produced by bradykinin and formalin, it is difficult to know to what extent its effects on nociceptive processing might be secondary to vascular effects in these studies.

In animal studies there are no clear indications that NO produces pain or hyperalgesia in normal tissue (15). However, in humans, solutions of NO produced pain when injected or perfused through a vascularly isolated hand vein segment (18). The concentrations necessary were high, in the millimole range, perhaps because of the short half-life of NO in body tissues. A further study from the same laboratory also showed that NO synthase inhibitors could block the pain of bradykinin in human veins (19). Therefore the possibility exists that NO may act directly to activate or sensitize nociceptors. In support of this hypothesis, it is known that cyclic guanosine monophosphate can be activated in primary sensory neurons in a NO-dependent manner (20).

NERVE GROWTH FACTOR

Nerve growth factor (NGF) is a member of a small family of neurotrophic factors known as neurotrophins. Other neurotrophins in mammals are brain-derived neurotrophic factor (BDNF), neurotrophin-3 (NT-3), and neurotrophin-4/5 (NT-4/5) (21). Nerve growth factor exerts its actions via specific receptors. The receptor that appears critical for most of the biological effects of NGF is a tyrosine kinase receptor known as trkA (other trks are responsible for mediating the effects of the other neurotrophins) (21).

Nerve growth factor has a well-established role in neuronal development. Essentially, all small-diameter primary sensory neurons in spinal nerves (and indeed the fifth cranial nerve) fail to survive through to the postnatal period in animals in which either the *NGF* or *trkA* gene is disrupted (22). These animals are, as a result, profoundly analgesic. In the adult animal, primary sensory nociceptors lose their dependence for survival on NGF, but several lines of evidence suggest that these nociceptive afferents continue to be responsive to this factor. Table 1 lists some of the evidence that is further discussed below.

TrkA receptors are still expressed on adult primary sensory nociceptors (and indeed on sympathetic postganglionic neurons). About 40% to 45% of spinal dorsal root ganglion neurons and trigeminal ganglion neurons are trkA positive (23). Specifically, it is the small-diameter cells (the classically defined B population of cells) that express this receptor, and these are known mostly to possess unmyelinated axons. Interestingly, an extremely high correlation exists between trkA expression and expression of the neuropeptide CGRP (greater than 90%) (23). Since other neuropeptides, such as substance P, are contained within the CGRP popula-

TABLE 1. *Evidence supporting the role of NGF as an inflammatory mediator*

trkA is expressed selectively on nociceptors
Exogenous NGF causes hyperalgesia
Exogenous NGF sensitizes nociceptors
Chronic sequestration of endogenous NGF results in hypoalgesia
NGF upregulates sensory neuropeptides
Exogenous NGF causes central sensitization
Endogenous NGF is upregulated in many inflammatory conditions
Acute sequestration of endogenous NGF prevents hyperalgesia in several inflammatory models

tion, these too must co-localize with trkA-positive neurons. In short, trkA continues to be expressed ubiquitously in the adult sensory system, and specifically on nociceptive afferents.

In adult animals, relatively modest doses of NGF produce hyperalgesia. Thus, small injections (in the order of 0.5 µg) of NGF into one footpad of freely moving rats produces a rapid onset (in the order of tens of minutes) and prolonged (in the order of many hours) thermal hyperalgesia (24). Similarly, injection-site hyperalgesia and spontaneous deep body pain have been reported in human volunteers subjected to very small doses (in the order of 1 µg/kg) of intravenous NGF (25). Recently, an electrophysiological analysis of nociceptive afferents in the rats confirmed that these fibers can be thermally sensitized by local peripheral administration of NGF (26). However, it is not clear if this activation and sensitization takes place because of an interaction between the exogenously administered NGF and trkA receptors expressed on nociceptor afferents, or whether the interaction is indirect. Evidence for the latter possibility has been produced in experiments in which other trkA-bearing peripheral cells are eliminated (in particular, mast cells and sympathetic postganglionic fibers) (24). Under these circumstances the rapid hyperalgesic effects of exogenously administered NGF are largely attenuated. It therefore seems possible that one of the rapid effects of NGF is to induce the release of more traditional algogenic mediators.

Nerve growth factor given to adult animals does bind to trkA receptors on nociceptors and, following internalization of the ligand-receptor complex, NGF is retrogradely transported to the cell somata of these afferents. There it exerts profound effects on gene expression. Most notably, chronic administration of exogenous NGF to normal adult animals leads to a dramatic upregulation of the neuropeptides CGRP and substance P, reflected in increased levels in the peripheral and central terminals of these nociceptors (27).

Another approach to the study of the putative nociceptive actions of NGF has been to remove endogenously produced protein. This task has not proved easy because of the relative lack of available tools. However, we have been able to use a synthetically produced recombinant protein, trkA-IgG, consisting of the extracellular domain of the trkA receptor fused to the FC portion of an IgG molecule (28). This synthetic protein is capable of binding NGF (with extremely high affinity), but not other neurotrophins. It is possible to use this sequestering receptor-body as a pharmacological "antagonist" of NGF. We have delivered this molecule chronically in vivo by osmotic minipumps to the skin of one hind limb of adult rats (29). We have monitored the behavior of the animals over a 2-week period of continuous NGF sequestration. Starting 4 to 5 days after delivery of the trkA-IgG fusion protein, the animals exhibited a progressive and then stable hypoalgesia of the treated skin region, that is, reduced sensitivity to thermal noxious stimuli.

Additionally, after 2 weeks of NGF sequestration, the animals exhibited greatly reduced sensitivity to the chemical algogen capsaicin. These effects were reversible, suggesting they were not due to destruction of unmyelinated nociceptive afferents. Further support for this suggestion has been obtained using electrophysiological techniques in which the response properties of individual cutaneous nociceptors, deprived of NGF as before, were studied (30). In this case, as expected from the behavioral data, nociceptive afferents showed reduced thermal and chemical sensitivity. These results strongly suggest that the absolute sensitivity of nociceptive systems is regulated by the available supply of NGF in peripheral targets.

The reason that these biological effects of NGF may be important is that NGF is known to be markedly upregulated in many animal models of inflammation. These increases have been seen using a variety of techniques, including reverse transcriptase polymerase chain reaction, in situ hybridization for NGF mRNA, and enzyme-linked immunosorbent assay, for NGF protein (31). The increases have also been seen in diverse tissues with diverse stimuli. Thus, carrageenan inflammation, adjuvant-induced arthritis, and turpentine-induced cystitis in the rat all produce rapid increases in NGF levels. A more limited data set suggests that NGF upregulation may be a common event in human inflammatory disorders. There are reports that synovial fluid contains increased levels of NGF in rheumatoid patients and that painful interstitial cystitis is associated with increased bladder levels of NGF in human patients (31). Thus, one might propose that the biological effects of exogenous NGF, described above, might be replicated by the actions of increased NGF protein levels in pathophysiological states of inflammation.

That this is the case has recently been demonstrated by several laboratories that have used different strategies to analyze the contribution of NGF upregulation to abnormal sensory function in different inflammatory pain models. We have found that the thermal hyperalgesia associated with carrageenan inflammation of the rat hind paw is largely attenuated if the inflammatory stimulus is given in the presence of the NGF-sequestering molecule trkA-IgG (29). Other recent reports confirm that anti-NGF strategies are effective in reducing the behavioral hyperalgesia seen in experimental inflammatory models induced by both carrageenan and Freund's adjuvant (32,33). We have recently studied (electrophysiologically) changes in excitability of primary afferent nociceptors innervating rat hind paw skin following carrageenan inflammation in the presence and absence of the NGF-sequestering molecule trkA-IgG. Inflammation induced by carrageenan induces spontaneous activity in many nociceptive afferents and an increase in the thermal sensitivity of these afferents to noxious heating. Nociceptors studied in animals treated in an identical fashion, except for the inclusion of the trkA-IgG fusion molecule along with the inflammatory agent, showed essentially no changes in spontaneous activity (compared with control un-inflamed skin) and no heat sensitization (34), that is, the acute effects of trkA-IgG, presumably by sequestering NGF, prevented the development of abnormal sensitivity in nociceptors following carrageenan inflammation. The importance of NGF as a mediator of inflammatory pain appears to extend beyond cutaneous systems. We have produced a body of experimental evidence also showing that NGF plays a critical role in the development of sensory abnormalities in an animal model of cystitis in the rat (35,36).

Thus, there is a growing and compelling body of evidence that NGF exerts potent biological effects specifically on nociceptive systems. Moreover, NGF appears to be a critical factor in the development of hyperalgesic states in a variety of models of experimental inflammation and injury.

Relevance to Vascular Headache

Presently, the role of NGF as a mediator of vascular headache pain remains mostly speculative. However, several pieces of circumstantial evidence suggest that the study of this molecule deserves more attention in the pathogenesis of headache. This evidence comes in three parts, as follows:

1. Exogenous NGF, administered at very low doses (less than 1 µg/kg i.v.), in humans, is known to produce headache, as well as more distributed pains. Some of these sensory abnormalities following NGF treatment develop very quickly and can persist for hours or even days (37).

2. It seems almost certain that the nociceptive innervation of perivascular structures will be rich in trkA. The evidence is itself somewhat circumstantial. We know that NGF receptors, i.e., trkA receptors, are very tightly co-expressed with the neuropeptide CGRP (23). We also know that CGRP is ubiquitously expressed in trigeminal afferents in general and in perivascular afferents in particular (38). It therefore seems likely that many perivascular afferents will be sensitive to NGF in the same way as other nociceptive afferents are known to be.

3. NGF levels are increased in spreading depression. Potassium-induced spreading depression is an experimental model often assumed to be relevant to the development of aura in vascular headaches. One report has documented changes in NGF mRNA levels in experimental spreading depression in the rat (39). In this case, neocortical expression of NGF mRNA was found to be dramatically upregulated within a few hours of the initiation of spreading depression. It is not clear whether the time course is appropriate to support the suggestion that NGF liberated in this way might sensitize perivascular afferents. The NGF upregulation seen in this experiment persisted for 24 hours.

Together these pieces of circumstantial evidence are consistent with the notion that NGF may be a sensitizing molecule produced in at least some situations that are relevant to the emergence of vascular headache.

ACKNOWLEDGMENTS

Some of the work reported in this chapter was supported by grants from the MRC of Great Britain, the Special Trustees of St. Thomas' Hospital, and the Wellcome Trust.

REFERENCES

1. Nichols FT, Mawad M, Mohr JP, Stein B, Hilal S, Michelsen WL. Focal headache during balloon distension in the internal carotid and middle cerebral arteries. *Stroke* 1990;21:555–559.
2. Meyer RA, Campbell JN, Raja SN. Peripheral neural mechanisms of nociception. In: Wall PD, Melzack R, eds. *Textbook of pain*. Edinburgh: Churchill Livingstone, 1994;13–44.
3. Koltzenburg M, Handwerker HO. Differential ability of human cutaneous nociceptors to signal mechanical pain and to produce vasodilatation. *J Neurosci* 1994;14:1756–1765.
4. McMahon SB. Mechanisms of cutaneous deep and visceral pain. In: Wall PD, Melzack R, eds. *Textbook of pain*, 2nd ed. Edinburgh: Churchill Livingstone, 1994;129–151.
5. Strassman AM, Raymond SA, Burstein R. Sensitization of meningeal sensory neurones and the origin of headaches. *Nature* 1996;384:560–564.
6. Dray A, Perkins MN. Bradykinin and inflammatory pain. *Trends Neurosci* 1993;16:99–104.
7. Bevan SJ, Geppetti P. Protons: small stimulants of capsaicin sensitive sensory neurones. *Trends Neurosci* 1994;17:509–512.
8. Levine J, Taiwo Y. Inflammatory pain. In: Wall PD, Melzack R, eds. *Textbook of pain*. Edinburgh: Churchill Livingstone, 1994;45–56.
9. Curtis R, Scherer SS, Somogyl R, et al. Retrograde axonal transport of LIF is increased by peripheral nerve injury: correlation with LIF expression in the distal nerve. *Neuron* 1994;12:191–204.
10. Dray A, Urban L, Dickenson AH. Pharmacology of chronic pain. *Trends Pharmacol Sci* 1994;15:190–197.
11. Dray A, Urban L. New pharmacological strategies for pain relief. *Annu Rev Pharmacol* 1996;36:253–280.
12. Moncada S, Palmar RMJ, Higgs EA. Endothelium-derived relaxing factor: identification as nitric oxide and role in the control of vascular tone and platelet function. *Biochem Pharmacol* 1988;37:2495–2501.
13. McMahon SB, Lewin GR, Wall PD. Central hyperexcitability triggered by noxious inputs. *Curr Opin Neurobiol* 1993;3:602–610.
14. Sung CP, Arleth AJ, Shikano K, Berkowitz BA. Characterization and function of bradykinin in vascular cells. *J Pharmacol Exp Ther* 1988;247:8–13.
15. Nakamura A, Fujita M, Shiomi H. Involvement of endogenous nitric oxide in the mechanism of bradykinin-induced peripheral hyperalgesia. *Br J Pharmacol* 1996;117:407–412.
16. Haley JE, Dickenson AH, Schachter M. Electrophysiological evidence for a role of nitric oxide in prolonged chemical nociception in the rat. *Neuropharmacology* 1992;31:251–258.
17. Kawabata A, Manabe S, Manabe Y, Takagi H. Effect of topical administration of L-arginine on formalin-induced nociception in the mouse: a dual role of peripherally formed NO in pain modulation. *Br J Pharmacol* 1994;112:547–550.
18. Holthusen H, Arndt JO. Nitric-oxide evokes pain at nociceptors of the paravascular tissue and veins in humans. *J Physiol* 1995;487:253–258.
19. Kindgen-Milles D, Arndt JO. Nitric-oxide as a chemical link in the generation of pain from veins in humans. *Pain* 1996;64:139–142.
20. McGhee DS, Goy MF, Oxford GS. Involvement of the nitric oxide-cyclic GMP pathway in the desensitization of bradykinin responses of cultured sensory neurons. *Neuron* 1992;9:315–324.
21. Barbacid M. The Trk family of neurotrophin receptors. *J Neurobiol* 1994;25:1386–1403.
22. Crowley C, Spencer SD, Nishimura MC, et al. Mice lacking nerve growth factor display perinatal loss of sensory and sympathetic neurons yet develop basal forebrain cholinergic neurons. *Cell* 1994;76:1001–1011.
23. Averill S, McMahon SB, Clary DO, Reichardt LF, Priestley JV. Immunocytochemical localisation of

trkA receptors in chemically identified subgroups of adult rat sensory neurons. *Eur J Neurosci* 1995; 7:1484–1494.
24. Andreev NY, Dmitrieva N, Koltzenburg M, McMahon SB. Peripheral administration of nerve growth factor in the adult rat produces a thermal hyperalgesia that requires the presence of sympathetic post-ganglionic neurones. *Pain* 1995;63:109–115.
25. Petty BG, Cornblath DR, Adornato BT, et al. The effect of systemically administered recombinant human nerve growth factor in healthy human subjects. *Ann Neurol* 1994;36:244–246.
26. Rueff A, Mendell LM. Nerve growth factor and NT-5 induce increased thermal sensitivity of cutaneous nociceptors in vitro. *J Neurophysiol* 1996;76:3593–3596.
27. Verge VMK, Richardson PM, Wiesenfeld-Hallin Z, Hokfelt T. Differential influence of nerve growth factor on neuropeptide expression in vivo: a novel role in peptide suppression in adult sensory neurons. *J Neurosci* 1995;15:2081–2096.
28. Shelton DL, Sutherland J, Gripp J, et al. Human trks: molecular cloning, tissue distribution, and expression of extracellular domain immunoadhesins. *J Neurosci* 1995;15:477–491.
29. McMahon SB, Bennett DLH, Priestley JV, Shelton D. The biological effects of endogenous NGF on adult sensory neurones revealed by a trkA-IgG fusion molecule. *Nature Med* 1995;1:774–780.
30. Koltzenburg M, Bennett DLH, Shelton D, Toyka KV, McMahon SB. Sequestration of endogenous NGF in adult rats reduces the sensitivity of nociceptors. In: *Proceedings of the 8th World Congress on Pain*. 1996;120 (abst).
31. McMahon SB, Bennett DLH. Growth factors and pain. In: Dickenson A, Besson J-M, eds. *Handbook of experimental pharmacology. The pharmacology of pain*. Berlin: Springer-Verlag, 1996.
32. Lewin GR, Ritter AM, Mendel LM. Nerve growth factor induced hyperalgesia in the neonatal and adult rat. *J Neurosci* 1993;13:2136–2148.
33. Woolf CJ, Safieh-Garabedian B, Ma Q-P, Crilly P, Winter J. Nerve growth factor contributes to the generation of inflammatory sensory hypersensitivity. *Neuroscience* 1994;62:327–331.
34. Bennett DLH, McMahon SB, Shelton D, Koltzenburg M. NGF sequestration using trkA-IgG fusion molecule prevents primary afferent sensitization to carrageenan inflammation. In: *Proceedings of the 8th World Congress on Pain*. 1996;120 (abst).
35. McMahon SB, Dmitrieva N, Koltzenburg M. Visceral pain. *Br J Anaesth* 1995;75:132–144.
36. Dmitrieva N, Shelton D, Rice A, McMahon SB. The role of nerve growth factor in a model of visceral inflammation. *Neuroscience* [*in press*].
37. Apfel SC, Adornato BT, Cornblath DR, et al. Clinical trial of recombinant human nerve growth factor in peripheral neuropathies. *Neurology* 1995;45:278–279.
38. Priestley JV. Neurochemistry of neuronal pathways implicated in the pathogenesis of migraine. In: Rose FC, ed. *Towards migraine 2000*. Amsterdam: Elsevier, 1996;185–200.
39. Herrera DG, Maysinger D, Gadient R, Boeckh C, Otten U, Cuello AC. Spreading depression induces c-fos-like immunoreactivity and NGF mRNA in the rat cerebral cortex. *Brain Res* 1993;602:99–103.

Headache Pathogenesis: Monoamines, Neuropeptides, Purines, and Nitric Oxide, edited by J. Olesen and L. Edvinsson. Lippincott–Raven Publishers, Philadelphia © 1997

10

Messenger Molecules Involved in Central Sensitization

Clifford J. Woolf

Department of Anatomy and Developmental Biology, University College London, London WC1E 6BT, United Kingdom

It is now widely recognized that clinical somatic pain is a manifestation of the modifiability of the nervous system. The issue for headache in general and migraine in particular is the extent to which its pathogenesis shares some of the features of other pain states or is somehow unique. Before addressing this specific issue I will begin by reviewing some of the general features of clinical pain and the specific role central sensitzation plays in its production.

NEURAL PLASTICITY AND PAIN

A major recent advance in our understanding of somatic pain has been the recognition that pain is not a unitary state. Although we use a range of similar words (unpleasant, uncomfortable, distressing, stabbing, burning, cramping) to describe pain, the mechanisms involved in different pain states are different. The first distinction we need to make is between physiological and clinical pain. Physiological pain is the sensation we experience, under normal circumstances, in response to noxious stimuli. This pain is only initiated by high-intensity stimuli and acts to warn of impending damage to tissue, initiating both reflex withdrawal responses and complex behavior to minimize exposure to the stimulus. This pain is nociceptive, resulting from the activation of a specialized subset of primary sensory neurons, the nociceptors (Fig. 1). The peripheral terminals of nociceptors have a high threshold and possess thinly myelinated (Aδ) or unmyelinated (C) axons. The nociceptors are quite distinct from low-threshold primary sensory neurons, which transduce mechanical stimuli (touch, vibration, pressure) or thermal stimuli (warmth or cold). The low-threshold mechanoreceptors have large myelinated axons (Aβ fibers) enabling rapid conduction of signals from the periphery to the central nervous system and never contribute to physiological pain. Activation of Aβ fibers normally results only in innocuous sensations (Fig. 2).

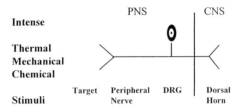

FIG. 1. Diagrammatic representation of a nociceptor. CNS, central nervous system; PNS, peripheral nervous system; DRG, dorsal root ganglion.

Clinical pain is quite unlike physiological pain in one key respect—it is characterized by pain in response to stimuli that would not normally evoke the sensation and by an exaggerated response to noxious stimuli. This hypersensitivity lies at the heart of clinical pain. Physiological pain is a localized, transient, high-threshold sensation in which the relationship between stimulus and response follows the general rules for all sensations up to the point at which tissue damage occurs. Clinical pain, in contrast, has a low threshold, it is more diffuse, the response may outlast the stimulus, and abnormal sensitivity spreads from the site of tissue damage to normal surrounding tissue. It is this change in sensitivity that is an expression of the modifiability or plasticity of the nervous system.

PERIPHERAL SENSITIZATION

Peripheral sensitization is an acute chemical-induced form of functional plasticity that mediates the conversion of the high-threshold nociceptor into a low-threshold sensory neuron. This form of plasticity manifests when sensory terminals are bathed in the products of tissue damage and inflammation (Fig. 3). A combination of inflammatory mediators and neuroactive cytokines act on the peripheral terminals of nociceptors to alter sensitivity by means of an alteration in ion channel properties. Sodium and calcium currents appear to be facilitated and potassium currents sup-

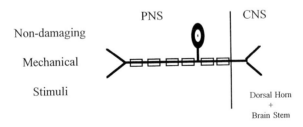

FIG. 2. Diagrammatic representation of a low-threshold neuron. CNS, central nervous system; PNS, peripheral nervous system.

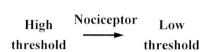

FIG. 3. Inflammation, by virtue of the inflammatory mediators it produces, can induce a localized increase in transduction sensitivity of nociceptors. ATP, adenosine triphosphate; 5-HT, serotonin; IL1-β, interleukin-1β; NGF, nerve growth factor; TNFα, tumor necrosis factor-α.

pressed. These changes are mediated by activation of G-protein-coupled receptors leading, via protein kinase A and C, to a phosphorylation of ion channel proteins. This explains why chemicals as diverse as prostaglandins, bradykinin, amines, purines, etc., may induce peripheral sensitivity changes and how they act synergistically (1,2). Apart from the classic inflammatory mediators, a more recent class of sensitizing agents has been recognized to be cytokines and growth factors, particularly nerve growth factor (NGF), which may act partly via the release of mediators from intervening inflammatory cells and partly from activation of the high-affinity trkA tyrosine kinase receptor on many nociceptors (3,4).

Peripheral sensitization is localized to sites of tissue damage (the zone of primary hyperalgesia) and mediates the increase in thermal sensitivity in sunburn and some localized changes in mechanical sensitivity by changing the transduction sensitivity of Aδ and C fibers (5). This form of pain hypersensitivity is nociceptive in that it is mediated by nociceptors. What has changed is the intensity of the stimulus necessary to activate the nociceptors. At its extreme, peripheral sensitization can convert so-called silent or sleeping nociceptors into low-threshold neurons. These sensory neurons have thresholds that are normally so high they cannot be activated by non-tissue-damaging stimuli (6).

CENTRAL SENSITIZATION

A second form of neural plasticity responsible for generating pain hypersensitivity, unlike peripheral sensitization, is activity-dependent rather than driven by an alteration in chemical milieu and is located within the central rather than the peripheral nervous system. This is central sensitization. In the early 1980s I demonstrated that an input in C nociceptors triggered a maintained increase in the excitability of spinal neurons that contributed to pain hypersensitivity, a phenomenon now known as central sensitization (7,8). Central sensitization results from an increase in the sensitivity of dorsal horn neurons to the excitatory amino acid glutamate (9,10). It is induced by the activation of protein kinase C in the central neuron (11,12) secondary to an increase in intracellular calcium (13). The elevation in calcium level in turn is evoked by metabotropic G-protein-coupled receptors (neurokinin and glutamate), by calcium entry through ligand-gated receptor ion channels, particularly the N-methyl-D-aspartic acid (NMDA) channel, and by activation of voltage-dependent ion channels (Fig. 4). The activated protein kinase C, by phosphorylating the NMDA receptor, removes its voltage-dependent magnesium ion block (14) (Fig. 5).

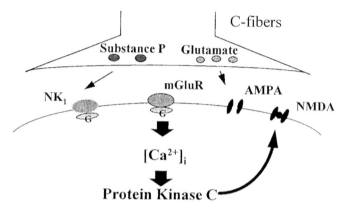

FIG. 4. Central sensitization is induced by the release from nociceptor synaptic terminals in the dorsal horn of glutamate and substance P. These transmitters, acting on a combination of ligand-gated ion channels and metabotropic receptors, increase intracellular calcium, which in turn activates protein kinase C, which phosphorylates cytoplasmic and membrane-bound ion channels.

Normally when glutamate binds to the NMDA receptor at resting membrane potential, it does not lead to intracellular passage of sodium and calcium ions because at this potential range, a Mg^{2+} ion sitting within the ion channel blocks such inward current. Once phosphorylation has attenuated this block by removing Mg^{2+} from the ion channel, at resting membrane potentials glutamate will begin to evoke a greater

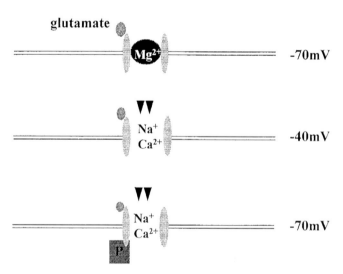

FIG. 5. Central sensitization is maintained as a result of the reduction in the voltage-dependent Mg^{2+} block of NMDA receptor ion channels. Normally at resting membrane potentials (~ −70 mV) glutamate fails to generate an inward current because of the ion channel block. Depolarization to ≤ −40 mV removes the MG^{2+} block. Phosphorylation of the NMDA receptor permits inward currents at resting membrane potentials, resulting in a substantial increase in glutamate sensitivity.

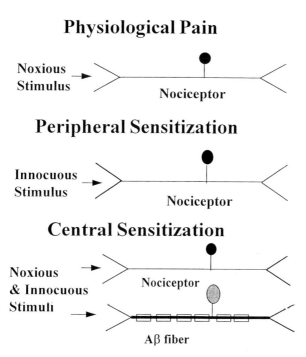

FIG. 6. Differential contribution of nociceptors and Aβ fibers to physiological and clinical pain.

response. It is this amplification that underlies central sensitization because it means that previously subthreshold inputs (15) can drive an output from the cell and this manifests as receptive field plasticity (16). The receptive fields of dorsal horn neurons expand, their threshold falls, and novel responses are recruited (17,18), changes that are remarkably similar to postinjury pain hypersensitivity changes in humans. A particular feature of the receptive field plasticity is that dorsal horn neurons, normally activated only by intense peripheral stimuli activating Aδ and C fibers, begin to respond to input from low-threshold Aβ mechanoreceptors (18). This is an example of non-nociceptive pain, pain generated by normal input in an innocuous-stimulus detection channel activating hyperexcitable central neurons. The recruitment of an Aβ-fiber-mediated component to postinjury cutaneous pain hypersensitivity can be demonstrated in human volunteers (19) as well as in patients (20,21). Figure 6 summarizes the difference between nociceptive and non-nociceptive pain.

PHENOTYPE SWITCHING

A more recent form of neural plasticity that has been elucidated is that of chemical-induced, transcription-dependent plasticity. This occurs in response to inflammation by which a number of neurally active growth factors and cytokines are released. These include the neurotrophin NGF (22), which acts on a subpopulation of

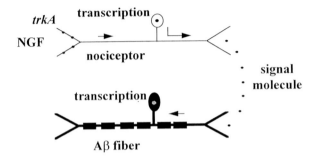

FIG. 7. Inflammation upregulates nerve growth factor (NGF) in the periphery, which acts on trkA-expressing nociceptors to induce transcription of a signal molecule that, by paracrine signaling, acts on Aβ fibers to alter their phenotype.

nociceptors expressing its high-affinity receptor trkA (23). The NGF-trkA complex is internalized and retrogradely transported from the periphery to the dorsal root ganglion, where, via specific signal transduction pathways, it alters the chemical phenotype of the cell in a transcription-dependent fashion (24). One effect of NGF is to increase the expression of the neuropeptides' substance P and calicitonin gene-related peptide (22). Another is to increase the levels of the growth-associated protein GAP-43 (25). We have recent evidence that transcription-dependent changes in primary sensory neurons are more than a matter of regulating the levels of protein/peptides but mediate a switch in the phenotype of these neurons (26). For example, substance P is normally found only in C and Aδ fiber trkA-expressing cells. After inflammation, however, the large myelinated low-threshold Aβ fiber also begins to express substance P. The mechanism responsible for this appears to be a paracrine signaling between the trkA Aδ and C fibers and the trkB/C Aβ fibers (Fig. 7). NGF, acting on the trkA cells, appears to induce a signal molecule that may be released from these cells in the dorsal root ganglion or from their terminals within the dorsal horn of the spinal cord, that then binds to a receptor on the Aβ fibers, and that after retrograde transport induces a change in the phenotype of the cells. This represents a novel form of signaling between different neurons operating over a fairly long time course that can produce profound modifications in function.

In the case of the novel expression of substance P in Aβ fibers after inflammation, what this means is that this neuropeptide is now released in the spinal cord in response to innocuous tactile stimuli in the periphery and provokes altered synaptic transmission and an increase in dorsal horn neuron excitability. In effect, these low-threshold sensory neurons, by switching phenotype, are acquiring some of the features and function of pain fibers (Fig. 8).

CENTRAL SENSITIZATION AND HEADACHE

Whenever cutaneous or muscle C fibers are activated, the consequent induction of central sensitization results in hypersensitivity manifesting as hyperalgesia, allodynia, and referred pain, with, in particular, the recruitment of pain responses to Aβ

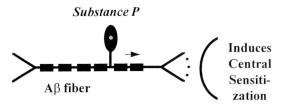

FIG. 8. The novel expression of the tachykinin substance P after inflammation leads to an alteration in the central synaptic drive generated by tactile stimuli, including increased excitability of dorsal horn neurons.

low-mechanothreshold afferent fiber inputs (27,28). This is equally true for the trigeminal system, in which cutaneous, muscle, and joint nociceptor activation results in central sensitization (29,30).

There are suggestions from human psychophysical studies that myofascial pains and tension-type headache have an altered threshold for pain that is very likely to be accounted for by an increase in the excitability or the gain of central sensory processing pathways (31–34). The question then is, what is the trigger for such central sensitization? Is it driven by peripheral C-fiber inputs, as is true for experimental secondary hyperalgesia and neuropathic pain, or is it a manifestation of an autonomous increase in excitability due to some predisposition for increased neuronal excitability (35)? This could occur by the removal of tonic or phasic inhibitory influences, as can be shown experimentally, or could be caused by some excessive neuronal excitability much like convulsive disorders (36). The answers to this important issue are simply unknown at this time.

Does central sensitization have a role in the pathogenesis of migraine? If migraine is associated with the activation of meningeal nociceptors, then this is likely to produce central sensitization in the spinal nucleus of the trigeminal pathway. There is little doubt that electrical activation of the trigeminal vascular pathway does activate brain stem neurons sufficiently to produce the expression of immediate-early genes like C-fos (37) and that cortical spreading depression has a similar effect (38). For the rest of the somatosensory system there is a remarkable correlation between C-fos expression evoked by C-fiber inputs and the induction of central sensitization (39). Functional imaging in a patient with spontaneous migraine attacks has recently revealed strong brain stem activation (40).

If central sensitization were induced by a trigeminovascular sensory inflow, what might result? One possibility is sensory hypersensitivity such that usually subthreshold or undetected sensory inputs from intracranial afferents begin to elicit pain; this might explain the sensitivity to alterations in intracranial pressure or the throbbing quality of the pain, which might be due to arterial pulsations activating low-threshold afferents adjacent to intracranial vessels. A second possibility is increased reflex responsiveness such that autonomic outflow initiated by sensory inputs are exaggerated; this might contribute to some of the blood flow changes characteristic of migraine.

Many unanswered questions remain. What activates meningeal afferents in migraine? Do they cause central sensitization? Can elimination of central sensitization reduce the clinical features of migraine?

A clue in favor of the latter is the observation that anticonvulsant agents do have some efficacy in reducing migraine (41,42) and that dihydroergotomine does prevent the central activation of brain stem neurons (37). If the messengers responsible for inducing central sensitization in the dorsal horn of the spinal cord are identical to those in the brain stem, then a number of novel targets for the treatment of migraine may emerge.

CONCLUSIONS

Based on the available evidence, there is a very strong likelihood that headache, both tension-type and migraine, is associated with the induction of central sensitization in neurons of the spinal nucleus of the trigeminal pathway. This offers new possibilities both for understanding the pathophysiology of these conditions and for therapeutic intervention.

ACKNOWLEDGMENTS

The support of the MRC and The Wellcome Trust is gratefully acknowledged.

REFERENCES

1. Treede R-D, Meyer RA, Raja SN, Campbell JN. Peripheral and central mechanisms of cutaneous hyperalgesia. *Prog Neurobiol* 1992;38:397–421.
2. Levine JD, Taiwo YO. Inflammatory pain. In: Wall PD, Melzack R, eds. *Textbook of pain*, 3rd ed. Edinburgh: Churchill Livingstone, 1994;45–56.
3. Lewin GR, Rueff A, Mendell LM. Peripheral and central mechanisms of NGF-induced hyperalgesia. *Eur J Neurosci* 1994;6:1903–1912.
4. Safieh-Garabedian B, Poole S, Allchorne A, Winter J, Woolf CJ. Contribution of interleukin-1β to the inflammation-induced increase in nerve growth factor levels and inflammatory hyperalgesia. *Br J Pharmacol* 1995;115:1265–1275.
5. Reeh PW. Chemical excitation and sensitization of nociceptors. In: Urban L, ed. *Cellular mechanisms of sensory processing. NATO ASI series. Cell biology*, vol 79. Berlin: Springer-Verlag, 1994; 119–131.
6. Schaible H-G, Schmidt RF. Effects of an experimental arthritis on the sensory properties of fine articular afferent units. *J Neurophysiol* 1985;54:1109–1122.
7. Woolf CJ. Evidence for a central component of post-injury pain hypersensitivity. *Nature* 1983;306: 686–688.
8. Woolf CJ, Wall PD. The relative effectiveness of C primary afferent fibres of different origins in evoking a prolonged facilitation of the flexor reflex in the rat. *J Neurosci* 1986;6:1433–1443.
9. Woolf CJ. A new strategy for the treatment of inflammatory pain: prevention or elimination of central sensitization. *Drugs* 1994;47:1–9.
10. Woolf CJ. Somatic pain—pathogenesis and prevention. *Br J Anaesth* 1995;75:169–176.
11. Chen L, Huang L-YM. Protein kinase C reduces Mg^{2+} block of NMDA-receptor channels as a mechanism of modulation. *Nature* 1992;356:521–523.
12. Yashpal K, Pitcher GM, Parent A, Quirion R, Coderre TJ. Noxious thermal and chemical stimulation induce increases in ^{3}H-phorbol 12,13-dibutyrate binding in spinal cord dorsal horn as well as persis-

tent pain and hyperalgesia, which is reduced by inhibition of protein kinase C. *J Neurosci* 1995;15: 3263–3272.
13. MacDermott AB, Mayer ML, Westbrook GL, Smith SJ, Baker JL. NMDA-receptor activation increase cytoplasmic calcium concentration in cultured spinal cord neurons. *Nature* 1986;321:519–522.
14. Mayer ML, Westbrook GL, Guthrie PB. Voltage-dependent block by MG^{2+} of NMDA responses in spinal cord neurones. *Nature* 1984;309:261–263.
15. Woolf CJ, King AE. Subthreshold components of the cutaneous mechanoreceptive fields of dorsal horn neurons in the rat lumbar spinal cord. *J Neurophysiol* 1989;62:907–916.
16. Woolf CJ, King AE. Dynamic alterations in the cutaneous mechanoreceptive fields of dorsal horn neurons in the rat spinal cord. *J Neurosci* 1990;10:2717–2726.
17. Cook AJ, Woolf CJ, Wall PD, McMahon SB. Dynamic receptive field plasticity in rat spinal cord dorsal horn following C primary afferent input. *Nature* 1987;325:151–153.
18. Woolf CJ, Shortland P, Sivilotti LG. Sensitization of high mechanothreshold superficial dorsal horn and flexor motor neurons following chemosensitive primary afferent activation. *Pain* 1994;58:141–155.
19. Torebjork HE, Lundberg LER, LaMotte RH. Central changes in processing of mechanoreceptor input in capsaicin-induced sensory hyperalgesia in humans. *J Physiol (Lond)* 1992;448:765–780.
20. Campbell JN, Raja SN, Meyer RA, McKinnon SE. Myelinated afferents signal the hyperalgesia associated with nerve injury. *Pain* 1988;32:89–94.
21. Koltzenburg M, Torebjork HE, Wahren LK. Nociceptor modulated central sensitization causes mechanical hyperalgesia in acute chemogenic and chronic neuropathic pain. *Brain* 1994;117:579–591.
22. Woolf CJ, Safieh-Garabedian B, Ma Q-P, Crilly P, Winter J. Nerve growth factor contributes to the generation of inflammatory sensory hypersensitivity. *Neurosci* 1994;62:327–331.
23. Averill S, McMahon SB, Clary DO, Reichardt LF, Priestley JV. Immunocytochemical localization of trkA receptors in chemically identified subgroups of adult rat sensory neurons. *Eur J Neurosci* 1995; 7:1484–1494.
24. Lindsay RM, Lockett C, Sternberg J, Winter J. Neuropeptide expression in cultures of adult sensory neurons: modulation of substance P and calcitonin gene-related peptide levels by nerve growth factor. *Neuroscience* 1989;33:53–65.
25. Leslie TA, Emson PC, Dowd PM, Woolf CJ. Nerve growth factor contributes to the upregulation of GAP-43 and preprotachykinin A mRNA in primary sensory neurons following peripheral inflammation. *Neuroscience* 1995;67:753–761.
26. Neumann S, Doubell TP, Leslie TA, Woolf CJ. Inflammatory pain hypersensitivity mediated by phenotypic switch in myelinated primary sensory neurones. *Nature* 1996;384:360–364.
27. Koltzenburg M, Lundberg LER, Torebjork HE. Dynamic and static components of mechanical hyperalgesia in human hairy skin. *Pain* 1992;51:207–220.
28. Kilo S, Schmelz M, Koltzenburg M, Handwerker HO. Different patterns of hyperalgesia induced by experimental inflammation in human skin. *Brain* 1994;117:385–396.
29. Yu XM, Sessle BJ, Hu JW. Differential effects of cutaneous and deep application of inflammatory irritant on the mechnoreceptive field properties of trigeminal brain stem nociceptive neurons. *J Neurophysiol* 1993;70:1704–1707.
30. Hu JW, Sessle BJ, Raboisson P, Dallel R, Woda A. Stimulation of craniofacial muscle afferents induces prolonged facilitatory effects in trigeminal nociceptive brain-stem neurones. *Pain* 1992;48: 53–60.
31. Bendtsen L, Jensen R, Olesen J. Qualitatively altered nociception in chronic myofascial pain. *Pain* 1996;65:259–264.
32. Jensen R. Mechanisms of spontaneous tension-type headaches: an analysis of tenderness, pain thresholds and EMG. *Pain* 1995;64:251–256.
33. Langemark M, Olesen J. Pericranial tenderness in tension headache. *Cephalalgia* 1987;7:249–255.
34. Schoenen J, Gerard P, De Pasqua V, Sianard Gainko J. Multiple clinical and paraclinical analyses of chronic tension-type headache associated or unassociated with disorder of pericranial muscles. *Cephalalgia* 1991;11:135–139.
35. Koltzenburg M, Wahren LK, Torebjork HE. Dynamic changes of mechanical hyperalgesia in neuropathic pain states and healthy subjects depend on the ongoing activity of unmyelinated nociceptive afferents. *Pflugers Arch* 1992;420:R52.
36. Sivilotti LG, Woolf CJ. The contribution of $GABA_A$ and glycine receptors to central sensitization: disinhibition and touch-evoked allodynia in the spinal cord. *J Neurophysiol* 1994;72:169–179.

37. Hoskin KL, Kaube H, Goadsby PJ. Central activation of the trigeminovascular pathway in the cat is inhibited by dihydroergotamine A c-Fos and electrophysiolgical study. *Brain* 1996;119:249–256.
38. Shimazawa M, Hara H, Watano T, Sukamoto T. Effects of Ca^{2+} channel blockers on cortical hypoperfusion and expression of c-Fos-like immunoreactivity after cortical spreading depression in rats. *Br J Pharmacol* 1995;115:1359–1368.
39. Coderre TJ, Katz J, Vaccarino AL, Melzack R. Contribution of central neuroplasticity to pathological pain: review of clinical and experimental evidence. *Pain* 1993;52:259–285.
40. Weiller C, May A, Limmroth V, et al. Brain stem activation in spontaneous human migraine attacks. *Nature Med* 1995;1:658–660.
41. Maizels M, Scott B, Cohen W, Chen W. Intranasal lidocaine for treatment of migraine: a randomized, double-blind, controlled trial. *JAMA* 1996;276:319–321.
42. McQuay H, Carroll D, Jadad AR, Wiffen P, Moore A. Anticonvulsant drugs for management of pain: a systematic review. *BMJ* 1995;311:1047–1052.

11

Messenger Molecules Involved in Sensitization at Supraspinal Levels

Mary M. Heinricher

Division of Neurosurgery, Oregon Health Sciences University, Portland, Oregon 97201

Over the past several decades, it has become increasingly evident that the encoding of afferent signals related to pain is shaped by well-defined supraspinal modulatory systems that modify the information at each stage of central processing, beginning at the dorsal horn. Recent considerations of headache mechanisms have raised the possibility that these supraspinal modulatory systems play a role in headache (1). The present paper will focus on the organization of a brain stem system implicated in pain modulation, with an emphasis on how activity in this system is regulated by different messenger molecules, both to enhance and to diminish processing of nociceptive information.

PERIAQUEDUCTAL GRAY MATTER-ROSTRAL VENTROMEDIAL MEDULLA PAIN-MODULATING NETWORK

Although the existence of descending controls of dorsal horn nociceptive processing had been recognized since the 1960s, the behavioral relevance of this modulatory influence was first demonstrated by Reynolds (2), in a report showing that electrical stimulation in the midbrain periaqueductal gray matter (PAG) surrounding the cerebral aqueduct inhibited behavioral responses to noxious stimulation in awake rats. Subsequent studies confirmed this observation, extended it to other species including humans, and ultimately led to the definition of a central nociceptive modulatory network with important links in the PAG and rostral ventromedial medulla (RVM) (Fig. 1) (3,4). The PAG itself has only sparse projections to the dorsal horn but sends a substantial output to the RVM, which in turn projects to spinal and trigeminal dorsal horns to influence nociceptive processing. As in the PAG, electrical stimulation in the RVM produces a behaviorally measurable antinociception, and both sites are important substrates for opioid analgesia (5–8). The PAG-RVM system receives inputs from ascending spinal afferent systems (including spinoreticular and spinomesencephalic tracts, as well as collaterals from spinothalamic tract axons) that converge with inputs from a wide range of supraspinal sites, including limbic

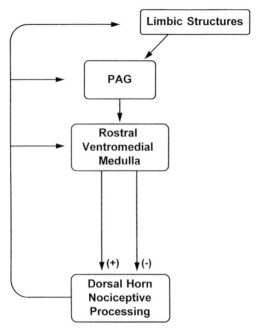

Fig. 1. Central pain-modulating network with links in the PAG and the RVM. The RVM receives a large input from the PAG and projects to spinal and medullary dorsal horns to modulate processing of nociceptive information. Processes organized in limbic forebrain can gain access to pain-modulating circuits via projections to the PAG.

forebrain structures, most notably the amygdala. This system is thus ideally situated to mediate a complex integration of sensory traffic with higher order, particularly limbic, influences. Although a number of other sites have now been implicated in descending modulation, this PAG-RVM system remains the best characterized.

The primary focus of investigators interested in pain modulation has understandably been on mechanisms of pain inhibition, yet there is increasing evidence that this system can enhance as well as depress pain processing. Recent painstaking investigations of the effect of electrical stimulation within the RVM reveal that this region exerts facilitating as well as inhibiting effects on nociception (9,10). However, the clearest demonstration of a facilitating outflow from RVM was provided in an experiment taking advantage of hyperalgesia induced as part of an acute opioid abstinence syndrome (11). In these experiments a rat was given morphine systemically to produce analgesia, and then the opioid antagonist naloxone. Following naloxone, there was a significant decrease in nociceptive threshold relative to premorphine baseline levels, i.e., a hyperalgesia. Importantly, this hyperalgesia was blocked by inactivation of the RVM using focal application of a local anesthetic. These observations demonstrated that the RVM can exert a facilitating, as well as inhibiting, effect on nociception, and there is increasing evidence that supraspinal modulation provides an ongoing bidirectional regulation of nociceptive processing under physiological conditions (12,13).

Studies of the activity of single RVM neurons in lightly anesthetized rats have revealed three physiologically, pharmacologically, and functionally distinct classes of neurons that provide a substrate for finely tuned modulation of nociception (14). Cells of one class, called off-cells, are likely to exert a net inhibitory effect on dorsal horn nociceptive processing. These neurons are characterized by an abrupt cessation of firing just prior to the occurrence of nocifensive reflexes (for example, the tail flick reflex, which is widely used as an index of nociceptive responsiveness in both anesthetized and awake animals), and they are invariably activated by systemic or local administration of opioids (15,16). Off-cell activation by opioids must be indirect, since these neurons do not respond to direct iontophoretic application of morphine (17). Cells of a second class, called on-cells, have properties complementary to those of off-cells. On-cells are characterized by a burst of activity associated with nocifensor reflexes. In itself, this burst of activity indicates that these neurons must not inhibit nociception, since the animal responds to the noxious input just when they are most active. In addition, administration of morphine by any of several routes, including systemically or by local infusion within the RVM, results in a depression of on-cell discharge (16,18). On-cells are also inhibited by direct iontophoretic application of opioids (17). Taken together, these observations suggest that the on-cell is a likely candidate for the pain-facilitating outflow from the RVM. Cells of a third class, called neutral cells, show no change in activity associated with nociceptive reflexes or opioid analgesic administration, and their role, if any, in nociception remains unknown. However, the fact that at least some neutral cells contain serotonin suggests that they may participate in some fashion (19).

REGULATION OF PAIN MODULATORY CIRCUITRY WITHIN THE ROSTRAL VENTROMEDIAL MEDULLA BY MESSENGER MOLECULES

The information gained from the study of direct and indirect actions of opioids within the RVM led to the model of RVM circuitry shown in Fig. 2. This model provides a useful framework for investigating the actions of other nonopioid, neuroactive compounds in pain-modulating systems. A number of neurotransmitters and neuropeptides have been shown to alter nociception when applied within the RVM, but only a subset of these have so far been studied at the single cell level in the context of on- and off-cells, among them norepinephrine and the neuropeptides cholecystokinin (CCK) and orphanin FQ (OFQ).

Norepinephrine

One neurotransmitter that has been of particular interest within the RVM is norepinephrine, since interfering with α-adrenergic transmission within the RVM in rats has been shown to produce changes in nociceptive thresholds (20). Interestingly, blockade of norepinephrine's actions at α_1- and α_2-receptors has opposite effects: focal administration of an α_2-antagonist within the RVM produces a decrease in

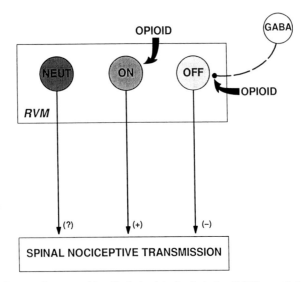

Fig. 2. Three classes of neurons identified physiologically in the RVM have distinct roles in pain modulation. All three project to the dorsal horn. On-cells are likely to exert a net facilitating effect on pain processes and are the only RVM neurons directly sensitive to opioids. These neurons are thus a means through which opioids can gain access to the modulatory circuitry of the RVM. Off-cells, likely to exert a net inhibitory effect on pain processing, are activated by opioids. This activation is indirect and is likely due to presynaptic suppression of γ-aminobutyric acid (GABA)-mediated inhibition. Neutral cells (NEUT) are not responsive to opioid analgesics; their role in pain modulation and their relationship to the other RVM classes are unknown.

threshold, whereas administration of an α_1-antagonist gives rise to an increase in threshold. Effects of α_1- and α_2-agonists are complementary to those of the antagonists, so that an α_2-agonist produces an increase in threshold and an α_1-agonist a decrease in threshold. These findings demonstrate that the pain-modulating circuitry of the RVM is differentially regulated by norepinephrine acting at two receptors. Investigations at the single cell level demonstrate that, as with opioids, this control is exerted at the level of the on-cell (21). On-cell firing is profoundly depressed by the α_2-agonist clonidine applied to individual neurons using iontophoresis; an α_1-mediated facilitation of on-cell firing by norepinephrine is also seen. Off-cells and neutral cells do not respond to norepinephrine or α-adrenergic agonists applied by iontophoresis. Thus, norepinephrine is capable of exerting bidirectional control of pain modulation via its action on the on-cell within the RVM.

Peptides

It is now well established that the analgesic actions of opioids can be modified by various endogenous peptides, among them neurotensin and CCK, and more recently

OFQ, the endogenous ligand for the "orphan" opioid receptor LC132. The role of CCK as a physiological opioid antagonist has received particular attention. Administration of CCK agonists can diminish opioid analgesia, whereas CCK antagonists enhance the antinociceptive effects of exogenous and endogenous opioids and can apparently slow or prevent the development of opioid tolerance in some paradigms (22). When microinjected into the RVM of lightly anesthetized rats, CCK has no effect on nociceptive threshold or on the firing of on- or off-cells or neutral cells. However, this peptide blocks the depression of on-cell firing and the activation of off-cells that normally follow systemic morphine administration and, at the same time, prevents the antinociceptive effects (23). The implication of this finding is that some outflow from the RVM, presumably the on-cell, prevents morphine from acting at other opioid-sensitive sites to produce analgesia. OFQ also blocks the antinociceptive actions of opioids acting within the RVM, but through a mechanism very different from that of CCK (24). Although OFQ potently suppresses the firing of all three classes of RVM neurons, activation of off-cells is the ultimate basis for RVM-mediated antinociception. Thus, the OFQ blockade of the antinociceptive actions of an opioid within the RVM is most easily explained by its inhibition of this cell class.

FOREBRAIN INFLUENCES ON ROSTRAL VENTROMEDIAL MEDULLA PAIN-MODULATING CIRCUITS

Recent investigations have pointed to forebrain regions as a source of inputs regulating pain-modulating functions of the RVM. Such connections could form the basis for modulation of pain responses by attention, stress, motivation, and learning processes. The role of the ventrolateral orbital cortex is particularly intriguing. Work of Dostrovsky and colleagues (25) has shown that electrical stimulation in this prefrontal cortical area produces a hyperalgesia. This stimulation also activates on-cells and suppresses off-cell firing. Although these results are correlative, they certainly raise the possibility that cortical influences could enhance nociception via the RVM.

A second forebrain region implicated in pain modulation is the amygdala. Antinociception can be elicited as a conditioned response to previously neutral cues that have been paired in a classical conditioning paradigm with noxious or aversive events (26). This phenomenon, termed conditional hypoalgesia, is blocked by lesions of the RVM (27). Stimuli that elicit conditional hypoalgesia apparently gain access to the modulatory circuitry of the RVM at least in part by means of fear-related processes organized in the amygdala (28). Direct local administration of morphine into the basolateral amygdala results in an antinociception, and, like systemic administration, activates off-cells and suppresses on-cell firing (29,30). The above findings demonstrate that one way in which the modulatory circuitry of the RVM is likely to be engaged physiologically to produce decreased pain responses in behaving animals is via activation of the amygdala.

CONCLUSIONS

A number of brain sites have been implicated in nociceptive modulating using stimulation, microinjection, and lesion techniques, but the system that has received the most attention to date is a network with links in the midbrain PAG and RVM. This system is now known to enhance as well as depress nociceptive processing. Recent studies of the pain-modulating circuitry within the RVM reveal that two physiologically identifiable classes of neurons, on- and off-cells, form the basis for this bidirectional control. On-cells likely facilitate, whereas off-cells inhibit, nociception. Messenger molecules now known to regulate activity of RVM neurons include opioids, norepinephrine, and neuropeptides. Further studies of these and other neurotransmitters and neuropeptides acting in RVM should provide potent tools for understanding and manipulating this system, knowledge that should ultimately provide a means through which central factors likely to contribute to pain, including headache, can be controlled.

ACKNOWLEDGMENTS

This work was supported by a grant from the NIDA (DA05608).

REFERENCES

1. Olesen J. Clinical and pathophysiological observations in migraine and tension-type headache explained by integration of vascular, supraspinal and myofascial inputs. *Pain* 1991;46:125–132.
2. Reynolds DV. Surgery in the rat during electrical analgesia induced by focal brain stimulation. *Science* 1969;154:444–445.
3. Barbaro NM. Studies of PAG/PVG stimulation for pain relief in humans. *Prog Brain Res* 1988;77:165–173.
4. Oliveras J-L, Besson J-M. Stimulation-produced analgesia in animals: behavioural investigations. *Prog Brain Res* 1988;77:141–157.
5. Mayer DJ, Price DD. Central nervous system mechanisms of analgesia. *Pain* 1976;2:379–404.
6. Willis WD Jr. Anatomy and physiology of descending control of nociceptive responses of dorsal horn neurons: comprehensive review. *Prog Brain Res* 1988;77:1–29.
7. Sessle BJ, Dubner R, Greenwood LF, Lucier GE. Descending influences of periaqueductal gray matter and somatosensory cerebral cortex on neurones in trigeminal brain stem nuclei. *Can J Physiol Pharmacol* 1976;54:66–69.
8. Yaksh TL, al-Rodhan NR, Jensen TS. Sites of action of opiates in production of analgesia. *Prog Brain Res* 1988;77:371–394.
9. Zhuo M, Gebhart GF. Characterization of descending inhibition and facilitation from the nuclei reticularis gigantocellularis and gigantocellularis pars alpha in the rat. *Pain* 1990;42:337–350.
10. Zhuo M, Gebhart GF. Characterization of descending facilitation and inhibition of spinal nociceptive transmission from the nuclei reticularis gigantocellularis and gigantocellularis pars alpha in the rat. *J Neurophysiol* 1992;67:1599–1614.
11. Kaplan H, Fields HL. Hyperalgesia during acute opioid abstinence: evidence for a nociceptive facilitating function of the rostral ventromedial medulla. *J Neurosci* 1991;11:1433–1439.
12. Barbaro NM, Heinricher MM, Fields HL. Putative nociceptive modulatory neurons in the rostral ventromedial medulla of the rat display highly correlated firing patterns. *Somatosens Mot Res* 1989;6:413–425.
13. Fields HL. Is there a facilitating component to central pain modulation? *APS J* 1992;1:71–78.

14. Fields HL, Bry J, Hentall I, Zorman G. The activity of neurons in the rostral medulla of the rat during withdrawal from noxious heat. *J Neurosci* 1983;3:2545–2552.
15. Fields HL, Vanegas H, Hentall ID, Zorman G. Evidence that disinhibition of brain stem neurones contributes to morphine analgesia. *Nature* 1983;306:684–686.
16. Heinricher MM, Morgan MM, Tortorici V, Fields HL. Disinhibition of off-cells and antinociception produced by an opioid action within the rostral ventromedial medulla. *Neuroscience* 1994;63:279–288.
17. Heinricher MM, Morgan MM, Fields HL. Direct and indirect actions of morphine on medullary neurons that modulate nociception. *Neuroscience* 1992;48:533–543.
18. Barbaro NM, Heinricher MM, Fields HL. Putative pain modulating neurons in the rostral ventral medulla: reflex-related activity predicts effects of morphine. *Brain Res* 1986;366:203–210.
19. Potrebic SB, Fields HL, Mason P. Serotonin immunoreactivity is contained in one physiological cell class in the rat rostral ventromedial medulla. *J Neurosci* 1994;14:1655–1665.
20. Sagen J, Proudfit HK. Evidence for pain modulation by pre- and postsynaptic noradrenergic receptors in the medulla oblongata. *Brain Res* 1985;331:285–293.
21. Heinricher MM, Haws CM, Fields HL. Opposing actions of norepinephrine and clonidine on single pain-modulating neurons in rostral ventromedial medulla. In: Dubner R, Gebhart GF, Bond MR, eds. *Pain research and clinical management,* vol 3. Amsterdam: Elsevier, 1988;590–594.
22. Stanfa L, Dickenson A, Xu XJ, Wiesenfeld-Hallin Z. Cholecystokinin and morphine analgesia: variations on a theme. *Trends Pharmacol Sci* 1994;15:65–66.
23. Heinricher MM, McGaraughty S. CCK modulates the antinociceptive actions of opioids by an action within the rostral ventromedial medulla: a combined electrophysiological and behavioral study. In: *Proceedings of the International Association for the Study of Pain 8th World Congress,* Vancouver, BC, Canada, 1996.
24. Heinricher MM, McGaraughty S, Grandy D. Circuitry underlying "anti-opioid" actions of orphanin FQ in the rostral ventromedial medulla [*in press*].
25. Hutchison WD, Harfa L, Dostrovsky JO. Ventrolateral orbital cortex and periaqueductal gray stimulation-induced effects on on- and off-cells in the rostral ventromedial medulla in the rat. *Neuroscience* 1996;70:391–407.
26. Fanselow MS. Conditioned fear-induced opiate analgesia: a competing motivational state theory of stress analgesia. *Ann NY Acad Sci* 1986;467:40–54.
27. Helmstetter FJ, Tershner SA. Lesions of the periaqueductal gray and rostral ventromedial medulla disrupt antinociceptive but not cardiovascular aversive conditional responses. *J Neurosci* 1994;14:7099–7108.
28. Helmstetter FJ. The amygdala is essential for the expression of conditional hypoalgesia. *Behav Neurosci* 1992;106:518–528.
29. Helmstetter FJ, Bellgowan PS, Tershner SA. Inhibition of the tail flick reflex following microinjection of morphine into the amygdala. *Neuroreport* 1993;4:471–474.
30. McGaraughty S, Heinricher MM. The effects of morphine in the basolateral nucleus of the amygdala on the ON, OFF, and neutral cells in the rostral ventromedial medulla of anesthetized rats. *Soc Neurosci Abstr* 1996;22:114.

12

An Epidemiological Study on the Activity of Cannabis in Idiopathic Headache

V. Amenta, G. M. Pitari, M. Caff, D. Impellizzieri, F. Giuliano, R. Costa, I. Sapuppo, and A. Bianchi

Department of Pharmacology and Toxicology, University of Catania Medical School, 95125 Catania, Italy

It is common belief in popular medicine that exogenous cannabinoids are active in the therapy of headache (1). Until a few years ago, there were no data about the existence of specific receptors to cannabinoids (2). The discovery of anandamide and other N-acyl-ethanolamines (3) as well as the relative endocannabinoid receptors CB_1 and CB_2 (4) opened new horizons in the study of the pharmacodynamics and relative clinical applications of exogenous cannabinoids. Endocannabinoids were found to be involved in the inflammatory response (through their immunological correlates) and in the modulation of pain (5). The aim of our study was to investigate whether migraineurs addicted to cannabinoids experience any particular variations of the clinical sypmtoms of migraine.

MATERIALS AND METHODS

We administered a specific questionnaire to 81 marijuana- or hashish-addicted people (60 men and 21 women; mean age, 29 years) to evaluate how many sufferers from migraine were among them (Table 1). The research was performed over several months at the Rehabilitation Center for the Addicted of Catania. We found that 48 subjects had a history of headache.

The intensity and frequency of headache were monitored and evaluated comparatively in all migraineurs who were habitual smokers of cannabinoids. Pain perceived by the subjects during the headache attack was evaluated according to an arbitrary verbal scale (rated from 0 to 4).

TABLE 1. *Demographic details of patients*

	Marijuana addicted	Hashish addicted
Sex (no.)		
Males	45	15
Females	16	5
Age (yr; mean and range)		
Males	30.7 (20–35)	28.5 (19–33)
Females	29.5 (19–36)	28.9 (24–34)
Headache sufferers (no.)		
Males	25	8
Females	11	4
Addiction history (yr; mean)		
Males	10.6	9.3
Females	7.9	7.5

TABLE 2. *Variations of clinical symptoms in 48 headache sufferers addicted to cannabinoids, after smoking the drug, at onset of the attack*

	Without cannabinoid smoking	After cannabinoids
Pain intensity (0–4) (mean±SE)	2.8±0.4	1.5±0.6
Attack duration (hr) (mean±SE)	15.6±2.8	10.1±1.9

TABLE 3. *Quality of response in 48 headache sufferers addicted to cannabinoids, after smoking the drug, at onset of the attack*

	No. of subjects
Worsening	2
No effect	15
Slight improvement	6
Considerable improvement	25

RESULTS

As shown in Tables 2 and 3, 31 of 48 subjects addicted to cannabinoids obtained pain relief when smoking the drug at the appearance of a headache attack. Moreover, the intensity of headache pain was significantly decreased in comparison with headache attacks not associated with cannabinoid smoking [pain score: 1.1 ± 0.2 vs. 3.1 ± 0.5 (mean ± SE); $p < 0.001$; Fig. 1].

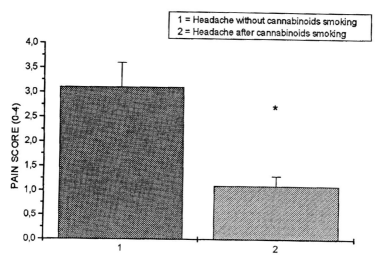

Fig 1. Pain variation induced by cannabinoids in 25 headache sufferers, after smoking the drug. *, $p < 0.0001$

CONCLUSIONS

Cannabinoids seem to exert an effect on pain in the addicted. Although such an effect may simply represent alleviation of cannabinoid abstinence, further study is warranted of the CB_1 and CB_2 receptors, as well as of their relative endocannabinoid agonists, anandamide and other N-acyl-ethanolamines.

REFERENCES

1. Martin BR, Compton DR, Thomas BF, Prescott WR, Little PJ, Razdan RK, Johnson MR, Melvin LS, Mechoulam R and Ward SJ. Behavioural, Biochemical and molecular modelling evaluations of cannabinoid analogs. *Pharmacol Biochem Behav* 1991;40:471–478.
2. Schimdt HH, Schmid PC and Natarajan V. N-acylated glicerophospholipids and their derivatives. *Prog Lipid Res* 1994;29:1–43.
3. Allison B and Miles H. Localization of cannabinoid receptors and nosaturable high-density cannabinoid binding sites in peripheral tissues of the rat: implications for receptor-mediated immune modulation by cannabinoids. *J Pharmacol Exp Ther* 1994;268:1612–1823.
4. Welch SP, Dunlow LD, Patrick GS and Razdan RK. Characterization of anandamide- and fluoro-anandamide-induced antinociception and cross-tolerance to Δ^9-THC after intrathecal administration to mice: blockade of Δ^9-THC induced antinociception. *J Pharmacol Exp Ther* 1995;273:1235–1244.
5. Abel E. *Marijuana: the first twelve thousand years.* New York: Plenum Press, 1982.

13

Activation of Cutaneous Afferent Neurons by Adenosine Triphosphate in the Neonatal Rat Tail-Spinal Cord Preparation In Vitro

Derek J. Trezise and Patrick P. A. Humphrey

Glaxo Institute of Applied Pharmacology, Department of Pharmacology, University of Cambridge, Cambridge, CB2 1QJ, United Kingdom

Somatosensory information is transmitted via primary afferent neurons to the spinal cord, where it is integrated, processed, and relayed to higher centers in the brain (1). Several lines of evidence suggest that extracellular adenosine 5´-triphosphate (ATP) may play an important role in the complex neurochemical events underlying these processes (2). For example, ATP excites certain dorsal horn neurons both in vitro and in vivo (3,4) and modulates glutamatergic synaptic transmission in the substantia gelatinosa of the spinal cord (5); it is thus a candidate as an excitatory transmitter at afferent synapses. This proposal is supported by the fact that antidromic stimulation of afferent fibers can release ATP from the peripheral nerve endings (6). Such ATP release, or that resulting from tissue damage and cell lysis, could act as an important local nociceptive stimulus at the level of the sensory nerve ending. Indeed, it is well established that both topical application of ATP to a blister base and subcutaneous injection are highly algogenic (7,8). However, activation of sensory nerve endings and nociceptors by ATP has not been extensively studied, and little is known about the mechanisms and nature of the purinoceptors involved. The recent cloning of a cDNA that encodes a novel ionotropic ATP receptor (P2X3) whose distribution is restricted to a subset of sensory, nociceptive neurons has heightened interest in the area (9,10).

In the present study we examined the effect of ATP and ATP analogs on cutaneous afferents in the neonatal rat tail-spinal cord preparation to understand further the excitatory effects of nucleotides on sensory neurons (11,12). In this preparation, activation of exposed sensory nerve endings in the tail in response to noxious stimuli is recorded indirectly via measurement of the evoked spinal motorneuron reflex.

MATERIALS AND METHODS

Neonatal rats (1 to 2 days old) were stunned and killed by decapitation and then placed in ice-cold modified physiological salt solution (PSS; mM in deionized water; NaCl 118, $NaHCO_3$ 25, KCl 4.7, $MgSO_4 \cdot 7H_2O$ 1.2, KH_2PO_4 1.2, D-glucose 11.1, $CaCl_2 \cdot 6H_2O$ 2.6), which was constantly gassed with 95% O_2/5% CO_2 to maintain pH 7.4. The most superficial layer of skin from the whole tail was gently removed, taking care not to damage the underlying tissue. The whole spinal cord was then carefully dissected out, complete with pelvic girdle and attached tail, and placed in a two-compartment recording chamber. The cord and tail were independently perfused with PSS at rates of 3 ml min^{-1} and 4 ml min^{-1}, respectively. All experiments were conducted at room temperature (22 to 28°C).

The potential difference across a spinal lumbar ventral root (L_3 to L_5) was recorded using a low-impedance, PSS-containing, glass microelectrode. The ventral root potential (VRP; d.c. with respect to the spinal cord that was earthed) was amplified (WPI Instruments), filtered (50 Hz), and displayed on an oscilloscope and a chart recorder (Lectromed M19). Drugs were applied to either the cord or the tail by addition to the appropriate perfusate. Preparations were left for 90 minutes for the VRP to stabilize and then tested for viability by addition of 5-hydroxytryptamine (5-HT; 100 μM for 30 seconds) to the cord. If depolarization responses to 5-HT amounted to less than 500 μV, or if baseline recording was unstable, preparations were rejected.

RESULTS

Application of ATP (0.3 to 100 μM; 30 seconds) to the exposed sensory nerve endings of the tail evoked concentration-related depolarization responses of the ventral root (Fig. 1A). The onset of these responses was rapid (<5 seconds) and the depolarization faded in the continued presence of the drug. The threshold concentration for excitation by ATP was 0.3 to 1μM, and the geometric mean EC_{50} value was 4.0 μM (95% confidence limits, 1.4 to 11.7 μM; n = 4). When expressed as a percentage of the maximal response evoked by bradykinin (1 μM), the maximal response to ATP amounted to 95.0 ± 6.7%. The ATP analogue, αβ-methylene ATP, also evoked concentration-related depolarization responses when applied to the tail. The mean EC_{50} value for αβ-methylene ATP was 0.43 μM (95% confidence limits, 0.27 to 0.67 μM; n = 4), and the maximal response amounted to 117.0 ± 3.8% of the response to bradykinin. Uridine 5′-triphosphate (UTP; n = 2), and L-βγ-methylene ATP (n = 3) produced only small responses when applied to the tail at concentrations up to 100 μM (see Fig. 1B).

When applied at 15-minute intervals, reproducible responses to αβ-methylene ATP (1 μM) could be obtained. The amplitude of successive depolarization responses amounted to 100 ± 0%, 102 ± 1%, 98 ± 4%, and 94 ± 5% of the initial response, respectively (n = 4). If the P_2 purinoceptor antagonist, pyridoxal 5-phos-

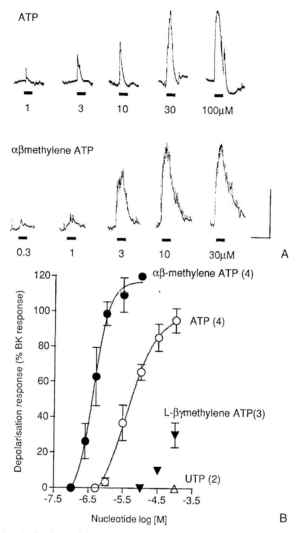

Fig. 1. Ventral root depolarizations of the neonatal rat spinal cord in response to cutaneous application of nucleotides in an in vitro tail-attached spinal cord preparation. **A:** Representative responses to ATP (*upper trace*) and to αβ-methylene ATP (*lower trace*) when applied to the tail for the duration indicated by the solid bar. In each case the vertical and horizontal calibration bars represent 0.5 mV and 1 minute, respectively. **B:** Mean data from several preparations (n values in parentheses). Data are plotted as a percentage of the response produced by 1 μM bradykinin against the log of the nucleotide concentration. Symbols represent the mean values and the vertical bars the SEM.

phate (P-5-P; 100 μM), was added to the perfusate immediately after the second exposure to αβ-methylene ATP (antagonist incubation time, 15 minutes), the subsequent agonist response was markedly reduced (16 ± 8% of the pre-antagonist control value; $n = 4$; $p < 0.01$ by Student's *t*-test; Fig. 2A). This inhibitory effect of P-5-P could be completely reversed on washout (100 ± 3% of pre-antagonist control

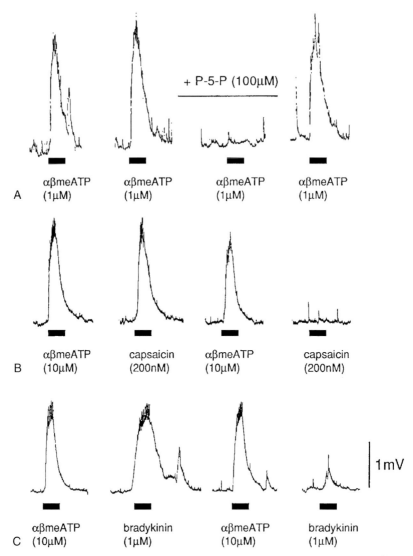

Fig. 2. Representative records of antagonist **(A)** and cross-desensitization **(B)** and **(C)** experiments in the neonatal rat tail-spinal cord preparation. In each panel drugs were applied for 30 seconds, the duration indicated by the solid bar. A period of 10 to 15 minutes was left between drug additions. In A note the marked reversible inhibitory effect of pyridoxal-5-phosphate (100 μM) on responses to αβmeATP. In B and C note that responses to αβmeATP could still be obtained after desensitization of responses to either capsaicin or bradykinin.

value). P-5-P (100 µM) did not attenuate responses to a submaximal concentration of capsaicin (100 nM), thus confirming the specificity of this agent for responses to αβ-methylene ATP (93 ± 4% of the pre-antagonist control value; $n = 3$, $p > 0.05$).

In the cross-desensitization experiments (Fig. 2B), addition of capsaicin (200 nM, 30 seconds) readily desensitized nerve endings to subsequent exposure to this agent, but did not modify the effects of αβ-methylene ATP ($10 > \mu$M). Similarly, bradykinin (1 µM, 30 seconds) produced prolonged self-desensitization, but responses to αβ-methylene ATP were unaffected (Fig. 2C). Even relatively long exposures (30 seconds) to a high concentration (10 µM) of αβ-methylene ATP did not produce cross-desensitization.

DISCUSSION

We have demonstrated that, when applied to exposed nerve endings in the skin of the neonatal rat, ATP produces excitation of motorneurons in the ventral horn of the spinal cord. The amplitude of these ventral root reflex responses was comparable to those produced by other extensively studied algesic substances (e.g., bradykinin, capsaicin), and the concentrations of ATP required were relatively low (12). Indeed, it is possible that even lower concentrations of ATP may be active in view of the well-documented inhibitory actions of cell surface ectoATPase enzymes that rapidly hydrolyze and inactivate certain nucleotides applied exogenously (13).

αβ-Methylene ATP, an analog that is resistant to ectoATPases, also activated the ventral root reflex and was more potent than ATP itself. Both UTP and L-βγ-methylene ATP were largely inactive. This agonist profile strongly suggests that ionotropic purinoceptors, possibly containing $P2X_3$ subunits, are involved (13). This conclusion is based on the known potent actions of αβ-methylene ATP on recombinant $P2X_3$ and $P2X_1$ receptors and the fact that L-βγ-methylene ATP (an agonist at the $P2X_1$ receptor) was inactive (9,10). $P2X_3$ channel proteins can heteropolymerize with P2X2 subunits to form functional αβ-methylene ATP-sensitive channels, and it is possible that such $P2X_{2/3}$ heteropolymers underlie the excitatory effects of purine nucleotides on cutaneous afferent nerves (10).

Pyridoxal-5-phosphate, at a concentration previously shown to antagonize P2X purinoceptor-mediated excitation of sensory neurons, produced specific, reversible inhibition of responses to αβ-methylene ATP (14). Desensitization of either capsaicin or bradykinin receptors did not inhibit the effects of this nucleotide. Together, these data confirm that responses to αβ-methylene ATP observed in the tail/spinal cord preparation are specifically purinoceptor mediated and do not involve the release of bradykinin or sensory neuropeptides.

In summary, we conclude that ATP activates functional ionotropic (P2X) purinoceptors on cutaneous afferent nerve endings. Although we have not provided definitive evidence that the ventral root depolarization responses result from activation of "nociceptive" fibers, we know that ATP is algogenic and that $P2X_3$ receptor mRNA is restricted to small-diameter nociceptive neurons (7–10,15). It would seem that activation of sensory nerves by ATP released either from inflammatory or damaged cells, or via antidromic stimulation, may be an important neurochemical mechanism for transmitting somatosensory information. Studies with potent and selective P2X purinoceptor antagonists in vivo are required to test this hypothesis.

REFERENCES

1. Salt TE, Hill RG. Neurotransmitter candidates of somatosensory primary afferent fibres. *Neuroscience* 1983;10:1083–1103.
2. Burnstock G, Wood JN. Purinergic receptors: their role in nociception and primary afferent transmission. *Curr Opin Neurobiol* 1996;6:526–532.
3. Jahr CE, Jessell TM. ATP excites a subpopulation of rat dorsal horn neurones. *Nature* 1983;304:730–733.
4. Salter MW, Henry JL. Effects of adenosine 5′-monophosphate and adenosine 5′-triphosphate on functionally identified units in the cat spinal dorsal horn. Evidence for a differential effect of adenosine 5′-triphosphate on nociceptive vs non-nociceptive units. *Neuroscience* 1985;15:815–825.
5. Li J, Perl ER. ATP modulation of synaptic transmission in the spinal substantia gelatinosa. *J Neurosci* 1995;15:3357–3365.
6. Holton P. The liberation of adenosine 5′-triphosphate on antidromic stimulation of sensory nerves. *J Physiol* 1959;145:494–504.
7. Coutts AA, Jorizzo JL, Eady RAJ, Greaves MW, Burnstock G. Adenosine triphosphate-evoked vascular changes in human skin: mechanism of action. *Eur J Pharmacol* 1981;76:391–401.
8. Bleehen T, Keele CA. Observations on the algogenic actions of adenosine compounds on human blister base preparation. *Pain* 1977;3:367–377.
9. Chen C-C, Akopian AN, Sivilotti L, Colqhuoun D, Burnstock G, Woo JW. A P2X purinoceptor expressed by a subset of sensory neurons. *Nature* 1995;377:428–431.
10. Lewis C, Neidhart S, Holy C, North RA, Buell G, Surprenant A. Coexpression of $P2X_2$ and $P2X_3$ receptor subunits can account for ATP-gated currents in sensory neurons. *Nature* 1995;377:432–435.
11. Yanagisawa M, Murakoshi T, Tamai S, Otsuka M. Tail-pinch method and the effects of some antinociceptive compounds. *Eur J Pharmacol* 1984;106:231–239.
12. Dray A, Bettaney J, Forster P. Actions of capsaicin on peripheral nociceptors of the neonatal rat spinal cord-tail in vitro: dependence of extracellular ions and independence of second messengers. *Br J Pharmacol* 1990;101:727–733.
13. Humphrey PPA, Buell G, Kennedy I, et al. New insights on P2X purinoceptors. *Naunyn Schmiedebergs Arch Pharmacol* 1995;352:585–596.
14. Trezise DJ, Bell NJ, Khakh BS, Michel AD, Humphrey PPA. P_2 purinoceptor antagonist properties of pyridoxal-5-phosphate. *Eur J Pharmacol* 1994;259:295–300.
15. Gold MS, Dastmalchi S, Levine JD. Coexpression of nociceptor properties in dorsal root ganglion neurones from the adult rat in vitro. *Neuroscience* 1996;71:265–275.

Headache Pathogenesis: Monoamines, Neuropeptides, Purines, and Nitric Oxide, edited by J. Olesen and L. Edvinsson.
Lippincott–Raven Publishers, Philadelphia © 1997.

14

Cortical Spreading Depression Does Not Activate Trigeminal C Fibers

Bente Krag Ingvardsen, *Henning Laursen, Uffe B. Olsen, and †Anker Jon Hansen

*Department of General Pharmacology and †Neuropharmacology, Novo Nordisk A/S, DK-2760 Maaloev, Denmark; and *Laboratory of Neuropathology and University Hospital, Rigshospitalet, DK-2100, Copenhagen, Denmark*

In the general population migraine has a prevalence of 10% to 20%. Ten percent experience migraine with aura (MA). The most common prodrome is scintillation scotomas, which propagate from the center to the periphery of the visual field. Clinical interest in cortical phenomena began when Lashley (1) scrutinized his own visual scotoma and calculated the speed of the advancing process to be about 3 mm/min. When Leão (2) later described a transient cortical depression of neuronal activity that moved at a velocity of 3 to 5 mm/min, he proposed that this cortical spreading depression (CSD) was the cause of the prodromal phase of MA. The theory has been supported by the findings that both the aura in humans and CSD in animals are associated with a reduction of regional cerebral blood flow (rCBF) (3). In patients the hypoperfusion is initiated in the occipital cortex and, like the aura, moves, as a spreading oligemia, across the cortex at a velocity of 2 to 3 mm/min. Oligemia is preceded by a short-lasting focal hyperemia (4); a brief neuronal excitation precedes the neuronal depression that characterizes CSD (2). Hence, CSD is the most likely cause of the prodromal phase of MA.

The cause of migraine headache, however, is still a matter of debate. The pain most likely involves an activation of trigeminal C fibers, which innervate dura mater and its blood vessels, the circle of Willis, and major cerebral arteries. Two hypotheses exist: (a) the vascular theory, stating that C fibers are activated by dilation of cerebral blood vessels (5); and (b) the neurogenic theory, stating that headache is due to neurogenic inflammation (NI) within the meningeal circulation (6). This response is characterized by vasodilation and protein extravasation mediated by neuropeptides [e.g., substance P (SP), calcitonin gene-related peptide (CGRP)] released from C fibers. NI is thought to sensitize C fibers and perpetuate pain after the stimulus has been removed (7).

Moskowitz et al. (8) have proposed a link between the prodrome of MA and headache that involves NI. They found that CSD elicited in rat neocortex was associated with c-fos expression in the trigeminal nucleus caudalis (TNC) of the brain stem, where C fibers end, and hence with an activation of trigeminal C fibers. C-fos expression was reduced by sumatriptan, which led to the conclusion that headache is induced by some events occurring in relation to CSD. The following scheme was suggested: CSD promotes the release of nociceptive substances from neocortex, which then activate meningeal C fibers, inducing NI and pain (headache). Moskowitz states that the time lapse (about 20 minutes) between the aura and headache reflects the time it takes for CSD to propagate and reach the blood vessels at the ventral surface of the brain that are most pain sensitive (6). The purpose of our study was to investigate further the proposed association between CSD and activation of trigeminal C fibers in rats.

METHODS

Elicitation of Cortical Spreading Depression

Male Wistar rats (250 to 400 g) were anesthetized with halothane. Four craniotomies were made, two on each side 2 mm lateral and 1 mm anterior to bregma, and 7 mm posterior and 3 mm lateral to bregma. DC potentials were recorded by glass micropipettes filled with 150 mM NaCl and positioned anteriorly. CSD was induced in the right occipital cortex by injection of 1 M KCl while 1 M NaCl was injected into the left, as control. Injections were made every 6 minutes for 1 hour. After another 1 hour the animals were killed by intracardiac perfusion fixation with saline (0.9%) followed by formalin buffer (4%). Serial vibratome sections (50 µm) of brain stem and upper cervical spinal cord were processed immunohistochemically for c-fos expression using the peroxidase-antiperoxidase method [primary antibody: c-fos (Ab-2) from Oncogene Science]. The following groups were studied: group 1: (n = 8) sumatriptan 0.3 mg/kg; group 2: (n = 3) morphine 3 mg/kg; and group 3: (n = 6) saline (control). All drugs were given i.v. 30 minutes before elicitation of CSD.

Electrical Stimulation of the Trigeminal Nerve

Male Sprague-Dawley rats were anesthetized by pentobarbital. Two craniotomies were made and two bipolar stimulating electrodes inserted in the right and left trigeminal ganglions, respectively. Only the right trigeminal nerve was stimulated electrically (5 Hz, 5 msec, 10 V) for 15 minutes. After another 1 hour and 45 minutes the animal was fixated and the brain stem and upper cervical spinal cord were processed for c-fos expression as described above. Three groups were studied: group 1: (n = 10) saline (control); group 2: (n = 6) sumatriptan (0.3 mg/kg); and group 3: (n = 4) morphine (1 mg/kg). Drugs were given i.v. 10 minutes before stimulation.

TABLE 1. *Fos-positive cells in the ipsilateral and contralateral TNC after CSD*

Group and treatment	Ipsilateral TNC (mean±SD)	Contralateral TNC (mean±SD)
1. sumatriptan (n=8)	39 ± 33	27±25
2. morphine (n=3)	18 ± 13	18±17
3. saline (n=6)	62 ± 10	40±9

TNC, 3 mm caudal to obex.

RESULTS

C-fos in Relation to Elicitation of Cortical Spreading Depression

C-fos expression was induced in lamina I and II, mainly in the ipsilateral (60%) but also in the contralateral (40%) TNC after elicitation of CSDs. Fewer Fos-positive cells were seen on both sides after sumatriptan (n.s.) and morphine pretreatment (ipsilateral: $p < 0.001$; contralateral: $p < 0.05$) (Table 1).

No positive correlation was seen between the number of CSDs elicited and the extent of c-fos expression in the ipsilateral or contralateral TNC. Instead there was a positive, linear correlation between the number of KC1 injections and the number of fos-positive cells in the ipsilateral TNC (Fig. 1).

C-fos Induced by Electrical Stimulation of the Trigeminal Nerve

Electrical stimulation of the trigeminal nerve induced an upregulation of c-fos expression in lamina I and II of TNC. C-fos expression was prominent on the ipsilateral side (80%) but sparse contralaterally (20%). The number of Fos-positive cells in the ipsilateral TNC correlated (linearly) with stimulus intensity. Morphine significantly reduced c-fos expression ($p < 0.01$) in the ipsilateral TNC, whereas sumatriptan was ineffective.

DISCUSSION

C-fos Expression in the Trigeminal Nucleus Caudalis

C-fos expression can be used to quantify the degree of pain in the trigeminal system as well as others following C-fiber stimulation, since the number of c-fos-expressing cells correlated with stimulus intensity and was reduced by morphine, in accordance with Presley et al. (9). Sumatriptan had no significant effect on c-fos expression, which is in agreement with Shepheard et al. (10), who showed that sumatriptan only reduces c-fos expression in TNC if the blood-brain barrier is disrupted.

The fact that elicitation of multiple CSDs increased c-fos expression in lamina I

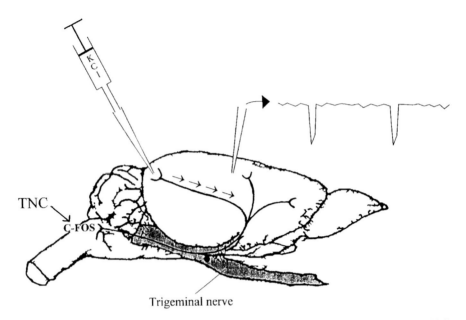

FIG. 1. C-fos expression in the trigeminal nucleus caudalis (TNC) following elicitation of multiple CSDs by KCl (1 M) injections into cortex. The algogen KCl, and not CSD, stimulates the meningeal nociceptors, thereby inducing c-fos upregulation in TNC, as described in the text.

and II of the ipsilateral TNC seems to prove that pain is involved. Again, morphine significantly reduced c-fos expression. However, the extent of c-fos expression was positively correlated with the number of KCl injections but not with the number of CSDs, demonstrating that the injection of the algogenic substance 1 M KCl rather than CSD stimulates the C fibers (Fig. 1). We suggest that 1 M KCl activated the nociceptors, causing c-fos expression in the ipsilateral TNC, while 1 M NaCl, a less potent algogen, induced c-fos staining in the contralateral TNC. Sumatriptan reduced the ipsilateral c-fos expression by 37% (n.s.) possibly by inhibiting local NI induced at the site of KCl injection. Hence, our results do not support the association between CSD and activation of trigeminal nerve fibers (8).

Spreading Depression and Migraine

There are two interesting aspects of a possible link between CSD and migraine headache. *First*, if the headache is induced by some event that takes place during the aura, it is expected that prophylactic drugs like dihydroergotamine, valproate, lignocaine, and acetylsalicylic acid would prevent or alter CSD. Kaube and Goadsby (11) showed in the cat that neither of these drugs inhibited or attenuated CSD after mechanical stimulation of the cortex. These findings argue against CSD being the initiating event for migraine headache (although it may still be the cause of the aura).

Second, neurogenic inflammation has been implicated in the pathogenesis of migraine headache (6). If episodes of CSD underlie headache, the question arises: do episodes of CSD induce NI? Electrical stimulation of the trigeminal nerve induces NI in rat dura mater that is reduced by sumatriptan (12). However, it has not yet been examined whether CSD causes NI within the animal dura mater, nor whether NI develops in human cranial blood vessels during a migraine attack. Plasma CGRP levels are elevated in jugular venous blood in migraineurs during headache and normalized after administration of sumatriptan and symptomatic relief (13). The same was seen after electrical stimulation of the superior sagittal sinus of cats (14) or the trigeminal ganglion in rats (15). Conflicting results exist regarding neuropeptide release after CSD. One study showed no elevation of CGRP in cat jugular venous blood either during the passage of a wave of CSD across the cortex nor 60 minutes later, during the period of post-CSD cortical oligemia (16). Another study suggests that CGRP is released in cats following CSD since application of a CGRP-receptor antagonist attenuated pial arteriolar dilation accompanying CSD (17). However, CGRP alone does not induce NI since protein extravasation is caused by SP. No study has shown that SP is released in relation to CSD. We conclude that at present there is no strong evidence to support the hypothesis that CSD is involved in migraine headache.

REFERENCES

1. Lashley KS. Patterns of cerebral integration indicated by the scotomas of migraine. *Arch Neurol Psychiatry* 1941;46:331–339.
2. Leão APP. Spreading depression of activity in cerebral cortex. *J Neurophysiol* 1944;7:359–390.
3. Lauritzen M. Cerebral blood flow in migraine and cortical spreading depression. *Acta Neurol Scand* 1987;76[suppl 113]:9–40.
4. Olesen J, Larsen B, Lauritzen M. Focal hyperemia followed by spreading oligemia and impaired activation of rCBF in classic migraine. *Ann Neurol* 1981;9:344–352.
5. Wolff HG. *Headache and other head pain*. New York: Oxford University Press, 1963.
6. Moskowitz MA. The neurobiology of vascular head pain. *Ann Neurol* 1984;16:157–168.
7. Fields HL. *Pain*. New York: McGraw-Hill, 1987.
8. Moskowitz MA, Nozaki K, Kraig RP. Neocortical spreading depression provokes the expression of c-fos protein-like immunoreactivity within trigeminal nucleus caudalis via trigeminovascular mechanisms. *J Neurosci* 1993;13:1167–1177.
9. Presley RW, Menetrey D, Levine JD, Basbaum AI. Systemic morphine suppresses noxious stimulus-evoked Fos protein-like immunoreactivity in the rat spinal cord. *J Neurosci* 1990;10:323–335.
10. Shepheard SL, Williamson DJ, Williams J, Hill RG, Hargreaves RJ. Comparison of the effects of sumatriptan and the NK_1 antagonist CP-99,994 on plasma extravasation in dura mater and c-fos mRNA expression in trigeminal nucleus caudalis of rats. *Neuropharmacology* 1995;34:255–261.
11. Kaube H, Goadsby PJ. Anti-migraine compounds fail to modulate the propagation of cortical spreading depression in the cat. *Eur Neurol* 1994;34:30–35.
12. Markowitz S, Saito K, Moskowitz MA. Neurogenically mediated leakage of plasma protein occurs from blood vessels in dura mater but not brain. *J Neurosci* 1987;7:4129–4136.
13. Edvinsson L, Goadsby PJ. Neuropeptides in migraine and cluster headache. *Cephalalgia* 1994;14:320–327.
14. Zagami AS, Goadsby PJ, Edvinsson L. Stimulation of the superior sagittal sinus in the cat causes release of vasoactive peptides. *Neuropeptides* 1990;16:69–75.
15. Buzzi MG, Moskowitz MA, Peroutka SJ, Byun B. Further characterization of the putative 5 HT re-

ceptor which mediates blockade of neurogenic plasma extravasation in rat dura mater. *J Pharmacol* 1991;103:1421–1428.
16. Piper RD, Edvinsson L, Ekman R, Lambert GA. Cortical spreading depression does not result in the release of calcitonin gene-related peptide into the external jugular vein of the cat: relevance to human migraine. *Cephalalgia* 1993;13:180–183.
17. Wahl M, Schilling L, Parsons AA, Kaumann A. Involvement of calcitonin gene-related peptide (CGRP) and nitric oxide (NO) in the pial artery dilatation elicited by cortical spreading depression. *Brain Res* 1994;637:204–210.

15

Systemic Nitroglycerin Activates Catecholaminergic, Neuropeptidergic, and Nitric Oxide Pathways in the Rat Brain

Cristina Tassorelli, *Shirley Anne Joseph, G. Sandrini, Alfredo Costa, and Giuseppe Nappi

*Neurological Institute "C. Mondino," University of Pavia, 27100 Pavia, Italy; *Division of Neurological Surgery, Strong Memorial Hospital, Rochester, New York 14642*

Nitroglycerin (NTG) is an organic nitrate ester that causes vasodilation via the release of nitric oxide (NO) in the wall of blood vessels. Several studies have suggested that NTG also acts on the central nervous system, although the exact mechanism and whether this is linked to NTG-derived NO is so far unknown. Our previous studies (1) have demonstrated that, following subcutaneous administration, NTG induces sustained expression of Fos protein, a marker of neuronal activation (2), in the hypothalamus, amygdala, periaqueductal gray, locus coeruleus, parabrachial nucleus, nucleus tractus solitarius, ventrolateral medulla, and spinal trigeminal nucleus caudalis of rats. The neurotransmission assets of these nuclei are fairly well known. The peculiar distribution of Fos-positive neurons within their anatomic boundaries prompted us to investigate the neurochemical characteristics of the neurons that respond to systemic administration of NTG.

EXPERIMENTAL PROCEDURES

Experiments were performed in two groups of male Sprague-Dawley adult rats (250 to 320 g.): in the *treated group* (n = 16), rats were injected subcutaneously with NTG 10 mg/kg of a 5-mg/ml solution containing alcohol, propylene glycol, and water as vehicle; in the *control group* (n = 8) rats received subcutaneously the vehicle alone.

Four hours after injection (time of maximal expression of Fos in response to NTG), animals were perfused through the ascending aorta, and brain sections were processed for immunohistochemical visualization of Fos using an antiserum directed against an in vitro translated product of the c-fos. A second incubation with other antisera was performed to demonstrate two antigens with contrasting colors in the same tissue section. Antisera used in this study were anti-rabbit dopamine β-hydroxylase (DβH), oxytocin (OT), arg^8-vasopressin (AVP), and corticotropin-releasing hormone (CRH). Details of the procedure we used have been described elsewhere (3).

A group of brain sections were processed for reduced nicotinamide adenine dinucleotide phosphate-diaphorase (NADPH-d) histochemistry to evaluate the distribution of Fos-immunoreactive cells within neurons containing NO synthase (4,5).

Data Analysis

The staining for Fos was typically limited to the nucleus of neurons, while all the neuronal markers we investigated in this study induced cytoplasmic staining. This facilitated the identification and count of neurons that contained both kinds of staining. Brain sections taken at comparable levels were used to index the number of Fos-immunoreactive neurons as well as of neurons that were double-labeled for another marker. The presence of NADPH-d-positive fibers and/or varicosities in close proximity (within 3 μm) to Fos-immunoreactive nuclei was evaluated as well.

RESULTS

Data on Fos expression in NTG-injected and vehicle-injected rats were in agreement with our previous findings (1). As regards the counts of neurons positive for the various transmitter markers, no significant differences were observed between the NTG-treated and the vehicle-treated groups.

Treated Group

Noradrenaline

In the *caudal ventrolateral medulla*, 80% of Fos-immunoreactive cells were positive for DβH, and almost 100% of DβH neurons were Fos positive. In the commissural and medial subdivisions of the *nucleus tractus solitarius*, 80% of DβH-positive neurons were labeled for Fos. The neurons double-labeled for Fos and DβH represented 30% of the total number of Fos-immunoreactive neurons observed in this nucleus. In the *locus coeruleus*, Fos-immunoreactive neurons represented 25% of the entire noradrenergic population, and virtually every Fos-positive neuron was also positive for DβH (Fig. 1).

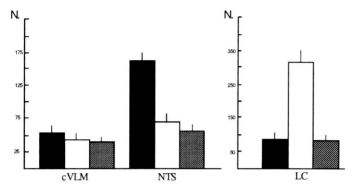

FIG. 1. Bar graphs summarizing the number of neurons (N) that stained for dopamine β-hydroxylase and for Fos in the caudal ventrolateral medulla (cVLM), nucleus tractus solitarius (NTS), and locus coeruleus (LC). Black columns represent the number of Fos-immunoreactive neurons, white columns the number of neurons positive for dopamine β-hydroxylase, and gray columns the neurons positive for both markers. Data are shown as mean ± SD.

Vasopressin and Oxytocin

In the *supraoptic nucleus* of the hypothalamus, 40% of the cells that expressed Fos following NTG administration were double-labeled for OT (Fig. 2). Fos/OT-positive neurons represented about 45% of the total number of OT-positive neurons in this nucleus. AVP immunoreactivity was observed in 60% of Fos-immunoreactive neurons in the same nucleus. The double-labeled neurons amounted to 65% of the total number of AVP-positive neurons in the nucleus. In the *paraventricular nucleus of*

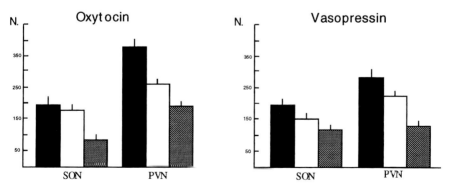

FIG. 2. Bar graphs summarizing the number of neurons (N) that stained for Fos and for oxytocin or arg-vasopressin in the supraoptic nucleus (SON) and paraventricular nucleus (PVN) of the hypothalamus. Black columns represent the number of Fos-immunoreactive neurons, white columns the number of neurons positive for the neuropeptide, and gray columns the number of neurons double-labeled for the neuropeptide and for Fos. Data are shown as mean ± SD.

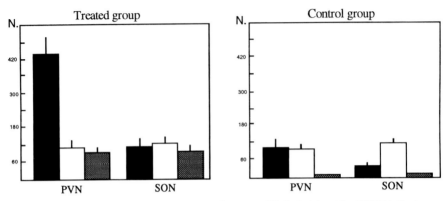

FIG. 3. Bar graphs summarizing the number of neurons (N) that stained for NADPH-diaphorase and for Fos in the supraoptic nucleus (SON) and paraventricular nucleus of the hypothalamus (PVN). Black columns show the number of Fos-immunoreactive neurons, white columns the number of neurons positive for NADPH-diaphorase activity, and gray columns the number of neurons labeled for both markers. Data are shown as mean ± SD. Student's *t* test for treated vs. control group: $p < .0001$; Chi-square test for treated vs. control group: $p < .0001$.

the hypothalamus, about 45% of Fos-positive cells in the lateral magnocellular and ventral subdivisions contained OT with double-labeled neurons representing 70% of OT population. Neurons double-labeled for Fos and AVP corresponded to 50% of Fos-immunoreactive neurons and to 60% of AVP-immunoreactive neurons.

Corticotropin Releasing Hormone

More than 80% of the neurons that expressed CRH in the parvocellular division of the *paraventricular nucleus of the hypothalamus* were also stained for Fos.

NADPH-Diaphorase

In the *paraventricular nucleus of the hypothalamus,* almost 80% of the NADPH-d-positive neurons were also labeled for Fos (Fig. 3). In the *supraoptic nucleus,* the

TABLE 1. *Number of Fos-positive neurons that received close appositions from NADPH-d-positive fibers in some nuclei of the brain stem[a]*

Area	Fos-positive neurons	Fos-positive neurons near NADPH-d fibers
Locus coeruleus	327.2±54.2	287.1±51.3
Parabrachial nucleus	214.7±86.4	168.1±59.3
Nucleus tractus solitarius	302.6±121.1	277.3±97.1
Spinal trigeminal n. caudalis	149.4±43.9	102.1±27.3

[a] Values are expressed as mean±SD.

co-localization rate of NADPH-d activity with Fos was above 90%. In the *locus coeruleus, parabrachial nucleus, nucleus tractus solitarius*, and *spinal trigeminal nucleus caudalis* a small portion of Fos-immunoreactive neurons co-localized with NADPH-d activity. In all these nuclei, however, the great majority of Fos-immunoreactive neurons (>70%) were found to be in close proximity to NADPH-d-positive neuronal processes (Table 1).

Control Group

The rate of co-localization of Fos with DβH, OT, AVP, and CRH in these rats was dramatically lower (<10% of Fos-immunoreactive neurons) than that observed in the treated group. As far as NADPH-d activity was concerned, co-expression with Fos was detected in about 10% of NADPH-d-positive neurons in the paraventricular nucleus of the hypothalamus and in less than 20% of NADPH-d-positive neurons in the supraoptic nucleus (Fig. 3). The few Fos-immunoreactive neurons observed in the brain stem did not show NADPH-d activity nor significant phenomena of vicinity with NADPH-d-positive fibers.

DISCUSSION

The dual immunocytochemical technique demonstrated that the noradrenergic structures in the brainstem were massively activated following NTG administration (6). The activation involved the noradrenergic neurons of the locus coeruleus, caudal ventrolateral medulla, A2 and C2 groups. Nitroglycerin is likely to activate these monoaminergic pathways partly because of vasodilation-induced hypotension. However, other mechanisms might be hypothesized when considering that the locus coeruleus does not play a significant role during hypotension. Other studies that evaluated Fos expression following hemorrhage- or sodium nitroprusside-induced hypotension pointed out a prominent involvement of the C1 group of neurons, which was scarcely involved in our model (7). The involvement of catecholaminergic neurons in the ventrolateral medulla that we observed rather resembles the pattern described by other authors following noxious stimulation (8).

In the hypothalamus, neurons containing AVP and OT were found to be simultaneously activated following NTG administration. Hypotension is known to induce Fos-immunoreactivity in AVP neurons in the supraoptic nucleus. More intriguing are the data regarding Fos expression in OT neurons in the supraoptic and paraventricular nuclei. Only severe hemorrhages, which involve a far greater degree of hypotension than that induced by the dose of NTG we used, are able to stimulate Fos expression in OT neurons located in these hypothalamic nuclei. These neurons have been shown to express Fos following specific stimuli, such as osmotic stress, administration of cholecystokinin and histamine, and parturition. The mechanism involved in their activation following NTG administration is so far unknown. It is well known that OT neurons in the hypothalamus receive noradrenergic afferents from the brain stem, and our data demonstrate that noradrenergic structures are massively activated by NTG, which suggests one possible mechanism for the recruitment of OT cells in this model.

The CRH neurons of the medial parvocellular part of the paraventricular nucleus of the hypothalamus were strongly activated by systemic NTG. The well-known bidirectional connectivity between CRH-containing neurons in the hypothalamus and the brain stem nuclei that were activated by NTG may provide a key to interpret the involvement of this peptidergic structure.

A subpopulation of NADPH-d-positive neurons in the paraventricular and supraoptic nuclei of the hypothalamus expressed Fos protein following systemic administration of NTG. This activation may be related to a direct effect of NTG, which has been found to induce marked increases in the levels of cyclic guanosine monophosphate (c-GMP) in the brain when subcutaneously administered (9). The NO-induced stimulation of the c-GMP pathway has been shown to induce the expression of c-fos (10). Thus, the interaction of NTG with NO-related metabolic mechanisms of NADPH-d neurons may explain the phenomenon we observed.

In most of the other areas that showed a strong Fos expression following NTG administration, such as the locus coeruleus, parabrachial nucleus, nucleus tractus solitarius, and spinal trigeminal nucleus caudalis, close appositions (within 3 μm from the Fos-positive nucleus) with NADPH-d-positive fibers were frequently observed. It is known that the ventral part of the paraventricular nucleus, where Fos-immunoreactivity was found co-localized with NADPH-d activity, contributes fibers to the locus coeruleus, parabrachial nucleus, and nucleus tractus solitarius. Future data on the connectivity of neurons containing NADPH-d activity will allow a more conclusive interpretation. However, the neurophysiological and neuroanatomical data gathered on the role of NO in these nuclei, along with the present data, seem to provide evidence of a possible role of NO in cell-to-cell signaling.

In conclusion, the systemic administration of NTG activates a specific set of brain structures that are involved in the control of vegetative, neuroendocrine, nociceptive, and behavioral functions. The neurochemical characterization of the neurons involved suggests an outstanding role for noradrenergic and neuropeptidergic systems, as well as for the pool of neurons that synthesize NO. The clinical implications of these data are quite intriguing, especially in the light of NTG-induced migraine headache, since they represent a neuroanatomical and neurochemical basis for the further study and comprehension of the phenomenon.

REFERENCES

1. Tassorelli C, Joseph SA. Systemic nitroglycerin induces Fos immunoreactivity in brainstem and forebrain structures of the rat. *Brain Res* 1995;682:67–178.
2. Dragunow M, Faull R. The use of c-*fos* as a metabolic marker in neuronal pathway tracing. *J Neurosci Methods* 1989;29:261–265.
3. Tassorelli C, Joseph SA. Systemic nitroglycerin activates peptidergic and catecholaminergic pathways in rat brain. *Peptides* 1996;17:443–449.

4. Vincent SR, Kimura H. Histochemical mapping of nitric oxide synthase in the rat brain. *Neuroscience* 1992;46:755–784.
5. Tassorelli C, Joseph SA. NADPH-diaphorase activity and Fos expression in brain nuclei following nitroglycerin administration. *Brain Res* 1995;695:37–44.
6. Guyenet PG. Central noradrenergic neurons: the autonomic connection. *Prog Brain Res* 1991;88:365–380.
7. Li Y-W, Dampney RAL. Expression of Fos-like protein in brain following sustained hypertension and hypotension in conscious rabbits. *Neuroscience* 1994;61:613–634.
8. Senba E, Matsunaga K, Tohyama M, Noguchi K. Stress-induced c-fos expression in the rat brain: activation mechanism of sympathetic pathway. *Brain Res Bull* 1993;31:329–344.
9. Torfgard K, Ahnler J, Axelsson KL, Norlander B, Bertler A. Tissue distribution of glyceryl trinitrate and the effect on cGMP levels in rat. *Pharmacol Toxicol* 1989;64:369–372.
10. Haby K, Lisovoski F, Aunis D, Zwiller J. Stimulation of the cyclic GMP pathway by NO induces expression of the immediate early genes c-*fos* and junB in PC12 cells. *J Neurochem* 1994;62:496–501.

16

Discussion Summary: Role of Messenger Molecules in Pain Processing

Clifford J. Woolf

Department of Anatomy and Developmental Biology, University College London, London WC1E 6BT, United Kingdom

The session brought up several important general issues. One was the relationship between headache and other general pain mechanisms. Is headache a special case or does it share common pathophysiological mechanisms with other pain states? Another issue is whether migraine and tension-type headaches are distinct in terms of their pathophysiological mechanisms. There is now a large body of evidence on the mechanisms involved in clinical pain states, indicating both peripheral and central sensitization, on top of which there is control mediated by descending mechanisms, which can both facilitate and inhibit pain transmission. The challenge is to try to see the extent to which these mechanisms contribute to the pathophysiology of headache.

Dealing first with the talk of Professor McMahon, what is clear is that high-threshold primary nociceptors can be sensitized in the periphery on exposure to a broad range of inflammatory mediators including cytokines and neurotrophins. Important issues remain to be resolved, however, such as, in the case of headache, what is the source of such sensitizing inflammatory mediators? Does cortical spreading depression represent a means whereby inflammatory mediators may be released or whereby other cells such as microglia or astrocytes may release inflammatory mediators that can act on sensory terminals? There is some evidence (to which Dr. McMahon alluded) from Claudio Cuello's laboratory indicating that nerve growth factor (NGF) levels do increase after cortical spreading depression in an animal model.

Another question relates to whether different inflammatory factors act synergistically together. Jes Olesen asked whether anything is known about the combination of NGF with other inflammatory mediators. At present, it is known that NGF does produce peripheral sensitization due to a combination of its action on the sympathetic nervous system, its capacity to degranulate mast cells, and its direct activation of trkA receptors on peripheral nociceptors; however, whether this neurotrophin interacts synergistically with other inflammatory mediators (such as the kinins, histamine, hydrogen and potassium ions, or purines) is simply not known at present.

Helen Connor enquired whether, given the fact that NGF has been administered systemically in human patients (by Genentech in a clinical trial to try to arrest diabetic neuropathy), and since it is known that these patients report pain, headache is experienced. This has not been reported, but it may be because NGF has not gained access to meningeal primary afferent terminals due to the blood-brain barrier.

Dr. Bach of the University of Copenhagen asked Dr. McMahon whether he could explain the nature of the different hyperalgesic phases following systemic NGF. At least three phases are apparent. The initial phase is entirely peripheral and seems to be mediated by the direct action of NGF on the nociceptors as well as by an interaction with sympathetic and mast cells. This is followed by a longer lasting phase acting for several hours that may be secondary to the activation by NGF of trkA receptors on sensory terminals, which may, through phosphorylation-dependent changes, produce a more persistent peripheral sensitization. Finally, the third phase reflects the retrograde transport of NGF bound to the trkA receptor to the cell body of the nociceptor, either in the dorsal root or the trigeminal ganglion, where it can induce transcription; these transcriptional changes may be responsible for the long-lasting hyperalgesic effects of NFG.

Troels Jensen of Aarhus University inquired about the relationship between NGF as an inflammatory mediator and its possible involvement in the production of neuropathic pain. Professor McMahon pointed out that a relative excess of NGF will, in some circumstances, produce pain by producing peripheral sensitization and by changing the phenotype of sensory neurons. In other circumstances it may be a cause of pain, as in neuropathic pain conditions in which a relative lack of neurotrophins (resulting from the disruption of contact of sensory neurons with their targets, which represent a source of neurotrophins) may result in a number of changes in sensory neurons, which manifest as pain. We have then the possibility that NGF antagonists may be useful clinically in some contexts, such as acute inflammation; in other contexts supplementation with NGF may be necessary, as in neuropathic pain conditions. Jim Lance asked Dr. McMahon whether, in view of the fact that calcitonin gene-related peptide (CGRP) is found to co-exist with trkA, the high-affinity NGF receptor, and given that CGRP levels are increased in patients with migraine, this could be an indication of the specific involvement of NGF in migraine. The answer, at the moment, must be that this is a distinct possibility, but its full evaluation must await the availability of NGF antagonists for use in humans, to see whether NGF actually contributes to migraine.

Dr. Peatfield of Charing Cross asked Dr. McMahon to comment on the fact that migraine is episodic, and how this relates to some of the prolonged changes in sensitivity that occur in the periphery. Dr. McMahon replied that, in fact, peripheral sensitization was usually relatively short-lived. Some of the effects were extremely short-lived and depended entirely on receptor binding by inflammatory mediators, and others were more long-lasting, presumedly involving phosphorylation of ion channels and other membrane-bound receptors on the peripheral terminal; all of these were reversible and were, therefore, compatible with an episodic condition such as migraine.

It was clear from the general discussion that sensitization of primary afferents may have an important role in the pathophysiology of headache and that factors such as NGF may contribute. An important issue that arose is whether, once sensitization of high-threshold nociceptors has occurred, this would be sufficient to account for the generation of pain signals in response to the dilation of cerebral vessels. If normally high-threshold mechanoreceptor afferents were sensitized such that dilation of the vessels would initiate an input to the brain, this may account for some of the pain that is experienced and also explain why vasoconstrictors have analgesic efficacy in the treatment of migraine. They may not alter the sensitization of the nociceptors, but by decreasing the diameter of blood vessels, they may decrease sensory input and therefore abort the sensory component of a migraine attack.

The next general issue discussed related to changes in sensitivity of neurons within the central nervous system and in particular whether there may be a predisposition in certain individuals for the development of central increased excitability. This would explain why a certain input may generate a full-blown attack in some patients but not in others. Such a correlation is being investigated in patients with myofascial pain syndrome and rheumatoid arthritis, in which central sensitization can be provoked using capsaicin (the pungent ingredient of chili peppers) which manifests as secondary hyperalgesia. In these patients, it appears that there is a differential capacity to generate central sensitization, and there may be a correlation between patients who suffer from rheumatoid arthritis or myofascial pain and an increased capacity to generate central sensitization. It will be intriguing if this turns out to be true for headache. Professor Jes Olesen pointed out that in patients with chronic tension-type headache who experience the pain on a daily basis, there is generalized tenderness, but this is not true in patients with migraine or intermittent tension-type headache, outside of the period of their headaches. Nevertheless, the distinct possibility remains that in these patients there is an increase of cerebral excitability. Cortical spreading depression in these patients may activate a degree of central sensitization and therefore pain that does not occur in other individuals; this may explain the mismatch, on some occasions, between the presence of aura and subsequent headache. This is an issue that is open to experimental investigation, and it is hoped that new data will emerge in the near future.

Helen Connor asked whether there was a possibility that migraineurs may have an ongoing state of central sensitization independent of a peripheral drive. This certainly seems unlikely. Like peripheral sensitization, the mechanisms of central sensitization are relatively short-lived; while central sensitization is due both to activity and some transcription-dependent changes, the re-establishment of a normal level of sensitivity can occur within a period of several hours. What is less certain is the extent to which the degree of central sensitization is under the control of descending inhibitory mechanisms. We do know that noxious inputs and peripheral inflammation can activate descending inhibitory controls; therefore, one of the ways in which one can potentially amplify or even produce central sensitization is by a partial reduction or removal of such inhibition. There are thus two general ways of generating central sensitization: an increase in excitability driven by primary afferent excitatory transmitters, or a decrease in either tonic or phasic inhibitory mechanisms by the blockade or partial antagonism of inhibitory transmitters such as γ-aminobutyric acid or glycine. There was some discussion about this, and the general consensus was that it is unlikely that migraine would be independent of primary afferent input (which at the very least is likely to trigger the headache and any associated central sensitization), but that the degree of inhibition that occurs may help to explain the predisposition in some individuals to a greater amount of headache for a certain amount of input.

This issue related to a question that Dr. Peatfield of Charing Cross asked: how does wind-up or central sensitization terminate? Is a negative feedback compensatory mechanism involved? The answer is that the processes involved are themselves short-lived, but also that central sensitization does not occur independent of inhibitory brain mechanisms. Activation of descending inhibitory mechanisms from the brain stem have the capacity both to facilitate and to depress sensory processing in the spinal trigeminal nucleus as well as in the dorsal horn of the spinal cord, and the latter may help damp down cerebral excitation.

A question was asked about the N-methyl-D-aspartate (NMDA) receptor and its blockade by magnesium, which appears to have a key role in the induction of central sensitization such that the removal of the normal magnesium block of the NMDA receptor-ion channel is associated with an increase in glutamate sensitivity. Does this open a possibility that magnesium treatment could be used for the treatment of either migraine or tension-type headaches? The answer, on theoretical grounds, is no, on the basis that the levels of magnesium present in extracellular fluid are sufficient to block the NMDA receptor fully and that additional magnesium should have no additional effect. There are anecdotal reports, however, that magnesium does have some analgesic and antihypersensitivity action. Dr. Bach asked Mary Heinricher whether anyone has recorded from neurons in the ventromedial reticular formation during cortical spreading depression as a way of seeing whether this nucleus has a positive role in the generation of migraine. The answer is that this has not yet been studied.

Further discussion raised the issue that migraine is a rather unique clinical condition, which has a class of highly efficacious drugs, the sumatriptan-like 5-HT$_{1D}$ agonists, originally designed to cause constriction of meningeal vessels; yet the specific pathophysiological mechanism that operates during migraine is unknown at the moment. This relates specifically to the possibility that this class of drugs may have an action not only on the vasculature but also on the nervous system. A further issue is whether their prime action is a prejunctional blockade of the release from the peripheral terminals of sensory neurons of vasoactive mediators, or whether some of their effect may be due to a prejunctional blockade of the release of transmitters centrally. The action of at least those members of this class of compounds that are lipophilic may be to block, therefore, the development of central sensitization by preventing release of centrally acting transmitters. A related issue is the extent to which neurogenic inflammation plays a role in the pathogenesis of migraine. There is increasing evidence that neurogenic extravasation by itself may be insufficient to explain the features of migraine fully and that there is a growing mismatch between the capacity of certain drugs to block extravasation and to have efficacy in treating migraine, at least those that act as postjunctional receptor blockers such as NKI and endothelin receptor antagonists. The issue remains of whether neurogenic inflammation, which consists of both vasodilation and an increase in capillary permeability, has any role in the pathogenesis of migraine and whether the vasodilator component can be used as a screen for the development of new compounds for the treatment of migraine.

The general conclusion is that changes in the nervous system, peripheral and cerebral sensitization, and the level of pain-modulating systems are likely to have a major role in the pathophysiology of headache. What needs to be evaluated is the extent to which currently available drugs interact with the nervous system as part of their action and whether drugs specifically targeted at preventing hypersensitivity in the nervous system may offer advantages in treating headache.

SECTION IV
Involvement of Amines and Amino Acids in Primary Headache

# 17

Amines and Amino Acids in Migraine

Vivette A. S. Glover

Department of Paediatrics, Queen Charlotte's Hospital, London W6 OXG, United Kingdom

Many studies have examined changes in monoamine and amino acid levels in migraine subjects in and out of an attack. Blood and urine, and to a lesser extent cerebrospinal fluid (CSF), have been used as the available peripheral sources.

Glutamate is the main excitatory neurotransmitter in the brain and γ-aminobutyric acid (GABA) the main inhibitory one. They are both in high concentrations in the cerebral cortex. Welch and co-workers (1) have suggested that patients who suffer from migraine with aura have a susceptibility to spontaneous neuronal discharge and subsequent spreading depression. This is based on release of the glutamate and supersensitivity of one of its receptors, the N-methyl-D-aspartate (NMDA) receptor. Nerve cells release nitric oxide in response to activation of the NMDA subtype of glutamate receptors (2).

Three independent studies have shown that glutamate levels in the blood are raised in subjects with migraine (Table 1). Two of these studies went on to examine levels during an attack, and both found increased levels here also. The study of Ferrari et al. (3) examined 23 different amino acids and found significant changes only in aspartic acid, glutamic acid (a rise), and aminobutyric acid (a fall). This is good evidence that the changes are reasonably specific to amino acids involved in neurotransmission, and not to amino acids in general. Where the studies disagree is whether the changes are specific to migraine with aura, or occur in other types of migraine also, and whether the changes are in the platelets or the plasma or both. These are problems that recur throughout the migraine literature. They are probably due to the logistical problems of having a study of sufficient power to distinguish changes in the two forms of migraine, and technical problems with separating plasma and platelets, without leakage from the latter. (A further confounding factor in many studies is a failure to exclude co-morbidity with other disorders such as anxiety and depression, which may also involve the same neurotransmitters.)

Few studies have been performed on the inhibitory amino acid GABA in migraine. An early study showed an increase in CSF levels during a migraine attack (4). A more recent one failed to find any differences in platelet levels between migraineurs and controls in between attacks (5).

TABLE 1. *Glutamate, aspartate, glycine, and GABA in migraine*

Between attacks	Headache	Reference
Raised platelet glutamic acid, glycine, and aspartic acid in patients with aura compared with other headache groups and controls	Glutamate further up in migraine with aura	D'Andrea et al. (32)
Migraine without aura, *high* plasma glutamate, normal platelet glutamate; in migraine with aura, glutamate levels were *high* in platelets but not plasma	Not studied	Cananzi et al. (33)
Measured all plasma amino acids in migraine; most normal, glutamic acid *raised* in migraine without aura, and *even more raised* with aura; aspartic acid *raised* in both	Glutamic acid *raised* in attack in both, with and without aura. Aspartic acid also *raised*	Ferrari et al. (3)
GABA measured in CSF in migraine—*undetectable*	*Raised*	Welch et al. (4)
Platelet GABA *same* in controls and migraine	Not studied	Kowa et al. (5)

GABA, γ-aminobutyric acid; CSF, cerebrospinal fluid.

There is no consensus as to what happens to peripheral levels of catecholamines and their metabolites in migraine (Table 2). One well-designed early study showed that in people waking with nocturnal migraine there was an increase in plasma noradrenaline in the period immediately before the attack (6). This would fit with the hypothesis that increased arousal or stress triggers the attack. Two more recent studies have found either no change or decreases in catecholamines and their metabolites in the attack phase. In general, no convincing differences in these parameters have been found between attacks (7–9).

Much of the work and the most convincing evidence concern changes in levels of serotonin (5-HT) in migraine. The platelet forms a reasonable model of the serotonergic nerve ending, with 5-HT present in storage granules, a specific uptake system, $5-HT_2$ receptors on the surface, and monoamine oxidase B present in the mitochondria; there is no other peripheral equivalent for other neurotransmitters. Thus it is easier to study peripheral 5-HT changes than those of other neurotransmitters, and this may contribute to the positive findings.

There is repeated evidence, from many studies, that 5-HT is released from the platelets of many, although not all, subjects during a migraine attack (10–16). It is less clear whether this occurs in all forms of migraine or only migraine without aura. Ferrari et al. (16) have claimed that the finding is specific to migraine without aura,

TABLE 2. *Catecholamines and metabolites in migraine*

Between attacks	Headache	Reference
Not studied	Plasma noradrenaline significantly *higher* in the 3 hr before subjects awoke with migraine	Hsu et al. (6)
24-hr urinary levels of total catecholamines, VMA, HMPG, and HVA compared with controls; only difference was *increase* in HVA in migraine	Not studied	Rao and Rao (7)
24-hr urinary levels of noradrenaline, adrenaline, dopamine, VMA, DOPAC, and HVA; only difference was *lower* dopamine in migraine	Urinary *decrease* in noradrenaline, adrenaline, and HVA	Ferrari and Odink (8)
Not studied	Adrenaline and noradrenaline in CSF and plasma compared with stressed controls; only difference was *lower* plasma noradrenaline in common migraineurs	Martinez et al. (9)

VMA, vanillylmandelic acid; HMPG, hydroxymethoxyphenylglycol; HVA, homovanillic acid; DOPAC, dihydrophenylacetic acid; CSF, cerebrospinal fluid.

but their number of migraines with aura subjects was small (n = 10), and their findings may have been subject to a type 11 error.

Ribeiro et al. (17) have shown that *serum* 5-HT rises over twofold in the first 3 hours of a migraine attack and that the effect is similar in both migraine with aura and migraine without aura. At first sight, this would be compatible with a release of 5-HT from platelets. However, as blood clots to make serum, the platelets release their 5-HT, and one would therefore expect the results with serum, whole blood, and platelets to be similar. The reason for the different findings in this study is unclear.

Several studies have also looked at urinary and plasma 5-hydroxyindoleacetic acid (5-HIAA) in migraine subjects both during and between attacks. Some have found increased excretion during an attack (8,10). Indeed, the study by Sicuteri et al. (18) in 1961 was one of the seminal papers that started investigation of the links between 5-HT and migraine. Others have failed to find such an increase (19). There are technical problems with examining urine, especially spot urines, as there is no adequate way to control for variation in volume. This can be overcome by examining 24-hour urines, but this may mask a more transient increase in output. It should also be noted that only a small proportion of an acute increase in urinary 5-HIAA is likely to come from the platelets, as they contain less than 10% of the body stores.

5-HT is predominantly metabolized by monoamine oxidase to 5-HIAA. However, when monoamine oxidase is inhibited, peripheral (urinary and blood) levels of 5-HIAA are little changed (20). [This is also true of the acids derived from tyramine and phenylethylamine parahydroxyphenyl acetic acid and phenylacetic acid (20).] This suggests that most of this 5-HIAA is not derived directly from endogenous 5-HT; it is not yet known what its source is. Thus interictal measurement of 5-HIAA is unlikely to reflect endogenous 5-HT metabolism, although increases during an attack may well be due to an increased release of the monoamine.

There is good evidence that the release of 5-HT can trigger headache. Reserpine (21), fenfluramine (22, and unpublished observations), or red wine (23) triggers a migraine attack in some but not all migraineurs. There is also evidence that intravenous injection of 5-HT itself or its precursors, tryptophan or 5-hydroxytryptophan, can abort or prevent an attack (24). All this provides a strong case for the involvement of 5-HT in the cause of migraine. However, it is not yet clear whether a release of 5-HT is a necessary, as opposed to a sufficient, cause of migraine.

It also remains unclear whether the release of 5-HT in a spontaneous migraine attack needs to be central, peripheral, or either. Lance (25) has described how hypothalamic symptoms are described by about 25% of patients. Recent studies using fenfluramine as a challenging agent have shown that it induces headache with associated migrainous symptoms in about half of the migraine subjects challenged with it, and a typical migraine attack in most but not all of these (unpublished observations) (Table 3). The induction of migrainous headache correlated very highly with the release of prolactin into the plasma (Table 4). This suggests an action via a central, hypothalamic release of 5-HT, as opposed to a peripheral one. Red wine can also induce migraine in susceptible subjects (23), and it too causes a release of 5-HT from platelets (26) and endogenous stores. However, with red wine-induced migraine there was no concomitant increase in plasma prolactin (unpublished observations), suggesting that it is possible to trigger a migraine attack without such a hypothalamic release.

Studies using positron emission tomography scanning during a spontaneous migraine attack have shown central activity in a region that includes the raphe nucleus (27). It may be that most spontaneous attacks are driven centrally, but triggering agents can act peripherally.

Fozard (28) has suggested that the release of 5-HT activates $5\text{-HT}_{2b/2c}$ receptors and that this in turn causes the cerebral vasculature to release nitric oxide. As glutamate acting on its NMDA receptors can also cause a release of nitric oxide, this

TABLE 3. *Fenfluramine-induced headache*

Treatment	Headaches with associated migrainous symptoms (no.)	Typical migraine (no.)
Fenfluramine (n=11)	6	4
Placebo (n=9)	1*	0

*$\chi^2=21$; $p=0.0000$.

TABLE 4. *Characteristics of migraines induced by different agents*

Agent	Action	Reference
Fenfluramine		
Time of onset	Starts within 2 hr	Unpublished observations
Peak	2–4 hr	
Correlation with plasma prolactin	0.85*	
Red wine		
Time of onset	Starts within 3 hr	Littlewood et al. (23)
Peak	3–6 hr	
Correlation with plasma prolactin	None	
m-CPP		
Time of onset	Starts after 5 hr	
Peak	5–8 hr	Gordon et al. (31)
	8–12 hr	Brewerton et al. (30)
Correlation with plasma prolactin	None	Gordon et al. (31)

*$p=0.0006$.
m-CPP, m-chlorophenylpiperazine.

could provide a final common pathway. Indeed, nitric oxide has been suggested as a key molecule in the initiation of migraine (29). However, this hypothesis does not explain why a fenfluramine-induced migraine starts within 2 hours and peaks within 4 hours, whereas an m-chlorophenylpiperazine (m-CPP)-induced migraine takes at least 5 hours to start and peaks after 5 to 12 hours (30,31) (Table 4). As m-CPP acts directly on $5\text{-HT}_{2b/2c}$ receptors, one would expect that it would induce an attack more rapidly than fenfluramine, and this remains a puzzle. It is possible that the *depletion* of 5-HT is of primary importance in the generation of a migraine attack, rather than its action on a specific receptor.

REFERENCES

1. Welch KM, Barkely GL, Ramadan NM, D'Andrea G. NMR spectroscopic and magnetoencephalographic studies in migraine with aura: support for the spreading depression hypothesis. *Pathol Biol (Paris)* 1992;40:394–454.
2. Fabricius M, Akgoren N, Lauitzen M. Arginine-nitric oxide pathway and cerebrovascular regulation in cortical spreading depression. *Am J Physiol* 1995;269:H23–29.
3. Ferrari MD, Odink J, Malessy MJA, Bruyn GW. Neuroexcitatory plasma amino acids are elevated in migraine. *Neurology* 1990;40:1582–1586.
4. Welch KM, Chabi E, Bartosh K, Achar VS, Meyer JS. Cerebrospinal fluid and gamma aminobutyric acid levels in migraine. *BMJ* 1975;3:516–517.
5. Kowa H, Shimomura T, Takahashi K. Platelet gamma-aminobutyric acid levels in migraine and tension-type headache. *Headache* 1992;32:229–232.
6. Hsu LKG, Crisp AH, Kalucy RS, et al. Early morning migraine. *Lancet* 1977:447–450.
7. Rao A, Rao SN. Urinary excretion of biogenic amine metabolites in migraine. *Biochem Arch* 1988;4:141–144.
8. Ferrari MD, Odink J. Urinary excretion of biogenic amines in migraine and tension headache. In: Clifford Rose F, ed. *New advances in headache research.* 1989;85–88.
9. Martinez F, Castillo J, Pardo J, Lema M, Noya M. Catecholamine levels in plasma and CSF in migraine. *J Neurol Neurosurg Psychiatry* 1993;56:1119–1121.
10. Curran DA, Hinterberger H, Lance JW. Total plasma serotonin, 5-hydroxyindoleacetic acid and p-hydroxy-m-methoxymandelic acid excretion in normal and migrainous subjects. *Brain* 1965;88:997–1010.

11. Anthony M, Hinterberger HJ, Lance JW. Plasma serotonin in migraine and stress. *Arch Neurol* 1967; 16:544–552.
12. Anthony M. The mechanisms underlying migraine. *Med J Aust* 1972;2[suppl]:11–15.
13. Hilton BP. 5-Hydroxytryptamine levels and platelet aggregation responses in subjects with acute migraine headache. *J Neurol Neurosurg Psychiatry* 1972;35:505–509.
14. Somerville BM. Platelet bound and free serotonin in jugular and forearm venous blood during migraine. *Neurology* 1976;26:41–45.
15. D'Andrea G, Toldo M, Cortelazzo S, Milone FF. Platelet activity in migraine. *Headache* 1982;22: 207–212.
16. Ferrari MD, Odink J, Tapparelli C, Van Kempen GMJ, Pennings EJM, Bruyn GW. Serotonin metabolism in migraine. *Neurology* 1989;39:1239–1242.
17. Ribeiro CA, Cotrim MD, Morgadino MT, Ramos MI, Santos ES, de Macedo T. Migraine, serum serotonin, and platelet 5-HT2 receptors. *Cephalalgia* 1990;10:213–219.
18. Sicuteri F, Test A, Anselmi B. Biochemical investigations in headache: increase in hydroxyindoleacetic acid excretion during migraine attacks. *Int Arch Allergy* 1961;19:55–58.
19. Curzon G, Theaker P, Phillips B. Excretion of 5-hydroxyindoleacetic acid (5-HIAA) in migraine. *J Neurol Neurosurg Psychiatry* 1966;29:85–90.
20. McKenna KF, Baker GB, Coutts RT. Urinary excretion of biogenic amines and their metabolites in psychiatric patients receiving phenelzine. *Neurochem Res* 1993;18:1023–1027.
21. Curzon G, Barrie M, Wilkinson MIP. Relationships between headache and amine changes after administration of reserpine to migrainous patients. *J Neurol Neurosurg Psychiatry* 1969;32:555–561.
22. Del Bene E, Anselmi B, Del Bianco PL, et al. Fenfluramine headache: a biochemical and monoamine receptorial human study. In: Sicuteri F, ed. *Headache: new vistas*. Florence: Biomedical Press, 1977; 101–109.
23. Littlewood JT, Gibb C, Glover V, Sandler M, Davies PTG, Clifford Rose F. Red wine as a cause of migraine. *Lancet* 1988;i:558–559.
24. Kimball RW, Friedman AP, Vallejo E. Effect of serotonin in migraine patients. *Neurology* 1969; 10:107.
25. Lance JW. The pathophysiology of migraine: a tentative hypothesis. *Pathol Biol* 1992;40:355–360.
26. Pattichis K, Jarman J, Glover V, Sandler M, Aislaitner G, Gorrod JW. Red wine as a migraine trigger: examination of its effects on ^{14}C-5-hydroxytryptamine release from platelets. In: Olesen J, Saxena PR, eds. *5–Hydroxytryptamine mechanisms in primary headaches*. Philadelphia: Lippincott–Raven, 1992;242–246.
27. Weller C, May A, Limmroth V, et al. Brain stem activation in spontaneous human migraine attacks. *Nature Med* 1995;1:658–660.
28. Fozard JR. The 5-hydroxytryptamine-nitric oxide connection: the key link in the initiation of migraine. *Arch Int Pharmacodyn* 1995;329:111–119.
29. Olesen J, Lykke Thomsen LL, Iversen H. Nitric oxide is a key molecule in migraine and other vascular headaches. *TIPS* 1994;15:149–153.
30. Brewerton TD, Murphy DL, Mueller A, Jimerson DC. Frequency of migraine-like headaches by the serotonin agonist m-chlorophenylpiperazine. *Clin Pharmacol Ther* 1988;43:605–609.
31. Gordon ML, Lipton RB, Brown S-L, et al. Headache and cortisol responses to m-chlorophenylpiperazine are highly correlated. *Cephalalgia* 1993;13:400–405.
32. D'Andrea G, Cananzi AR, Joseph R, et al. Platelet glycine, glutamate and aspartate in primary headache. *Cephalalgia* 1991;11:197–200.
33. Cananzi AR, D'Andrea G, Perini F, Zamberlan F, Welch KM. Platelet and plasma levels of glutamate and glutamine in migraine with and without aura. *Cephalalgia* 1995;15:132–135.

18

Amines, Purines, and Amino Acids in Tension-Type Headache and Cluster Headache

László Vécsei, János Tajti, and Délia Szok

Department of Neurology, Szent-Györgyi University Medical School, Szeged 6725, Hungary

TENSION-TYPE HEADACHE

In the International Headache Classification, tension-type headache (TTH) was included without indications of specific pathophysiological mechanisms (1). Epidemiological study provides strong support for the pathogenic importance of peripheral muscular factors in TTH. Secondary changes in the central pain-modulating system may be involved when a chronic form of the disease develops (2). Disturbances in peripheral (myofascial) tissue and defective function of antinociceptive systems have also been suggested as possible mechanisms.

Serotonin

Ferrari (3) recently summarized the biochemistry of TTH. In earlier studies two groups found reduced levels of platelet serotonin (5-HT) (4,5), whereas two other studies did not (6,7). The different methodologies used in these investigations make a comparison of results difficult. Shimomura et al. (8) reported that under stress the absorbance of 5-HT into the platelets in patients with TTH is reduced. It has been suggested that, in patients with TTH, abnormalities of 5-HT uptake into platelets and factors exist that cause release of 5-HT from platelets. Furthermore, it was reported that during headaches a desensitization phenomenon takes place, with complete loss of high-affinity binding sites for 5-HT to lymphocytes and monocytes (9). Recent studies suggest the participation of 5-HT and substance P in the development of migraine and TTH as well (10). The platelet-rich plasma 5-HT fluctuations observed in TTH are related more to the pathogenic mechanisms of headache than to those of depression (11). Marazziti and coworkers (12) reported similar biochemical abnormalities in patients with "migraine without aura" and TTH and suggested that, at least for platelet markers, a continuum exists between these two forms of primary headache. Jensen and Hindberg (13) performed controlled studies of 5-HT in platelet-poor plasma during and between episodes of TTH. The 5-HT concentration in patients free of headaches was not different from controls, whereas an increase in 5-HT was observed during headaches. This finding is attributed to the release of 5-HT from platelets or disordered 5-HT metabolism during headache attacks. However, D'Andrea et al. (14) reported that the increased platelet 5-HT secretion may be due to substantially increased basal platelet 5-HT levels, which in turn may be related to increased platelet 5-HT uptake. Apart from differences in methodology, these studies also differ with regard to clinical selection criteria and timing of blood sampling, rendering a comparison difficult. The salivary substance P and 5-HT levels in patients with TTH during active headache periods were higher than those in healthy controls (15). These data suggest that substance P is released from afferent fibers of trigeminal nerves and is secreted from the salivary gland. With the abnormalities in 5-HT uptake by platelets and in factors that cause release of 5-HT from platelets, 5-HT was released into saliva (Table 1).

Drugs Influencing the 5-HT System

Nappi et al. (16) demonstrated that ritanserin, a highly selective and long-acting antagonist of 5-HT_2 receptors, shows high efficacy in the treatment of chronic headache with depression. The 5-HT_{1D}-like receptor agonist sumatriptan was more effective than a placebo in the treatment of chronic TTH (17), but the drug has no clinically relevant effect in the treatment of episodic TTH (18). It was suggested that antidepressant drugs (fluvoxamine and mianserine) can induce or potentiate analgesia by direct action on the central nervous system, probably by blocking 5-HT reuptake and therefore enhancing the action of 5-HT at the central terminals of the opioid-mediated intrinsic analgesia systems (19). The modest overall improvement for paroxetine (a 5-HT reuptake inhibitor) and sulpiride (a dopamine antagonist) indicates that neither of the two approaches is ideal for the treatment of chronic TTH (20) (Table 2).

Catecholamines and Amino Acids

Gallai et al. (21) suggested that a sympathetic hypofunction exists in patients suffering from TTH and migraine even during headache-free intervals. However, no significant variations of neuropeptide Y (co-stored and co-secreted with norepinephrine) concentrations were observed between headache-free periods and attacks in TTH patients (22), but plasma catecholamine (epinephrine, norepinephrine, and dopamine) levels were lower in patients than in controls (23). Ferrari et al. (24) investigated plasma concentrations of amino acids in migraine patients using TTH and

TABLE 1. *Serotonin in tension-type headache*

Results with TTH patients	Sample	Reference
Decreased platelet 5-HT concentration	Platelet	Anthony and Lance (4); Rolf et al. (5)
Normal platelet 5-HT concentration	Platelet	Ferrari et al. (6); Shukla et al. (7)
Before cold stimulation, 5-HT contents in platelets of TTH patients were lower than those found in controls; 1 minute after the start of cold stimulation, control levels of 5-HT rose, and TTH levels fell	Platelet	Shimomura and Takahashi (8)
Impairment of 5-HT binding to lymphocytes and monocytes in TTH	Lymphocytes, monocytes	Giacovazzo et al. (9)
Concentration of platelet 5-HT was lower and SP/5-HT ratio higher than in controls	Platelet	Nakano et al. (10)
PRP 5-HT levels were higher in TTH than in controls; a decrease in PRP 5-HT was observed in patients with TTH to similar levels after treatment with amitryptiline as the depressed group	PRP	Leira et al. (11)
Migraine and TTH patient groups exhibited a lower number of ^{3}H-imipramine binding sites and lower activity of the thermolabile form of sulphontransferase	Platelet	Marazziti et al. (12)
Plasma 5-HT increased during episodes of TTH; 5-HT concentration in patients free of headache did not differ from controls	Plasma (PPP)	Jensen and Hindberg (13)
Platelet 5-HT content increased, and hypersecretion was present from dense and alpha-granules *in vitro*	Platelet	D'Andrea et al. (14)
SP and 5-HT levels during active headache periods are higher	Saliva	Marukawa et al. (15)

TTH, tension-type headache; 5-HT, serotonin; SP, substance P; PRP, platelet-rich plasma; PPP, platelet-poor plasma.

healthy normal individual controls. Glutamic acid and aspartic acid were elevated in migraine headaches, but no abnormalities could be demonstrated in TTH. D'Andrea et al. (25) studied platelet glycine, glutamic acid, and aspartic acid in primary headaches. High levels of these amino acids were found in patients with migraines with aura compared with normal subjects and other headache groups (including TTH). Taken together, these data suggest indirectly that there is glutamate release during migraine headaches, but not during TTH. However, flupirtine (partly an N-methyl-D-aspartate antagonist) is effective and safe in the treatment of chronic TTH (26). Furthermore, it was suggested that glutamate plays a role in headaches related to cerebrovascular disease (27) (Table 3).

TABLE 2. *Drugs influencing the serotonin system in tension-type headache*

Results with TTH patients	Patients	Reference
Antiheadache and antidepressive properties of ritanserine (a 5-HT$_2$ antagonist) were proved	Chronic headache with depression	Nappi et al. (16)
Sumatriptan (5-HT$_{1D}$-like agonist) has a significant effect in chronic TTH	Chronic TTH	Brennum et al. (17)
Sumatriptan (50HT$_{1D}$-like agonist) has no clinically relevant effect in episodic TTH	Episodic TTH	Brennum et al. (18)
The therapeutic activity of fluvoxamine (specific 5-HT reuptake inhibitor) and mianserine unrelated to direct antidepressant activity	Chronic TTH	Manna et al. (19)
Neither paroxetine (5-HT reuptake inhibitor) nor sulpiride (dopamine agonist) improved headache more than one score-point on average	Chronic TTH	Langemark and Olesen (20)

TTH, tension-type headache; 5-HT, serotonin.

CLUSTER HEADACHE

Cluster headache (CH) falls into group 3 of the International Headache Society classification (CH and chronic paroxysmal hemicrania) and is coded 3.1.

Histamine and Serotonin

Bogucki (28) studied nitroglycerine- and histamine-provoked CH attacks. The constant latency time in individual patients during nitroglycerine and histamine provocation suggested that the same mechanism is involved in both methods of headache induction. Aubineau and co-workers (29) investigated whether 5-HT and histamine were released in the vicinity of the superficial temporal artery (STA) during CH attacks (using the microdialysis method). No histamine was detected in any sample from any patient during or outside attacks. The large amounts of 5-HT in the vicinity of the STA noted during CH attacks are probably due to local release. The origin of this release needs to be identified, but its time course indicates a rapid activation-inactivation cycle of secretory cells. These results indicate that 5-HT is probably involved, at a local level, in the pathogenesis of CH (29). Mathiau et al. (30) found that 5-HT induced classic dose-dependent constriction in arteries from non-CH patients but systematically triggered rhythmic contractions in arteries from episodic CH patients. Furthermore, clinical findings with sumatriptan stress the involvement of 5-HT in CH mechanisms (31,32).

TABLE 3. *Catecholamines and amino acids in tension-type headache*

Results with TTH patients	Patient/sample	Reference
Serum DBH activity significantly lower in TTH (and migraine) patients than in the control group (due to sympathetic hypoactivity)	TTH, migraine/serum	Gallai et al. (21)
Lower plasma levels of NPY observed in young migraine patients with aura; no significant reduction in young TTH patients	TTH, migraine/plasma	Gallai et al. (22)
Plasma catecholamine levels lower in patients than in controls	TTH/plasma	Castillo et al. (23)
Glutamic acid and aspartic acid elevated during migraines but not during TTH	Migraine, TTH/plasma	Ferrari et al. (24)
High levels of glutamate, aspartate, and glycine found in patients with migraines with aura compared with normal subjects and other headache groups (TTH); platelet glycine levels in TTH patients lower than in the control group	TTH, migraine/platelet	D'Andrea et al. (25)
Flupirtine effective and safe in the treatment of chronic TTH	Chronic TTH	Wörz et al. (26)
Glutamate in CSF higher in patients with headaches than in patients without headache	Cerebrovascular ischemic disease/ plasma, CSF	Castillo et al. (27)

TTH, tension-type headache; DBH, dopamine-β-hydroxylase; NPY, neuropeptide Y; CSF, cerebrospinal fluid.

Catecholamines and Amino Acids

CH sufferers had lower platelet levels of norepinephrine and epinephrine in all phases of the syndrome. Tyrosine levels were increased during CH attacks. These results provide biochemical evidence of sympathetic nervous system hypofunction in CH (33). In observing cortisol and adrenocorticotropic hormone changes on the insulin tolerance test, it was found that in both remission and cluster period patients these responses were reduced; a reduced norepinephrine increase was also noted in the cluster period (34). According to Drummond (35), the central sympathergic drive is not impaired in CH patients; thus a peripheral lesion probably induces a sympathetic deficit on the symptomatic side of the face. Recent results confirm the hypothesis that chronic CH patients have changed vascular reactivity due to permanent sympathicoplegia unilaterally in the middle fossa, in contrast to episodic CH patients who may exhibit nonpermanent sympathicoplegia unilaterally in the same region (36) (Table 4). Platelet glycine levels were higher in migraine with aura sufferers than in normal subjects, but levels in CH, TTH, and migraine without aura pa-

TABLE 4. *Amines and amino acids in cluster headache*

Results with CH patients	Patient/sample	Reference
Nitroglycerin and histamine provoked CH attacks (the underlying mechanism of both is at least partially the same)	CH	Bogucki (28)
Release of 5-HT only in painful area during CH attacks	CH (microdialysis)	Aubineau et al. (29)
5-HT systematically triggered rhythmic contractions in arteries from episodic CH patients	CH (superficial temporal arteries)	Mathiau et al. (30)
Findings using sumatriptan stress the involvement of 5-HT in CH mechanisms	CH/plasma	Sumatripan Cluster Headache Study Group (31)
Secondary CH (injury to the vertebral artery) responsive to sumatriptan	CH	Cremer et al. (32)
CH sufferers had lower platelet levels of norepinephrine and epinephrine	CH/platelet	D'Andrea et al. (33)
Reduced norepinephrine surge in the cluster period	CH/serum	Leone et al. (34)
The sympathetic deficit in CH is unlikely to be of central origin and is not a primary source of pain	CH	Drummond (35)
Chronic CH patients have changed vascular reactivity due to permanent sympathicoplegia; episodic CH patients have nonpermanent sympathicoplegia	CH	Hannerz and Jogestrand (36)
Platelet glycine levels in the CH patient group lower than normal	CH/platelet	D'Andrea et al. (25)

CH, cluster headache; 5-HT, serotonin.

tient groups were lower than normal. During headaches, platelet aspartic acid and glycine levels did not change from interictal values in any headache group (CH, TTH, or migraine) (25). However, it is known that excitatory amino acids play an important role in the pathogenesis of several neurological disorders (37).

Adenosine Receptors

The adenosine A3 receptor facilitates degranulation of mast cells (38), while the A1 receptor potentiates histamine H_1 receptor responses (39). Thus, adenosine-provoked pain is probably mediated by histamine, a known precipitating factor of CH. Adenosine-receptor antagonist purines counteract adenosine-provoked pain (40).

REFERENCES

1. Headache Classification Committee of the International Headache Society (Olesen J, et al.). Classification and diagnostic criteria for headache disorders, cranial neuralgias and facial pain. *Cephalagia* 1988; 8[Suppl 7]:1–96.
2. Jensen R. Pathogenic importance of muscular disorders in tension-type headache. *Funct Neurol* 1994;9:175–182.
3. Ferrari MD. Biochemistry of tension-type headache. In: Olesen J, Schoenen J, eds. *Tension-type headache: classification, mechanisms, and treatment*. Philadelphia: Lippincott–Raven, 1993;115–126.
4. Anthony M, Lance JW. Platelet serotonin in patients with chronic tension headaches. *J Neurol Neurosurg Psychiatry* 1989;52:182–184.
5. Rolf LH, Wiele G, Brune GG. 5-Hydroxytryptamine in platelets of patients with muscle contraction headache. *Headache* 1981;21:10–11.
6. Ferrari MD, Odink J, Tapparelli C, Van Kempen GMJ, Pennings EJM, Bruyn GW. Serotonin metabolism in migraine. *Neurology* 1989;39:1239–1242.
7. Shukla R, Shanker K, Nag D, Verma M, Bhargava KP. Serotonin in tension headache. *J Neurol Neurosurg Psychiatry* 1987;50:1682–1684.
8. Shimomura T, Takahashi K. Alteration of platelet serotonin in patients with chronic tension-type headache during cold pressure test. *Headache* 1990;30:581–583.
9. Giacovazzo M, Bernoni RM, Di Sabato F, Martelletti P. Impairment of 5-HT binding to lymphocytes and monocytes from tension-type headache patients. *Headache* 1990;30:220–223.
10. Nakano T, Shimomura T, Takahashi K, Ikawa S. Platelet substance P and 5-hydroxytryptamine in migraine and tension-type headache. *Headache* 1993;33:528–532.
11. Leira R, Castillo J, Martinez F, Prieto JM, Noya M. Platelet-rich plasma serotonin levels in tension-type headache and depression. *Cephalalgia* 1993;13:346–348.
12. Marazziti D, Bonuccelli U, Nuti A, et al. Platelet ^{3}H-imipramine binding and sulphotransferase activity in primary headache. *Cephalagia* 1994;14:210–214.
13. Jensen R, Hindberg I. Plasma serotonin increase during episodes of tension-type headache. *Cephalagia* 1994;14:219–222.
14. D'Andrea G, Hasselmark L, Alecci M, Perini F, Welch KMA. Increased platelet serotonin content and hypersecretion from dense and alpha-granules in vitro in tension-type headache. *Cephalalgia* 1993;13:349–353.
15. Marukawa H, Shimomura T, Takahashi K. Salivary substance P, 5-hydroxytryptamine, and gamma-aminobutyric acid levels in migraine and tension-type headache. *Headache* 1996;36:100–104.
16. Nappi G, Sandrini G, Granella F, et al. A new 5-HT2 antagonist (Ritanserin) in the treatment of chronic headache with depression. A double-blind study vs. amitryptiline. *Headache* 1990;30:439–444.
17. Brennum J, Kjeldsen M, Olesen J. The 5-HTl-like agonist sumatriptan has a significant effect in chronic tension-type headache. *Cephalagia* 1992;12:375–379.
18. Brennum J, Brinck T, Schriver L, et al. Sumatriptan has no clinically relevant effect in the treatment of episodic tension-type headache. *Eur J Neurol* 1996;3:23–24.
19. Manna V, Bolino F, Di Cicco L. Chronic tension-type headache, mood depression and serotonin: therapeutic effects of fluvoxamine and mianserine. *Headache* 1994;34:44–49.
20. Langemark M, Olesen J. Sulpiride and paroxetine in the treatment of chronic tension-type headache. An explanatory double-blind trial. *Headache* 1994;34:20–24.
21. Gallai V, Gaiti A, Sarchielli P, Coata G, Trequattrini A, Paciaroni M. Evidence for an altered dopamine-hydroxylase activity in migraine and tension-type headache. *Acta Neurol Scand* 1992;86:403–406.
22. Gallai V, Sarchielli P, Trequattrini A, Paciaroni M, Usai F, Palumbo R. Neuropeptide Y in juvenile migraine and tension-type headache. *Headache* 1994;34:35–40.
23. Castillo J, Martínez F, Leira R, Lema M, Noya M. Plasma monoamines in tension-type headache. *Headache* 1994;34:531–535.

24. Ferrari MD, Odink J, Bos KD, Malessy MJA, Bruyn GW. Neuroexcitatory plasma amino acids are elevated in migraine. *Neurology* 1990;40:1582–1586.
25. D'Andrea G, Cananzi AR, Joseph R, et al. Platelet glycine, glutamate and aspartate in primary headache. *Cephalalgia* 1991;11:197–200.
26. Wörz R, Lobisch M, Gessler M, et al. Flupirtine versus placebo in chronic tension-type headache. *Headache Q* 1996;7:30–38.
27. Castillo J, Martínez F, Corredera E, Aldrey JM, Noya M. Amino acid transmitters in patients with headache during the acute phase of cerebrovascular ischemic disease. *Stroke* 1995;26:2035–2039.
28. Bogucki A. Studies on nitroglycerin and histamine-provoked cluster headache attacks. *Cephalalgia* 1990;10:71–75.
29. Aubineau P, Cunin G, Brochet B, Louvet-Giendaj C, Henry P. Release of serotonin only in painful area during cluster headache attacks. *Lancet* 1992;339:1294–1295.
30. Mathiau P, Brochet B, Boulan P, Henry P, Aubineau P. Spontaneous and 5-HT induced cyclic contractions in superficial temporal arteries from chronic and episodic cluster headache patients. *Cephalagia* 1994;14:419–429.
31. The Sumatriptan Cluster Headache Study Group (Ekbom K, et al.). Treatment of acute cluster headache with sumatriptan. *N Engl J Med* 1991;325:322–326.
32. Cremer PD, Halmagyi GM, Goadsby PJ. Secondary cluster headache responsive to sumatriptan. *J Neurol Neurosurg Psychiatry* 1995;59:633–634.
33. D'Andrea G, Cananzi AR, Morra M, et al. Platelet catecholamines in cluster headache. *J Neurol Neurosurg Psychiatry* 1992;55:308–309.
34. Leone M, Zappacosta BM, Valentini S, Colangelo AM, Bussone G. The insulin tolerance test and the ovine corticotrophin-releasing hormone test in episodic cluster headache. *Cephalagia* 1991;11:269–274.
35. Drummond PD. The site of sympathetic deficit in cluster headache. *Headache* 1996;36:3–9.
36. Hannerz J, Jogestrand T. Chronic cluster headache: provocation with carbon dioxide breathing and nitroglycerine. *Headache* 1996;36:174–177.
37. Vécsei L, Freese A, Swartz KJ, Beal MF. *Neurological disorders: novel experimental and therapeutic strategies.* Chichester: Horwood, 1992.
38. Linden J. Cloned adenosine A3 receptors: pharmacological properties, species differences and receptor functions. *Trends Pharmacol Sci* 1994;15:298–306.
39. Dickenson JM, Hill SJ. Interactions between adenosine A1- and histamine H1-receptors. *Int J Biochem* 1994;26:959–969.
40. Sylven C. Mechanism of pain in angina pectoris—a critical review of the adenosine hypothesis. *Cardiovasc Drugs Ther* 1993;7:745–759.

19

Effects of Migraine Treatments on Amines and Amino Acid Messenger Molecules

Helen E. Connor

Glaxo-Wellcome Research and Development, Stevenage, Herts SG1 2NY, United Kingdom

There is an extensive literature on the levels of endogenous amines and amino acids during migraine, including 5-hydroxytryptamine (5-HT) (1), noradrenaline (2), glutamate (3), and glycine (4). This topic is reviewed in Chapter 17 by Glover (*this volume*). The purpose of the present review is to focus on changes in levels of these endogenous substances following administration of antimigraine drugs and to consider whether any of these changes may be relevant to antimigraine activity.

ACUTE TREATMENT: SUMATRIPTAN/SEROTONIN RECEPTOR AGONISTS

Sumatriptan is a selective agonist at 5-HT_{1B} and 5-HT_{1D} receptors, and its action in constricting cranial blood vessels and inhibiting trigeminal nerve activity is now well documented (5). Sumatriptan is highly effective in the acute treatment of migraine (6). Other drugs of this class are now being developed and have a similar biological profile of action (e.g., 311C90) (7).

Serotonin and Noradrenaline

Considering first the possibility that $5\text{-HT}_{1B/1D}$ receptor agonists could modify peripheral levels of 5-HT or noradrenaline, no real evidence suggests that this occurs at physiologically relevant doses, although sumatriptan-sensitive prejunctional inhibitory 5-HT_1 receptors have been found on sympathetic nerves in some tissues (e.g., dog saphenous vein) (5). Direct evidence is provided by the lack of effect of sumatriptan (1 μM) on platelet 5-HT levels, on platelet 5-HT uptake, or on reserpine-induced 5-HT release from platelets in migraineurs or nonheadache controls in vitro (8). Indirect evidence comes from the observation that sumatriptan, over a wide dose range, has no effect on arterial blood pressure in anesthetized dogs (9).

Inhibitory $5\text{-HT}_{1B/1D}$ prejunctional receptors occur on both serotonergic and other neurons in the central nervous system (CNS). Hence this provides an alternative mechanism by which 5-HT$_{1B/1D}$ agonists could modify endogenous amine (or amino acid) levels. However, to have such an effect, drugs would need to gain access to these central sites. The possibility that sumatriptan could modify brain extracellular levels of 5-HT was investigated in the frontal cortex of anesthetized guinea pigs using intracerebral dialysis (10). Sumatriptan (10 to 100 nM), infused directly into the brain via the dialysis loop, dose-dependently reduced extracellular levels of 5-HT. This effect is probably due to stimulation of 5-HT terminal and/or somatodentritic autoreceptors. However, when administered peripherally, even at relatively high doses (up to 0.5 mg/kg i.p.), sumatriptan had no effect on extracellular 5-HT levels (10). This finding suggests that sumatriptan only poorly penetrates the CNS and, after peripheral administration, cannot gain access to these central sites to a sufficient degree to have an effect.

Some 5-HT$_{1B/1D}$ receptor agonists in development are more lipophilic than sumatriptan and may therefore more readily gain access to central sites. Indeed, after peripheral administration of [^{3}H]311C90 to anesthetized cats, binding of labeled drug was demonstrated in the hindbrain and spinal cord (trigeminal nucleus caudalis, dorsal horn) using an ex vivo autoradiography technique (11). Although the receptor subtype(s) involved was not determined, these data demonstrate that 311C90 can reach central sites, and it has been postulated that this action may provide additional benefit in the treatment of migraine (12).

An area of brain stem activation, which may coincide with the anatomical location of the dorsal raphe nucleus (DRN), has recently been found to occur during spontaneous migraine attacks (13). However, sumatriptan (6 mg s.c.) had no effect on this area of brain stem activation (13). Interestingly, experiments in guinea pig DRN slices suggest that functional 5-HT$_{1B/1D}$ autoreceptors are present in this brain region: electrical stimulation-evoked release of 5-HT was measured by fast cyclic voltametry, and sumatriptan inhibited 5-HT release with 50% inhibition at 40 nM. This effect of sumatriptan was inhibited by the selective 5-HT$_{1B/1D}$ antagonist GR127935 (14). Such receptors may regulate the amount of neuronally released 5-HT in the dorsal raphe nucleus and may decrease the firing rate of serotonergic neurons projecting from the DRN region.

The effect of sumatriptan on brain monoamines has been investigated by Mitsikostas et al. (15) in rats. Sumatriptan, at a dose of 0.6 mg/kg s.c., decreased levels of 5-HT and increased the ratio of 5-hydroxyindoleacetic acid (5-HIAA)/5-HT and dihydrophenylacetic acid (DOPAC)/dopamine in some brain regions (hypothalamus and striatum) with no effect in other regions (frontal cortex). These data are indicative of increased turnover and/or metabolism of 5-HT and dopamine in certain brain regions, but the mechanism of this effect was not established. Such a change is opposite to what might be expected if sumatriptan was acting at central inhibitory 5-HT$_{1B/1D}$ autoreceptors to inhibit release. Sumatriptan 0.6 mg/kg s.c. is a high dose relative to clinical doses for migraine, and using higher or lower doses, no dose-response relationship was found (15). Hence this central effect of sumatriptan seems unlikely to be relevant to its antimigraine activity.

Excitatory and Inhibitory Amino Acids

No data are available to show whether changes in either excitatory or inhibitory amino acid levels are modified by sumatriptan/other 5-HT$_{1B/1D}$ agonists in vivo, although in vitro studies indicate that 5-HT$_{1B/1D}$ inhibitory receptors are present on glutaminergic and γ-aminobutyric acid (GABA)-ergic neurons (16,17). Again, because of poor CNS penetration, this is likely to be of little relevance to the clinical activity of sumatriptan.

PROPHYLACTIC DRUGS: SODIUM VALPROATE

Sodium valproate/valproic acid (valproate) has been shown in several double-blind placebo-controlled trials to have efficacy in the prophylactic treatment of migraine. This has recently been reviewed by Silberstein (18). Valproate causes a reduction in the number of attacks. Migraine duration and intensity is also reduced in some trials. Despite the extensive use of valproate as an anticonvulsant drug for many years, a conclusive mode of action has not been defined. Similarly, the mechanism by which valproate has benefit in the treatment of migraine is not known.

γ-Aminobutyric Acid

Many animal studies show that valproate increases concentrations of the inhibitory amino acid neurotransmitter GABA in whole brain, discrete brain regions, and synaptosomes (19,20). It has been suggested that GABA elevation in response to valproate is primarily due to enhancement of GABA synthesis, and this would explain why valproate is more effective at increasing GABA in nerve terminals rather than in whole brain (19,20). However, conversely, valproate-induced reductions in extracellular GABA in brain have also been described and attributed to enhanced GABA-ergic transmission leading, via a negative feedback, to presynaptic suppression of release (21). One possible mechanism of action of valproate in migraine is therefore to increase GABA-ergic transmission in specific brain regions and thus to counter neuronal hyperexcitability (22), which has been suggested to predispose to migraine (23). It seems unlikely that valproate-induced GABA-ergic transmission blocks cortical spreading depression, which is possibly involved in the initiation of a migraine attack, since valproate was recently shown to be without effect on cortical spreading depression evoked in anesthetized cats (24).

With regard to anticonvulsant activity, it is difficult to explain the whole spectrum of activity of valproate in terms of GABA-ergic mechanisms, and hence other potential biological actions have been investigated. Unlike epilepsy, in which seizure models in animals are relatively well established, it is much more difficult to model migraine in animals in order to correlate biological activity with disease benefit. However, studies investigating effects of valproate on other neurotransmitter systems may well have relevance to the prophylactic activity of this drug in migraine patients.

Excitatory Amino Acids

Valproate has been reported to reduce levels of certain excitatory amino acids in brain (e.g., aspartate) (20), although little effect on glutamate levels has been found (19,20). Thus decreased excitatory neurotransmission in the brain could underlie the activity of this drug in migraine. No changes in plasma levels of amino acids (including aspartate) were found in rats after valproate treatment (20).

Serotonin, Noradrenaline, and Dopamine

In addition to effects on brain amino acid levels, valproate can also modify levels of 5-HT, noradrenaline, and dopamine in specific brain regions. For example, in rats in which brain extracellular levels of 5-HT and dopamine were measured using microdialysis, valproate caused a significant, dose-dependent elevation of 5-HT in hippocampus and caudate putamen (25). Levels of dopamine were also increased. In ventral hippocampus, levels of both neurotransmitters were only transiently increased after valproate administration, but in anterior caudate putamen, a sustained increase in 5-HT levels above basal occurred (25). The increase in levels of 5-HT and dopamine is thought to reflect increased release of 5-HT and dopamine. Another study looking at levels in brain tissue after chronic administration of valproate to rats showed increased 5-HT levels in some brain regions (e.g., 80% increase in the brain stem) and decreases in other regions (21% decrease in hypothalamus) (26). Differential changes in brain levels of noradrenaline and dopamine were also found (26). Increased levels of 5-HIAA (the major metabolite of 5-HT) are found in the cerebrospinal fluid (CSF) of animals and humans after valproate (27,28); this could reflect increased neuronal synthesis and/or metabolism of 5-HT, or interference by valproate with transport of 5-HIAA out of the CSF (27). However, taken together, the data point to valproate increasing 5-HT function in the brain. Changes in 5-HT neuronal pathways have been proposed as a putative pathological deficit underlying migraine, and hence it is possible that valproate could act to normalize and restore this deficit (1).

Valproate: Summary

It is clear from the data given above that the effects of valproate on endogenous levels of amines and amino acids in brain are complex and sometimes contradictory. Most data are derived from animal experiments rather than human studies and can therefore involve the use of high doses, which are not clinically relevant. Some animal studies have used acute rather than chronic dosing and may thus report changes that are not relevant to long-term use, in which up- or downregulation of neurotransmitter systems may occur. Since valproate is a prophylactic treatment for migraine, chronic dosing is obviously more relevant for trying to dissect out its mechanism of action in this disease.

NEW ANTICONVULSANT DRUGS AS ANTIMIGRAINE TREATMENTS

Several of the new antimigraine drugs, such as lamotrigine, gabapentin, and vigabatrin, are being evaluated for efficacy in the prophylactic treatment of migraine: in a double-blind placebo-controlled trial, lamotrigine was found to be ineffective (29), whereas an open-label study with gabapentin showed indications of efficacy (30). These drugs differ from valproate in their biological profile of action (31) and may therefore also differ in their effects on brain levels of neurotransmitter substances. When more extensive clinical data are available for these drugs, it may be possible to correlate efficacy as a migraine prophylactic with a particular biological profile of action and hence draw some conclusions about which mechanism(s) is important.

CONCLUSIONS

The effect of antimigraine drugs on levels of endogenous amines and amino acids is of most relevance to prophylactic treatments: valproate has effects on brain levels of several neurotransmitter substances, including GABA, 5-HT, and noradrenaline, and such changes may be relevant to its clinical efficacy in migraine. For sumatriptan, an acute migraine treatment, the few animal studies to date indicate no direct effect on central amine levels at clinically relevant doses. $5-HT_{1B/1D}$ receptor agonists that have greater CNS penetration could potentially cause changes in central levels of these substances, but no data exist to show this, and whether such an action would have relevance to clinical efficacy is unknown.

To gain a better understanding of changes in amine/amino acid levels that are relevant to the action of antimigraine drugs, more information is needed on changes that occur in the CNS, particularly in humans. Animal studies are hampered by the lack of appropriate models. Whereas data on CSF levels in humans can be generated, it remains debatable how relevant this is to changes that may be going on at a synaptic level in a discrete brain region. Plasma levels are probably even less predictive of discrete neuronal changes. New noninvasive technology offers one approach to gaining more insight into events occurring within the human brain. For example, noninvasive measurements of GABA and glutamate have recently been performed in human occipital lobe using [^{1}H] nuclear magnetic resonance and showed significant increases in GABA and decreases in glutamate following treatment with vigabatrin (33). Measurement of endogenous transmitter levels in migraine patients before and after drug treatment will be a challenge but could provide valuable insight into disease and/or treatment mechanisms.

REFERENCES

1. Ferrari MD, Saxena PR. On serotonin and migraine: a clinical and pharmacological review. *Cephalalgia* 1993;13:151–165.
2. Ferrari MD, Odink J. Urinary excretion of biogenic amines in migraine and tension headache. In: Rose C, ed. *New advances in headache research*. London: Smith-Gordon, 1989;85–88.
3. Ferrari MD, Odink J, Bos KD, Malessy MJA, Bruyn GW. Neuroexcitatory plasma amino acids are elevated in migraine. *Neurology* 1990;40:1582 1586.
4. Rothrock JF, Mar KR, Yaksh TL, Goldbeck A, Moore AC. Cerebral spinal fluid analyses in migraine patients and controls. *Cephalalgia* 1995;16:489–493.
5. Beattie, DT, Connor HE, Feniuk W, Humphrey PPA. The pharmacology of sumatriptan. *Rev Contemp Pharmacother* 1994;5:285–294.
6. Pilgrim A, Blakeborough P. The clinical efficacy of sumatriptan in the acute treatment of migraine. *Rev Contemp Pharmacother* 1994;5:295–309.
7. Martin GR. Pre-clinical profile of the novel 5-HT1D receptor agonist 311C90. In: Rose C, ed. *New advances in headache research*, 4th ed. London: Smith-Gordon, 1994;3–4.
8. Feniuk W, Humphrey PPA, Perren MJ. The selective carotid vasoconstrictor action of sumatriptan in anaesthetised dogs. *Br J Pharmacol* 1989;96:83–90.
9. Anthony M, Regaglia F, Yang M. The effect of sumatriptan on platelets. In: Rose C, ed. *New advances in headache research*, 4th ed. London: Smith-Gordon, 1994;179–182.
10. Sleight AJ, Cervenka A, Peroutka SJ. In vivo effects of sumatriptan (GR43175) on extracellular levels of 5-HT in the guinea-pig. *Neuropharmacology* 1990;29:511–513.
11. Knight YE, Goadsby PJ. Central nervous system distribution of [^{3}H]-311C90 in cat. *Cephalalgia* 1995;15[Suppl 14]:214.
12. Goadsby PJ, Edvinsson L. Peripheral and central trigeminovascular activation in cat is blocked by the serotonin (5-HT)-1D receptor agonist 311C90. *Headache* 1994;7:394–399.
13. Weiller C, May A, Limmroth V, et al. Brain stem activation in spontaneous human migraine attacks. *Nature Med* 1995;1:658–660.
14. Starkey SJ, Skingle M. 5-HT$_{1D}$ as well as 5-HT$_{1A}$ autoreceptors modulate 5-HT release in the guinea-pig dorsal raphe nucleus. *Neuropharmacology* 1994;33:393–402.
15. Mitsikostas DD, Papadopoulou-Daifotis Z, Sfikakis A, Varonos D. The effect of sumatriptan on brain monoamines in rats. *Headache* 1996;36:29–31.
16. Maura G, Raiteri M. Serotonin 5-HT$_{1D}$ and 5-HT$_{1A}$ receptors respectively mediate inhibition of glutamate release and inhibition of cGMP production in rat cerebellum in vitro. *J Neurochem* 1996;66:203–209.
17. Feuerstein TJ, Huring H, Velthoven VV, Lucking CH, Landwehrmeyer GB. 5-HT$_{1D}$-like receptors inhibit the release of endogenously formed [^{3}H]GABA in human, but not rabbit, neocortex. *Neurosci Lett* 1996;209:210–214.
18. Silberstein SD. Divalproex sodium in headache: literature review and clinical guidelines. *Headache* 1996;36:547–555.
19. Biggs CS, Pearce BR, Fowler LJ, Whitton PS. The effect of sodium valproate on extracellular GABA and other amino acids in the rat ventral hippocampus: an in vivo microdialysis study. *Brain Res* 1992; 594:138–142.
20. Loscher W, Hostermann D. Differential effects of vigabatrin, γ-acetylenic GABA, aminooxyacetic acid, and valproate on levels of various amino acids in rat brain regions and plasma. *Naunyn Schmiedebergs Arch Pharmacol* 1994;349:270–278.
21. Wolf R, Tscherne U. Valproate effect on γ-aminobutyric acid release in pars reticulata of substantia nigra: combination of push-pull perfusion and fluorescence histochemistry. *Epilepsia* 1994;35:226–233.
22. Mathew N, Sabhina A. Valproate in the treatment of persistant chronic daily headache. An open label study. *Headache* 1991;31:71–74.
23. Welch KMA, D'Andrea G, Tepley N, Barkley G, Ramadan NM. The concept of migraine as a state of neuronal hyperexcitability. *Neurol Clin* 1990;8:817–828.

24. Kaube H, Goadsby PJ. Anti-migraine compounds fail to modulate the propagation of cortical spreading depression in the cat. *Eur Neurol* 1994;34:30–35.
25. Biggs CS, Pearce BR, Fowler LJ, Whitton PS. Regional effects of sodium valproate on extracellular concentrations of 5-hydroxytryptamine, dopamine and their metabolites in the rat brain: an *in vivo* microdialysis study. *J Neurochem* 1992;59:1702–1708.
26. Baf MHM, Subhash MN, Lakshmana KM, Rao BSSR. Sodium valproate induced alterations in monoamine levels in different regions of the rat brain. *Neurochem Int* 1994;24:67–72.
27. MacMillan V, Leake J, Chung T, Bovell M. The effect of valproic acid on the 5-hydroxyindolacetic, homovanillic and lactic acid levels of cerebrospinal fluid. *Brain Res* 1978;420:268–276.
28. Fahn S. Post-anoxic action myoclonus: improvement with valproic acid. *N Engl J Med* 1978;299:313–314.
29. Steiner TJ, Findley LJ, Yuen AWC. Lamotrigine versus placebo in the prophylaxis of migraine with and without aura. *Cephalalgia* 1997;17:103–108.
30. Mathew N. Gabapentin in migraine prophylaxis. Presentation at 11th Migraine Trust meeting, London 1996.
31. Upton N. Mechanisms of action of new anti-epileptic drugs: rational design and serendipitous findings. *Trends Pharmacol Sci* 1994;15:456–463.
32. Petroff OAC, Rothman DL, Behar KL, Mattson RH. Initial observations on effect of vigabatrin in in vivo ^{1}H spectroscopic measurements of γ-aminobutyric acid, glutamate and glutamine in human brain. *Epilepsia* 1995;36:457–464.

20

Systemic Administration of *m*-Chlorophenylpiperazine Does Not Induce Fos Expression in the Rat Trigeminal Nucleus Caudalis

Renée S. Martin and Graeme R. Martin

Department of Molecular Pharmacology, Roche Bioscience, Center for Biological Research, Palo Alto, California 94304

The observation that several drugs used for migraine prophylaxis are high-affinity antagonists for the 5-hydroxytryptamine (5-HT)$_{2B}$ and 5-HT$_{2C}$ receptor subtypes has led to the hypothesis that these receptors are important in the initiation of attacks (1,2). In support of this theory, the 5-HT$_{2B/2C}$ receptor agonist 1-(*m*-chlorophenylpiperazine) (m-CPP) has been shown both to induce migraine-like headache in migraineurs (3) and to evoke plasma protein extravasation in rat dura mater (Johnson and Nelson, Lilly Research Laboratories, personal communication, 1996).

Intravenous infusion of glyceryl trinitrate has also been found to induce migraine-like headache in migraineurs (4). In addition, histamine has been shown to evoke headache by H$_1$ receptor-mediated stimulation of nitric oxide (NO) synthesis (5). The observation that 5-HT$_{2B/2C}$ receptors in a variety of blood vessels mediate endothelium-dependent vasorelaxation via NO synthesis provides a potential link between 5-HT$_{2B/2C}$ receptor involvement and NO in the induction of migraine headache (6). Messenger RNA (mRNA) for both the endothelial nitric oxide synthase enzyme and the 5-HT$_{2B}$ receptor has been found in mammalian and human cerebral vasculature (7,8).

To investigate whether 5-HT$_{2B/2C}$ receptor activation can lead to excitation of the trigeminovascular system, we have determined the effect of m-CPP on Fos expression in the trigeminal nucleus caudalis (TNC) of anesthetized rats. The dose used, 100 µg·kg^{-1} i.v., is the same as that reported to evoke vascular leakage in rat dura (Johnson and Nelson, personal communication) and is similar to the dose that induces migraine-like headache [0.5 mg·kg^{-1} p.o., reaching a peak plasma concentration of 41.3 ± 28.1 ng·ml^{-1} 2 to 3 hours later (3)]. As the onset of head pain was reported to commence 4 hours after the oral dose, we have investigated a time course of Fos expression at 2, 4, and 6 hours after intravenous injection.

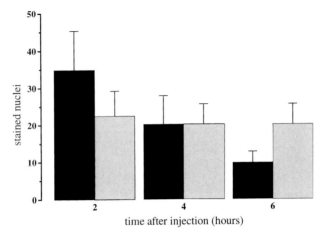

FIG. 1. Time course for the effect of intravenous administration of 100 µg·kg^{-1} m-CPP (black bars) on Fos-LI in rat brain stem TNC. Control animals were given a time-matched injection of an equivalent volume of saline (0.1 ml·kg^{-1}; gray bars) (n = 5 animals for every time point in both groups).

MATERIALS AND METHODS

Male Sprague-Dawley rats (250 to 300 g) were anesthetized with pentobarbitone (60 mg·kg^{-1} i.p., initially, followed by 20 mg·kg^{-1}hr^{-1} i.p. infusion). Following surgery animals were maintained at 37°C in the supine position, where they breathed spontaneously. After a 10-minute stabilization period, m-CPP (100 µg·kg^{-1} dissolved in 0.9% saline) or an equivalent volume of saline (0.1 ml·kg^{-1}) was administered via an indwelling cannula in the femoral vein. Two, 4, or 6 hours later the animals were perfused with phosphate-buffered saline followed by 4% formalin through the left ventricle (50 ml·min^{-1} for 1.5 and 3 minutes, respectively). Fos-like immunoreactivity (Fos-LI) was localized in free-floating sections (40 µm) from brain stem TNC by the avidin-biotin-peroxidase method (Vectastain). The number of stained nuclei in either left or right TNC, taken as the mean of 16 to 24 sections, was averaged for each treatment group (n = 5).

In separate experiments, bipolar electrodes were placed in the left and right trigeminal ganglia. Three hours later the right ganglion alone was stimulated electrically (0.6 mA, 5 msec, 5 Hz, for 5 minutes). The animals were perfusion-fixed 2 hours later.

RESULTS

Intravenous injection of m-CPP (100 µg·kg^{-1}) had no significant effect on Fos-LI in the TNC at any of the 2-, 4-, or 6-hour time points compared with saline (Fig. 1). This dose also had no significant effect on Fos-LI in either the nucleus tractus soli-

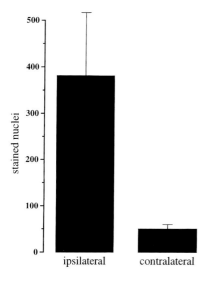

FIG. 2. Effect of unilateral electrical stimulation of the trigeminal ganglion in rat brain stem showing the significant elevation of Fos-LI in the ipsilateral TNC relative to the contralateral side (n = 3 animals).

tarius or the reticulate nucleus in these sections (data not shown). By contrast, a profound unilateral elevation in Fos-LI in the TNC following electrical stimulation of the ipsilateral trigeminal ganglion was observed (Fig. 2).

CONCLUSIONS

No elevation in Fos-LI was observed 2 to 6 hours following intravenous administration of m-CPP (100 µg·kg^{-1}), suggesting that 5-HT$_{2B/2C}$ receptor stimulation does not trigger TNC activation in the brain stem of the rat either directly or indirectly. These data contrast with the observations that a similar dose of m-CPP induces plasma protein extravasation from blood vessels in the rat dura mater (1 and 100 µg·kg^{-1}) (Johnson and Nelson, personal communication). From these findings it can be inferred that m-CPP-induced extravasation does not involve trigeminovascular activation. Since m-CPP-evoked plasma protein extravasation has been reported to be blocked by methysergide (Johnson and Nelson, personal communication, 1996), it is conceivable that the drug acts at an undefined vascular receptor to mediate this effect directly. The observation that extravasation can occur in the absence of trigeminal nerve activation questions both the relevance of vascular leakage to the pathophysiology of migraine and its utility as a model of the disease.

Although the induction of plasma protein extravasation without elevation in Fos expression may suggest that the former can be assayed with higher sensitivity, there is no evidence as yet to suggest that this is the case. Comparatively intense electrical stimulation of the trigeminal ganglion is required to evoke plasma protein extravasation (9). Under these conditions Fos expression in the TNC is also elevated.

However, Fos expression is also induced by mechanical micromanipulation of the superior sagittal sinus, arguably a more physiological stimulus (10).

In addition to stimulating the 5-HT_{2A}, 5-HT_{2B}, and 5-HT_{2C} receptor subtypes, m-CPP has been found to bind to other receptors/enzymes with moderate to high affinity (≤ 1 µM) (11,12). Hoyer (12) and Shen et al. (13) reported that m-CPP binds to the 5-HT_3 and the recombinant rat 5-HT_7 receptors, respectively. Higher concentrations of m-CPP (1 to 10 µM) bind to the 5-HT_{1A}, $5\text{-HT}_{1B/D}$, α_2-adrenergic, and recombinant 5-ht_6 receptors (12,14,15) and evoke release of 5-HT from rat hypothalamus (16). As it is not possible to predict either the concentration of m-CPP in a particular tissue or the prevailing drug receptor-mediated effects in a given species, we cannot assume that the behavior of m-CPP in the rat is representative of its actions in humans. Nonetheless it is interesting that orally administered m-CPP in humans evokes migraine-like headache, yet an analogous systemic concentration in rats appears to induce vascular leakage but not trigeminal nerve stimulation.

ACKNOWLEDGMENTS

This work was supported by the generous funding of Glaxo-Wellcome Medicines Research Centre, Stevenage, United Kingdom, in association with King's College, University of London.

REFERENCES

1. Fozard JR, Gray JA. 5-HT_{1C} receptor activation: a key step in the initiation of migraine? *TIPS* 1989; 10:307–309.
2. Kalkman HO. Is migraine prophylactic activity caused by 5-HT_{2B} or 5-HT_{2C} receptors? *Life Sci* 1994;54:641–644.
3. Brewerton TD, Dennis LM, Mueller EA, Jimerson DC. Induction of migraine-like headaches by the serotonin agonist m-CPP. *Clin Pharmacol Ther* 1988;42:605–609.
4. Iversen HK, Olesen J, Tfelt-Hansen P. Intravenous nitroglycerin as an experimental headache model. Basic characteristics. *Pain* 1989;38:17–24.
5. Iversen HK, Olesen J. The effect of histamine H_1 blockade on nitroglycerin-induced headache in vascular responses. *Cephalalgia* 1993;13[Suppl 13]:P82.
6. Martin GR, Bolofo ML, Giles HG. Inhibition of endothelium-dependent vasorelaxation by arginine analogues: a pharmacological analysis of agonist and tissue dependence. *Br J Pharmacol* 1992;105: 643–652.
7. Nemade RV, Lewis AI, Zuccarello M, Keller JT. Immunohistochemical localization of endothelial nitric oxide synthase in vessels of the dura mater of the Sprague-Dawley rat. *Neurosci Lett* 1995; 197:78–80.
8. Schmuck K, Ullmer C, Kalkman HO, Probst A, Lubbert H. Activation of meningeal 5-HT_{2B} receptors: an early step in the generation of migraine headache? *Eur J Neurosci* 1996;8:959–967.
9. Shepheard SL, Williamson DJ, Williams J, Hill RG, Hargreaves RJ. Comparison of the effects of sumatriptan and the NK_1 antagonist CP-99,994 on plasma extravasation in the dura mater and c-*fos* m-RNA expression in the trigeminal nucleus caudalis of rats. *Neuropharmacology* 1995;34:255–261.
10. Hoskin KL, Kaube H, Goadsby, PJ. Fos-expression in trigeminal neurons evoked by mechanical stimulation of the superior sagittal sinus in the cat is reduced by sumatriptan. In: Rose CF, ed. *New advances in headache research*. vol. 4. London: Smith-Gordon; 1994.
11. Wainscott DB, Cohen ML, Schenck KW, et al. Pharmacological characteristics of the newly cloned rat 5-hydroxytryptamine$_{2F}$ receptor. *Mol Pharmacol* 1992;43:419–426.

12. Hoyer D. 5-HT receptors and effector coupling mechanisms in peripheral tissues. In: Fozard JF, ed. *The peripheral actions of 5-HT*. New York: Oxford University Press; 1989:72–88.
13. Shen Y, Monsma FJ, Metcalf MA, Jose PA, Hamblin MW, Sibley DR. Molecular cloning and expression of a 5-hydroxytryptamine$_7$ serotonin receptor subtype. *J Biol Chem* 1993;268:18200–18204.
14. Hamik A, Peroutka SJ. 1-(m-Chlorophenyl)piperazine (mCPP) interactions with neurotransmitter receptors in the human brain. *Biol Psychiatry* 1989;25:569–575.
15. Monsma FJ, Shen Y, Hamblin MW, Sibley DR. Cloning and expression of a novel serotonin receptor with high affinity for tricyclic psychotropic drugs. *Mol Pharmacol* 1992;43:320–327.
16. Pettibone DJ, Williams M. Serotonin-releasing effects of substituted piperazines *in vitro*. *Biochem Pharmacol* 1984;33:1531–1535.

21

Release of Histamine from Dural Mast Cells by Substance P and Calcitonin Gene-Related Peptide and Effect of Sumatriptan

Anders Ottosson and *Lars Edvinsson

*Department of Forensic Medicine, University of Lund, S-221 85 Lund, Sweden; and
Department of Internal Medicine, Lund University Hospital, S-221 85 Lund, Sweden

Histamine has long been implicated in the pathogenesis of various types of headache, as have the neuropeptides substance P (SP) and calcitonin gene-related peptide (CGRP). The trigeminovascular system seems to be the final common pathway for the transmission of vascular headaches (1). Histamine-containing mast cells are numerous in the dura mater, and dural mast cells are found adjacent to unmyelinated nerves (2). Furthermore, SP and CGRP have been demonstrated in the dura mater and in the middle meningeal artery (3). Figure 1 presents a model for the possible role of sensory neuropeptides in mast cell activation and vasoregulation.

The aim of the present study was to examine if SP and CGRP can stimulate histamine release from mast cells in the dura mater, and if this release is affected by the antimigraine drug sumatriptan.

MATERIALS AND METHODS

Dural samples were obtained from male Sprague-Dawley rats weighing between 250 and 350 g. The rats were exsanguinated during general anesthesia, and the carotid arteries were cannulated and perfused by saline. The skull was opened by a horizontal cut from the foramen magnum to the eye region, thereby allowing the vertex of the skull to be lifted off. The dura was divided into six segments by a scalpel blade while still attached to the skull and then gently removed. The samples were placed in a buffered salt solution (containing 145 mM NaCl, 2.7 mM KCl, and 10% v/v Sörensen phosphate buffer, 67 mM) in polystyrene centrifuge tubes. Histamine release from the mast cells was determined fluorometrically by the use of *o*-phthaldialdehyde (4). Dose-response curves were constructed for each drug and each animal. Histamine release was expressed as percent of the total histamine content. Stimulated histamine release was determined by correcting for spontaneous release,

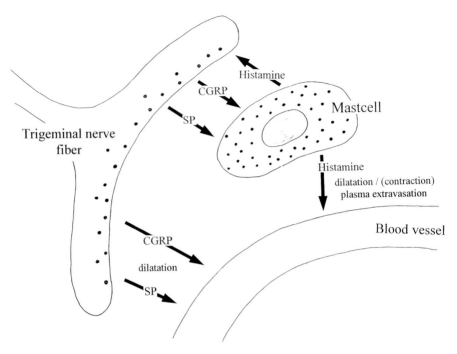

FIG. 1. A model for the possible role of the sensory neuropeptides substance P (SP) and calcitonin gene-related peptide (CGRP) in mast cell activation and vasoregulation.

which was determined by parallel incubation without histamine-releasing stimulus. Blocking agents were administered to the samples 15 minutes before the histamine-releasing agent. The results are expressed as mean values ± SEM.

RESULTS

Substance P released histamine in a concentration-related manner from rat dural mast cells. The highest release (at 100 μM) was 37 ± 4% of total mast cell histamine content (Fig. 2). The neurokinin$_1$ (NK$_1$) receptor antagonist FK888 blocked the SP-evoked histamine release significantly ($p = 0.008$, Kruskal-Wallis test; Fig. 3). Calcitonin gene-related peptide also released histamine in a concentration-dependent fashion from the dural mast cells, with a maximum release of 33 ± 3% of total mast cell histamine content at a CGRP-concentration of 10 μM (Fig. 2). The CGRP receptor antagonist CGRP$_{8-37}$ blocked the CGRP-evoked histamine release ($p = 0.001$); the effects of the antagonists were concentration dependent (Fig. 3).

Capsaicin at a concentration of 10^{-5} M did not induce any histamine release from rat dural mast cells (n = 20). Sumatriptan at a concentration of 10^{-6} M had no histamine-releasing effect per se. The CGRP-evoked histamine release was significantly

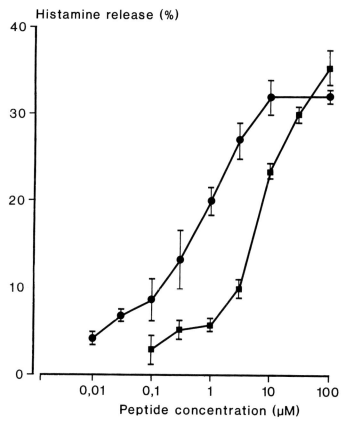

FIG. 2. Histamine release from rat dura mater induced by substance P (■) and CGRP(●), (n = 4–10). Values represent mean ± SEM.

blocked by sumatriptan ($p = 0.01$, n = 4) (Fig. 4). The SP-evoked histamine release was not significantly blocked by sumatriptan ($p = 0.07$, n = 4) (Fig. 4).

DISCUSSION

The neuropeptides CGRP and SP readily release histamine from rat dural mast cells. The response to SP was blocked by the selective NK_1 receptor antagonist FK888, suggesting that SP activates NK_1 receptors. The blocking effect of $CGRP_{8-37}$ on the CGRP-evoked histamine release suggests a $CGRP_1$ receptor-coupled activation of dural mast cells. Histamine release by these neuropeptides indicates a coupling between the trigeminovascular system and histamine through mast cell degranulation. Neurogenic inflammation (manifested as vasodilation and plasma protein extravasation) has long been implicated in the pathogenesis of

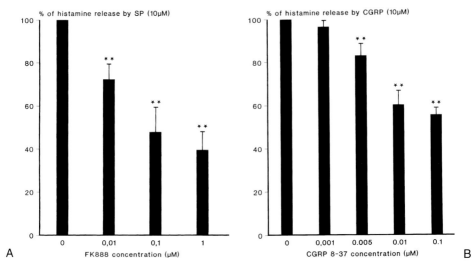

FIG. 3. A: Inhibition of substance P (SP)-induced histamine release from rat dura mater by the substance P antagonist FK888 (n = 4). **B:** Inhibition of calcitonin gene-related peptide (CGRP)-induced histamine release from rat dura mater by the CGRP antagonist $CGRP_{8-37}$ (n = 4–5). Values represent mean ± SEM. ★★, $p < 0.01$, by the Mann-Whitney U-test.

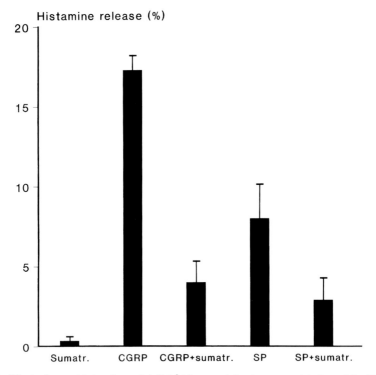

FIG. 4. Effect of sumatriptan (sumatr.) (10^{-6} M) on calcitonin gene-related peptide (CGRP)-induced (10^{-5} M) and substance P (SP)-induced (10^{-5} M) histamine release from rat dura mater. The inhibition of CGRP-induced histamine release was significant ($p = 0.01$), whereas the effect on the SP-induced histamine release was not significant. Values represent mean ± SEM, n = 4.

headache (5,6). Studies in patients have demonstrated increased levels of CGRP in venous outflow during attacks of migraine and cluster headache (7,8). The present results suggest an additional pathway for the possible involvement of SP and CGRP in cranial vasoregulation and in neurogenic inflammation, besides their direct vasodilatory effect (3). However, it should be noted that SP and CGRP histamine release occurs at much higher concentrations than those that cause vasodilation (3).

Capsaicin, a neurotoxin that may selectively cause release of sensory neuropeptides, had no histamine-releasing effect. A probable explanation is that the C-fiber content of SP and CGRP is low in the present samples, conceivably because of release during the sampling procedure. Alternatively, capsaicin may only cause release of subthreshold concentrations of SP/CGRP, not high enough to cause histamine release.

The CGRP-evoked histamine release was blocked by sumatriptan. If this also applies in humans, the antimigrainous effect of sumatriptan might be partly mediated through inhibition of CGRP-evoked histamine release, by a presently unknown mechanism.

REFERENCES

1. Moskowitz MA. The trigeminovascular system. In: Olesen J, Tfelt-Hansen P, Welch KMA, eds. *The Headaches*. Philadelphia: Lippincott–Raven, 1993:97–104.
2. Dimlich RVW, Keller JT, Strauss TA, Fritts MJ. Linear arrays of homogenous mast cells in the dura mater of the rat. *J Neurocytol* 1991;20:485–503.
3. Jansen I, Uddman R, Ekman R, Olesen J, Ottosson A, Edvinsson L. Distribution and effects of neuropeptide Y, vasoactive intestinal peptide, substance P, and calcitonin gene-related peptide in human middle meningeal arteries: comparison with cerebral and temporal arteries. *Peptides* 1992;13:527–536.
4. Rönnberg AL, Håkanson R. A simplified procedure for the fluorometric determination of histamine in rat stomach. *Agents Actions* 1984;14:195–199.
5. Moskowitz MA, Romero J, Reinhard JF, Melamed E, Pettibone DJ. Neurotransmitters and the fifth cranial nerve: is there a relation to the headache phase of migraine? *Lancet* 1979;2:883–884.
6. Moskowitz MA. Basic mechanisms of headache. *Neurol Clin* 1990;8:801–815.
7. Edvinsson L, Goadsby PJ. Neuropeptides in migraine and cluster headache. *Cephalalgia* 1994;14:320–327.
8. Goadsby PJ, Edvinsson L. Human in vivo evidence for trigeminovascular activation in cluster headache. Neuropeptide changes and effects of acute attacks therapies. *Brain* 1994;117:427–434.

22

Variability of Vascular Receptors on the Human Cerebral Arteries as Determined in Vitro

Peer Tfelt-Hansen, *Inger Jansen-Olesen, †A. Mortensen, and ‡Lars Edvinsson

*Department of Neurology, Bispebjerg Hospital, DK-2400 Copenhagen, Denmark; *Department of Biological Sciences, The Royal Danish School of Pharmacy, DK-2100 Copenhagen Ø, Denmark; †Department of Neurosurgery, Glostrup Hospital, DK-2600 Glostrup, Copenhagen, Denmark; and ‡Department of Internal Medicine, Lund University Hospital, S-221 85 Lund Sweden*

Clinical experience has shown that the amount of drug necessary to treat a disorder varies considerably among patients; interindividual differences in sensitivity to drugs is probably due to a large extent to pharmacodymamic variability, which is less recognized than pharmacokinetic variability among subjects (1). Thus, both in vitro and in vivo results support the hypothesis that a considerable dynamic variability, mainly variability in sensitivity, exists in human vascular receptors (see Ch. 23, *this volume*). Probably the most relevant vessels for migraine therapy are human intracranial arteries, but these vessels are difficult to obtain and have only been studied in limited numbers in vitro (2). In these studies concentration-response curves are mostly presented as means ± SEM, thereby inherently concealing the variability among subjects to some extent. In this reanalysis of previous in vitro results, we examined variability among subjects.

MATERIALS AND METHODS

Human small cerebral arteries obtained during neurosurgery (diameter, 0.3 to 0.6 mm) were cut into ring segments with intact endothelium; agonist activity of drugs was then tested in an in vitro system. For technical details, solutions, and drugs used, see refs. 3 and 4.

For each subject one to five segments were tested. E_{max} (maximum contractile or inhibitory effect) and EC_{50} [median (molar) effective concentration] or IC_{50} [inhibitory concentration (molar) of 50%] values were calculated for each segment. In the previous analysis the geometric mean ± SEM of the pEC_2 or pIC_{50} (negative log of the molar concentration at which half-maximum effect occurs) of all the segments were calculated (4). In this reanalysis, for each subject either one or the mean of several values of E_{max}, EC_{50}, or IC_{50} was used in the estimation of variability. Because the data were skewed, medians and ranges were calculated.

RESULTS

The geometric means ± SEM for pIC_{50} and pEC_{50}, as well as the medians and ranges for EC_{50} and IC_{50} values are given in Table 1. For substance P [N (number of subjects) = 11, n (total number of segments) = 18] the median E_{max} was 93% (of potassium) and the range was 61% to 100%. For human β-calcitonin gene-related peptide (CGRP) (N = 7, n = 11) the median E_{max} was 93% (of potassium) and the range was 29% to 101%. For human α-CGRP (N = 11, n = 25) the median E_{max} was 92% (of potassium) and the range was 54% to 99%. For histamine (N = 5, n = 11) the median E_{max} was 87% (of potassium) and the range 75% to 98%. For 5-hydroxytryptamine (5-HT) (N = 8, n = 21) the median E_{max} was 42% (of potassium) and the range was 16% to 133%. For 5-carboxamidotryptamine (5-CT) (N = 6, n = 13) the median E_{max} was 50% (of potassium) and the range was 22% to 205%. For sumatriptan (N = 3, n = 10) the median E_{max} was 63% (of potassium) and the range was 59% to 79%. For 8-hydroxy-dipropylaminotetralin (8-OH-DPAT) (N = 4, n = 6) the median E_{max} was 57% (of potassium) and the range was 35% to 78%.

Note that whereas E_{max} in most cases varied relatively little, the exception being an eightfold difference among subjects for 5-HT, ranges for sensitivity, IC_{50}, and EC_{50} demonstrate an up to 1,000-fold difference among subjects for this pharmacodynamic parameter (Table 1).

DISCUSSION

Methodological Considerations

Giving the geometric means for pIC_{50}/pEC_{50} values is probably a reasonable way of presenting the results for the logarithmic values. However, as demonstrated in Table 1, presenting the variability by giving the SEM tends to conceal the real variability. This concealment effect is further increased when the n used in the calculation of SEM is increased by using several segments from each patient as independent results. Presenting the variability of the results with range (or alternatively with percentiles) for EC_{50} or IC_{50} discloses a huge variability in sensitivity among subjects (Table 1).

Clinical Implications

As in a previous analysis of in vitro results (see Ch. 23) the E_{max} (intrinsic activity) varied relatively little among subjects, whereas the sensitivity parameters, IC_{50}

TABLE 1. Geometric means (GM) ± SEM for pIC_{50} and pEC_{50} and medians and ranges for IC_{50} and EC_{50}: effect of drugs on human pial arteries[a]

	GM±SEM	Median	Range	Drug	N/n[b]
IC_{50}					
Substance P 11/25	9.49±0.23[c]	3×10^{-10} M	2×10^{-12}–3.5×10^{-9} M	Human α-CGRP	
	10.03±0.25[c]	3×10^{-10} M	7×10^{-13}–2×10^{-9} M	5-HT	8/22
Human β-CGRP	9.35±0.24[c]	5×10^{-10} M	8×10^{-11}–5×10^{-9} M	Histamine	5/11
	7.84±0.17[c]	7×10^{-8} M	6×10^{-9}–1.5×10^{-7} M	5-CT	6/13
EC_{50}					
Substance P	7.10±0.14[d]	15×10^{-8} M	2×10^{-8}–3×10^{-6} M		
	6.15±0.14[d]	3.6×10^{-7} M	3×10^{-7}–3.5×10^{-6} M	Sumatriptan	3/10
Human β-CGRP	7.45±0.19[d]	2×10^{-8} M	1×10^{-8}–1×10^{-6} M	8-OH-DPAT	4/6
	5.2±0.42	6.7×10^{-5} M	1.2×10^{-6}–1.3×10^{-4} M		

[a]For details on calculations, see Materials and Methods.
[b]N/n, number of subjects/total number of segments.
[c]pIC_{50}.
[d]pEC_{50}.
CGRP, calcitonin gene-related peptide; 5-CT, 5-carboxamidotryptamine; EC_{50}, median effective concentration; 5-HT, 5-hydroxytryptamine; IC_{50}, inhibitory concentration of 50%; 8-OH-DPAT, 8-hydroxy-dipropylaminotetrolin; pEC_{50} and pIC_{50}, negative log of the molar concentration at which half-maximum effect or inhibition occurs.

and EC_{50}, showed a huge interindividual difference. This large observed variability, up to 1,000-fold among subjects, could in some minor extent be due to problems in calculating the IC_{50} and EC_{50} from the concentration-response curves, but the magnitude of the variability must reflect a considerable, real pharmacodynamic variability among subjects. Such variability should be taken into account when drugs are used in the treatment of migraine. Doses of vasoactive drugs should be tailored to the individual patient. This general statement is supported by new results showing that patients differ in their choice of doses of sumatriptan for the treatment of migraine attacks (5).

REFERENCES

1. Rowland M, Sheiner LB, Steimer J-L, eds. *Variability in drug therapy. Description, estimation, and control*. Philadelphia: Lippincott–Raven, 1985:167–184.
2. Edvinsson L, Skärby T, Tfelt-Hansen P, Gjerris F, Olesen J. Presence of alpha-adrenoreceptors in human temporal arteries. Comparison between migraine patients and controls. *Cephalalgia* 1983;3:219–224.
3. Jansen I. *Sensory neuropeptides in the cerebral circulation: role in cerebrovascular disorders* [Dissertation]. Lund, Sweden: Lund University, 1991.
4. Armitage P, Berry G. *Statistical methods in medical research*. 3rd ed. Oxford: Blackwell Scientific Publications, 1994.
5. The S2BM11 Study Group. Patient preference between 25, 50 and 100 mg oral doses of sumatriptan. *Eur J Neurol* 1996;3[Suppl 5]:86.

23

Variability of the Vascular α-Adrenoceptor on Human Omental Vessels: An In Vitro Study

Peer Tfelt-Hansen and *Lars Edvinsson

*Department of Neurology, Bispebjerg Hospital, DK-2400 Copenhagen, Denmark; and *Department of Internal Medicine, Lund University Hospital, S-221 85 Lund, Sweden*

Clinical experience reveals that the amount of drug necessary to treat a disorder varies considerably among patients even when the disease treated seems fairly uniform, e.g., with regard to severity. This interindividual variability in doses needed could be due to interindividual differences in *pharmacokinetic parameters* such as bioavailability and clearance, or to interindividual differences in *pharmacodynamic parameters* such as intrinsic activity and sensitivity, or to both (1). Previously, interindividual differences in doses have been ascribed mainly to the often observed variability in kinetics, probably because it is easier to measure plasma levels of drugs than to measure relevant dynamic parameters in humans (2).

In vivo, when investigating the vasoconstrictor effect of parenteral ergotamine, we observed a large interindividual variability in this effect in migraine patients (3,4), in previous ergotamine abusers (3), and in normal volunteers (3). This variability (e.g., the sensitivity to ergotamine varied 30-fold) (4) was much larger than would be expected from the approximately threefold variation in kinetics parameters after parenteral ergotamine (5). Part of this estimated variability could be due to variability in measuring the effect or to the necessary modeling for obtaining the estimation of sensitivity (3). We therefore wanted to estimate the variability of a vasoconstrictor in vitro. Previously, a comparison of the α-adrenoceptor in human temporal arteries showed no difference between migraine patients (n = 6) and normal subjects (n = 6), but a considerable interindividual difference in sensitivity was observed in both groups (6). These arteries are, however, difficult to obtain and we therefore chose to study omental arteries and veins, since these vessels are easily obtainable during surgery.

MATERIALS AND METHODS

Twenty-nine biopsies from omental arteries and 26 biopsies from omental veins were obtained during surgery (in most cases, on the gallbladder), immediately placed in ice-cold Krebs-Ringer solution, and brought to the laboratory within 2 hours. In the laboratory, 1- to 3-mm-long circular vessel segments were mounted on a system of L-shaped metal holders immersed in a tissue bath. Isometric tension was continuously recorded by a force displacement transducer connected to a Grass polygraph. The contractile capacity was tested by exposure to a potassium-rich (120 mmol/L) buffer solution, and contraction by noradrenaline (NA) was expressed in percent of the potassium-induced contraction. EC_{50} [median (molar) effective concentration] and E_{max} (maximum contractile effect) were determined for each concentration-response relationship. The contractile response to NA was tested in two-vessel segments from the same patient; the means of these two determinations are given. For technical details, solutions, and drugs used, see ref. 6.

RESULTS

Noradrenaline contracted both types of omental vessels in a concentration-dependent manner. The coefficient of variations (calculated from the double measurements) for EC_{50} determinations was 6% for arteries and 7% for veins. The EC_{50} and E_{max} for omental arteries are given in Table 1. The EC_{50} values for arteries and veins within the 10% to 90% percentiles are further illustrated in Fig. 1. Note that whereas E_{max} only varied approximately twofold, the EC_{50} values varied considerably more for both arteries and veins, e.g., approximately 20-fold when the results are cut off at the 2.5% and 97.5% percentiles (Table 1). When the whole range of values is taken into account, the EC_{50} values varied up to 60-fold for arteries and 150-fold for veins (Table 1).

DISCUSSION

A large, at least 20-fold, interindividual variability in the sensitivity (EC_{50}) of human omental arteries and veins is the main result of this in vitro study (Table 1). By contrast, in an in vitro study with feline mesenteric arteries, the 95% confidence interval for the EC_{50} for NA was 3.5 to 24 $\times$ 10^{-7} M (n = 28) and thus varied sevenfold (7). These in vitro results support the previous in vivo results that demonstrated a huge interindividual difference in sensitivity of human leg arteries to ergotamine when tested in vivo (3,4). A similar large variability was found for the dose of locally infused NA necessary to bring the diameter of dorsal hand veins to half. [The dose varied 35-fold when only results between the 10% and 90% percentiles were considered (8)].

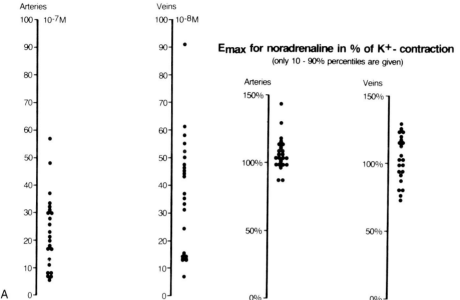

FIG. 1. EC_{50} (**A**) and E_{max} (**B**) values for the effect of noradrenaline on human omental arteries and veins. Note that only the values within the 10% and 90% percentiles are given (for medians and ranges, see Table 1).

Thus both in vitro and in vivo the sensitivity of human vessels to agonists varies considerably, and therefore a considerable dynamic variability should be anticipated when vasoactive drugs are used. The use of one standard dose of a drug should be discouraged, and there is a good scientific basis for tailoring the dose to the individual patient.

TABLE 1. EC_{50} and E_{max} for the effect of noradrenaline on human omental arteries (n=29) and veins (n=26)

	Arteries		Veins	
	EC_{50} (10^{-7} M)	E_{max} (% of K^+)	EC_{50} (10^{-8} M)	E_{max} (% of K^+)
Median	21	105	40	102
2.5–97.5% percentiles	4–100	81–149	6–110	71–131
Range	3–200	74–151	2–320	58–141

EC_{50}, median effective concentration; E_{max}, maximum contractile effect.

REFERENCES

1. Rowland M, Sheiner LB, Steimer J-L, eds. *Variability in drug therapy. Description, estimation, and control.* Philadelphia: Lippincott–Raven, 1985:167–184.
2. Smith SE, Rawling MD. *Variability in human drug response.* London: Butterworth, 1973.
3. Tfelt-Hansen P. The effect of ergotamine on the arterial system in man. *Acta Pharmacol Toxicol* 1986; 59[Suppl 3]:1–30.
4. Tfelt-Hansen P, Paalzow L. Intramuscular ergotamine: plasma levels and dynamic activity. *Clin Pharmacol Ther* 1985;37:29–35.
5. Ibraheem JJ, Paalzow L, Tfelt-Hansen P. Kinetics of ergotamine after intravenous and intramuscular administration to migraine sufferers. *Eur J Clin Pharmacol* 1982;23:235–240.
6. Edvinsson L, Skärby T, Tfelt-Hansen P, Gjerris F, Olesen J. Presence of alpha-adrenoreceptors in human temporal arteries. Comparison between migraine patients and controls. *Cephalalgia* 1983;3:219–224.
7. Skärby TVC, Andersson K-E, Edvinsson L. Pharmacological characterization of postjunctional alpha-adrenoceptors in isolated feline cerebral and peripheral arteries. *Acta Physiol Scand* 1983;117:63–73.
8. Martin SA, Alexieva S, Carruthers SG. The influence of age on dorsal hand vein responsiveness to norepinephrine. *Clin Pharmacol Ther* 1986;40:257–260.

24

A Study on Hormonal Responses and Painful Attacks Induced by *m*-Chlorophenylpiperazine in Cluster Headache Patients during Cluster Period

*Massimo Leone, *Domenico D'Amico, *Licia Grazzi,
*Angelo Attanasio, †Danilo Croci, *Giuseppe Libro,
†Angelo Nespolo, and *Gennaro Bussone

*Headache Center, †Biochemistry and Pharmacology Laboratory, Neurological Institute
"C. Besta," 20133 Milan, Italy

Male preponderance, the cyclical clinical pattern, and the efficacy of lithium suggest the involvement of the hypothalamus in the pathogenesis of cluster headache (CH). Neuroendocrinology has been used to investigate the hypothalamus in this condition, and some anomalies were observed, in particular of the hypothalamic-hypophyseal-adrenal (HPA) axis (1). Several transmitter systems modulate responses of the HPA axis; the serotoninergic system seems of particular interest in view of its roles in pain control and the regulation of biological rhythms (2,3), both of which have been shown to be altered in CH (1,4). To investigate the serotoninergic system in CH we administered the direct central serotoninergic agonist *m*-chlorophenylpiperazine (m-CPP) to CH patients.

MATERIALS AND METHODS

Twenty-three episodic CH patients, diagnosed according to International Headache Society criteria as being in a cluster period, and 17 sex- and age-matched controls were studied (5). No subject took any medication for at least the 2 weeks prior to testing. Sumatriptan, oxygen, or nonsteroidal anti-inflammatory drugs (NSAIDs) were employed to abort cluster attacks in CH patients in the days prior to testing. Testing began between 8 and 9 AM after overnight fasting. Blood samples were taken at –30, 0, 30, 60, 90, 120, 150, and 180 minutes. At time 0 m-CPP, 0.5 mg/kg was administered orally.

Cortisol was determined by fluorescence polarization immunoassay. Prolactin

(PRL) levels were determined by microparticle enzyme immunoassay. Plasma levels of m-CPP were determined by high-performance liquid chromatography (6). Means of plasma levels of the two hormones and of m-CPP were calculated at each sampling. The δ-maximum values for each patient of cortisol and PRL were calculated [δ-maximum=maximum response−baseline level (at T0)/baseline level (at T0)].

RESULTS

The plasma levels of m-CPP increased significantly following oral administration in both CH patients and controls (Fig. 1). The mean values in blood sampled from +30 to +180 minutes were 14.32 ± 4.16, 33.07 ± 7.4, 40.24 ± 7.12, 44.24 ± 7.54, 39.37 ± 6, and 37.79 ± 7.33 in CH patients and 14.92 ± 4.2, 33.19 ± 6.59, 46.43 ± 10.72, 45.41 ± 8.08, 39.76 ± 8.63, and 33.93 ± 6.44 in controls (ng/mL; mean ± SEM). Cortisol data were unavailable in four subjects (two from each group).

Baseline cortisol levels were higher in CH patients than controls at time −30 minutes (17.43 ± 1.21 and 14.13 ± 1.48 in patients and controls, respectively; µg/dL; mean ± SEM; Student's t test, $p = 0.09$) and at time 0 (13.21 ± 0.87 and 10.43 ± 1.03, respectively; Student's t test, $p < 0.05$). The timing of the cortisol peak did not differ in the two groups, occurring between +60 and +90 minutes in both cases. Cortisol δ-maxima were significantly reduced in CH patients (Student's t test, $p < 0.02$) (Fig. 2).

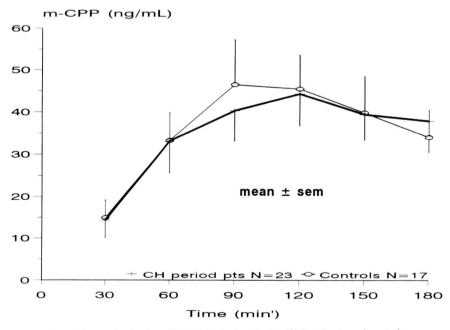

FIG. 1. Plasma levels of m-CPP in cluster headache (CH) patients and controls.

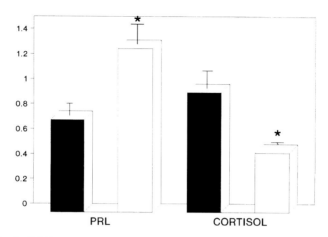

FIG. 2. Prolactin (PRL) and cortisol δ-maxima after m-CPP administration. ■, controls; □, CH patients.

Baseline PRL levels were lower in CH patients than controls, but the difference was not significant. At –30 minutes the PRL concentrations were 9.91 ± 1.11 and 13.47 ± 1.68, respectively (Student's t test, $p = 0.07$), and at time 0 they were 7.69 ± 0.94 and 10.51 ± 1.73, respectively (Student's t test, $p = 0.06$) in patients and controls (ng/mL; mean ± SEM). The PRL peaks occurred between 90 and 150 minutes with no between-group difference in time of occurrence of the peak. Values of PRL δ-maxima were significantly increased in CH (Student's t test, $p < 0.05$) (Fig. 2).

As expected, there was a good correlation between m-CPP and cortisol plasma levels in CH ($r = 0.83$, $p = 0.03$, df = 6) and in controls ($r = 0.77$, $p = 0.08$, df = 6). Values of m-CPP also correlated with PRL plasma levels in patients ($r = 0.9$, $p = 0.03$, df = 6) and controls ($r = 0.75$, $p = 0.08$, df = 6). Cortisol and PRL levels did not correlate with each other in either of the two groups ($r = 0.1$, $p = 0.81$, df = 8 and $r = 0.43$, $p = 0.2$, df = 8 in patients and controls, respectively).

Two of the 17 CH patients (9%) and 2 of the controls (12%) had a migrainous headache after m-CPP. Nine of the 23 CH patients (39.13%) developed a typical CH attack after m-CPP at a mean of 93.18 ± 49.21 minutes (mean ± SD; range 43 to 144 minutes) (Fig. 3). These patients showed increased m-CPP plasma levels after 90 minutes compared with the patients who did not develop the attack. In the latter group m-CPP levels decreased after 90 minutes while in the former they did not (Fig. 3). No differences were observed in baseline values or δ-maxima of cortisol or PRL.

DISCUSSION

The neuropeptide m-CPP is known to stimulate the secretion of cortisol mainly through interaction with cerebral 5-hydroxytryptamine $(5\text{-HT})_{2A/C}$ receptors (7),

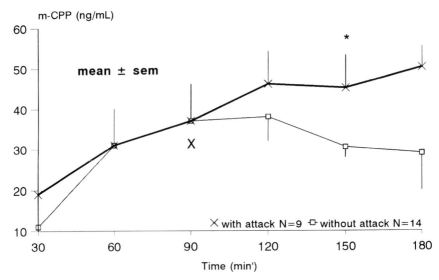

FIG. 3. m-CPP (0.5 mg/kg PO) plasma levels in cluster headache (CH) patients with or without attack during the test.

while PRL secretion is also mediated by 5-HT$_{1A}$ receptor stimulation (8). In humans, administration of the 5-HT$_2$ blocker ritanserin increases the PRL response to L-tryptophan, suggesting that 5-HT$_2$ receptors have an inhibitory action on 5-HT$_{1A}$-induced PRL secretion (8). Overstimulation of 5-HT$_2$ receptors could explain the increased baseline levels of cortisol and reduced levels of PRL as well as the altered hormonal responses to m-CPP in our CH patients (Fig. 4), suggesting a deranged central serotoninergic tone. Several other neurotransmitters are involved in the modulation of cortisol and PRL secretion, and a role for these in the alterations observed cannot be excluded (9).

None of the subjects had a personal or family history of migraine, and this might explain the low incidence of migrainous headache after m-CPP administration among our subjects. About 39% of our patients developed typical CH attacks following m-CPP administration. Such attacks appeared outside the usual time of occurrence and when m-CPP plasma levels were at their peak, suggesting that this substance precipitated the attacks. Administration of m-CPP may trigger "vascular"

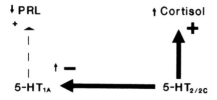

FIG. 4. Possible effects of 5-hydroxytryptamine (5-HT)$_{2/2c}$ receptor overstimulation on *basal* cortisol and prolactin (PRL) plasma levels in CH.

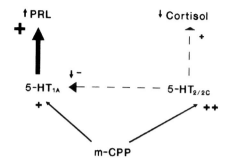

FIG. 5. Possible effects of 5-hydroxytryptamine (5-HT)$_{2/2c}$ receptor overstimulation on cortisol and PRL *responses* to m-CPP test in CH.

headaches as a consequence of release of nitric oxide (10) by activation of nitric oxide synthetase or by acting on 5-HT$_{2C/2B}$ receptors located on the endothelial cells of the craniovascular bed (11).

In conclusion, we suggest that the reduced cortisol and increased PRL responses to m-CPP challenge in CH patients could be the expression of an alteration in the cerebral serotoninergic system, in particular of 5-HT$_2$ and 5-HT$_{1A}$ receptors (Fig. 5). It is interesting to note that stimulation of these two receptors may produce opposing effects in the pain-controlling system: 5-HT$_2$ stimulation is correlated with activation of pain circuits, while stimulation of 5-HT$_{1A}$ receptors increases the pain threshold (3). Assuming downregulation of 5-HT$_2$ receptors, one may speculate that the neuronal system concerned with the transmission of pain stimuli may be hyperactive in the cluster period, while upregulation of 5-HT$_{1A}$ receptors could indicate a reduced ability to inhibit pain stimuli, since in fact CH patients have been reported to have a reduced pain threshold (4).

REFERENCES

1. Leone M, Bussone G. A review of hormonal findings in cluster headache. Evidence for hypothalamic involvement. *Cephalalgia* 1993;13:309–317.
2. Clarke DE. A synopsis of the pharmacology of clinically used drugs at 5HT receptors and uptake sites. In: Olesen J, Saxena PR, eds. *Frontiers in headache research*. vol 2. *5-Hydroxytryptamine mechanism in primary headaches*. Philadelphia: Lippincott–Raven, 1992:118–128.
3. Eide PK, Hole K. Review: the role of 5-hydroxytryptamine (5-HT) receptor subtypes and plasticity in the regulation of nociceptive sensitivity. *Cephalalgia* 1993;13:75–85.
4. Sandrini G, Alfonsi G, Pavesi G, et al. Corneal reflex and pain perception in cluster headache. In: Rose C, ed. *New advances in headache research and therapy*. London: Smith and Gordon, 1989: 209–212.
5. Headache Classification Committee of the International Headache Society. Classification and diagnostic criteria for headache disorders, cranial neuralgias and facial pain. *Cephalalgia* 1988;8[Suppl 7]:1–96.
6. Suckow RF, Cooper TB, Kahn RS. HPLC methods for the analysis of plasma m-CPP. *J Chromatography* 1990;528:228–234.
7. Fiorella D, Rabin RA, Winter JC. The role of the 5-HT2A and 5-HT2C receptors in the stimulus effects of m-chlorophenylpiperazine. *Psychopharmacology* 1995;119:222–230.
8. Lee MA, Nash JF, Barnes M, Meltzer HY. Inhibitory effects of ritanserin on the 5-hydroxytrypto-

phan-mediated cortisol, ACTH and prolactin secretion in humans. *Psychopharmacology* 1991;103: 258–264.
9. Gordon M, Lipton RB, Brown SL, et al. Headache and cortisol responses to m-chlorophenylpiperazine are highly correlated. *Cephalalgia* 1993;13:400–405.
10. Olesen J, Thomsen LL, Lassen LH, Jansen-Olesen I. The nitric oxide hypothesis of migraine and other vascular headaches. *Cephalalgia* 1995;15:94–100.
11. Fozard JR. 5-Hydroxytryptamine and nitric oxide: the causal relationship between two endogenous precipitants of migraine. In: Sandler M, Ferrari M, Harnett S, eds. *Migraine: Pharmacology and genetics*. London: Chapman & Hall, 1996:167–179.

ary: Monoamines, Neuropeptides, Purines, and Nitric Oxide*, edited by J. Olesen and L. Edvinsson.
Lippincott–Raven Publishers, Philadelphia © 1997.

25

Discussion Summary: Involvement of Amines and Amino Acids in Primary Headache

James W. Lance

Institute of Neurological Sciences, Wales Medical Center, Randwick, New South Wales 2031, Australia

Many studies aimed at elucidating the pathophysiology of migraine over the past 30 years have relied on biochemical investigations of blood platelets, plasma, or serum. The most robust of all these findings has been the discovery that platelets discharge their content of serotonin [5-hydroxytryptamine (5-HT)] at the onset of a migraine attack and that free serotonin increases in the plasma. Other studies have shown elevation of aspartic and glutamic acid and a decrease in the level of γ-aminobutyric acid (GABA). Catecholamine studies have given variable results and do not permit a consistent interpretation. There was general discussion about the relevance of blood studies to changes in the central nervous system, with agreement that platelets themselves played no part in the pathophysiology of headache.

Fenfluramine, a 5-HT-releasing agent, induces migraine headaches, an effect correlated with release of prolactin into the plasma, unlike the headaches induced by red wine. This is consistent with a hypothalamic action inducing migraine. *m*-Chlorophenylpiperazine (m-CPP), a central serotonin agonist, induced cluster headache in 9 of 23 episodic cluster headache patients, those in whom m-CPP levels remain high 90 minutes after administration. Prolactin levels increased from a reduced baseline level to an elevated level after m-CPP but were not significantly higher in those patients who developed headache. The base level of cortisol, which was elevated, fell after m-CPP. This finding suggests precipitation of cluster headache through a serotonergic hypothalamic mechanism. The concentration of serotonin around the superficial temporal artery was found to be elevated in cluster headache. Studies of arteries taken from patients with episodic cluster headache showed that 5-HT causes rhythmic contractions instead of the usual dose-dependent constriction.

Estimations of platelet and plasma 5-HT in tension-type headache have produced conflicting results, possibly because some patients examined had 15 or more headaches in a month but nevertheless had had days of headache freedom, while other patients studied suffered chronic daily headache with no remission. The finding of a low platelet content of 5-HT in chronic tension-type headache may be related to the daily ingestion of analgesics or ergotamine rather than the chronic daily headache itself. There is some evidence for sympathetic hypofunction in tension-type headache, migraine, and cluster headache patients even in headache-free intervals. The 5-HT$_{2B/2C}$ agonist m-CPP induces migraine-like headaches as well as cluster headaches, and antagonists of those receptors have been used in prophylaxis. Administration of m-CPP to rats did not increase Fos expression in the trigeminal nucleus, whereas electrical stimulation of the trigeminal ganglion caused a marked increase in Fos. This finding indicates that peripheral stimulation of 5-HT$_{2B/2C}$ receptors did not stimulate pain fibers. The fact that m-CPP induces migraine in human subjects suggests that a central mechanism is involved.

Histamine is released from rat dural mast cells by 48/80, substance P (SP), and calcitonin gene-related peptide (CGRP), the effect of the latter two agents being blocked by SP and CGRP receptor antagonists; neuropeptide Y and vasoactive intestinal peptide had little effect. Histamine release correlated with maximum dilation of the blood vesssels. The relevance of this to migraine is uncertain because similar changes could not be demonstrated in human dural mast cells.

A wide range of variability in response of human pial arteries to 5-HT, CGRP, SP, histamine, and sumatriptan has been demonstrated; for example, vascular constriction after administration of sumatriptan varied from 59% to 79% of potassium-induced constriction. Arteries from human omentum were constricted by noradrenaline in a concentration-dependent manner similar to responses previously demonstrated in human temporal arteries. Here too there was a wide variability in that the EC$_{max}$ ranged from 3% to 200% of the maximal potassium-induced constriction.

Electrical stimulation of dural vessels in the rat through a bony window induced dilation that was mediated by the release of CGRP, as the administration of a CGRP antagonist diminished the response by 81%. Since sumatriptan diminished the same response by 50%, it appears that sumatriptan partially blocks CGRP release, probably by acting on prejunctional receptors on trigeminal nerve endings. No direct constriction of the vessels was observed when sumatriptan was administered intravenously. Substance P produced dilation of the dural vessels, but this effect was largely blocked by a neurokinin 1 receptor antagonist, whereas this agent had no effect at all on the dilation induced by electrical stimulation. In the experimental model of Moskowitz, whereby stimulation of the trigeminal system in the rat produces extravasation of protein from dural vessels by antidromic release of peptides, CP 122,288 blocks extravasation with an IC$_{50}$ of 0.3 ng/kg i.v. However, it is much less effective in the electrical stimulation model, in which CP 122,288 does not inhibit the neurogenic vasodilation mediated by CGRP until a dose of more than 3 mg/kg i.v. is administered. This activity is in line with its affinity at 5-HT$_{1B/1D}$ receptors, which is comparable with the effect of sumatriptan and is in the same dose range, as it is active as a vasoconstrictor. Clinical trial results of CP 122,288 are eagerly awaited as a guide to the pathological mechanism responsible for the vasodilation of migraine headache.

In studies of human coronary artery strips, the constriction produced by 5-HT is mediated by $5\text{-}HT_2$ and $5\text{-}HT_{1B/1D}$ receptors. The latter are stimulated by sumatriptan, which causes some 40% of the constriction produced by 5-HT. This confirms earlier work. Nevertheless, sumatriptan produces only about 20% of the maximal constriction of the coronary arteries produced by thromboxane A2. In vivo studies of coronary arteries have shown a 14% reduction in diameter caused by therapeutic doses of sumatriptan. The receptors in platelets are of the $5\text{-}HT_2$ subtype and are not altered by administration of sumatriptan. The direct injection of sumatriptan into the guinea pig brain stimulates $5\text{-}HT_{1B/1D}$ autoreceptors and thus inhibits the release of 5-HT in the central nervous system but has no central effect when given intravenously. The prophylactic action of valproate is probably achieved by increasing GABA synthesis, but 5-HT levels are increased in parts of the central nervous system such as the hippocampus and basal ganglia. The effect of the newer anticonvulsants has yet to be assessed, but lamotrigine does not appear to have any preventive action in migraine. There are uncontrolled reports that gabapentin may be useful, and vigabatrin is also being studied.

SECTION V

Involvement of Neuropeptides in Primary Headaches

26
Opioid Peptides in Primary Headaches

Flemming W. Bach

Department of Neurology, The National University Hospital, Rigshospitalet, DK-2100 Copenhagen, Denmark

The discovery of the endogenous opioid peptides and their receptors in the 1970s was followed by a mass of literature aiming to relate changes in the function of these systems to pain. Mostly because of the hypotheses of Federigo Sicuteri (1), headache disorders are probably the most extensively studied group of painful conditions. He emphasized that hypernociception, anhedonia, and dysautonomia occur in both primary headaches and morphine abstinence; based on these similarities, he speculated that migraine is a "hypoendorphin syndrome" (1). This idea initiated a series of studies using the approach of measuring endogenous opioid peptides first in plasma, then in cerebrospinal fluid (CSF), and recently in immune cells. This chapter will review these studies in a critical light from the perspective of what may be learned about headache mechanisms from the data.

ENDOGENOUS OPIOID PEPTIDES

Traditionally, the endogenous opioid peptides are divided into three groups or families, the endorphins, enkephalins, and dynorphins. This classification is mainly based on the production of the peptides from three different genes and protein precursors (Table 1), but it is also meaningful because of different anatomy and binding properties to different opioid receptors. Before evaluating studies presenting measurements of concentrations of endogenous opioid peptides in relation to headache, it seems relevant to summarize the location and physiology of endogenous opioid peptides.

Studies on headache patients have focused on β-endorphin, Met-enkephalin, and dynorphin. β-Endorphin is found in highest concentrations in the anterior pituitary, and almost all β-endorphin circulating in the blood is secreted by the pituitary (2,3). Concentrations of β-endorphin in plasma do not correlate with those in CSF (3,4), β-endorphin administered intravenously is not analgesic centrally (5) or in the periphery (6), and plasma concentrations of β-endorphin do not correlate with pain perception (7). Thus, it is unlikely that circulating β-endorphin is directly involved in pain

TABLE 1. *Schematic table of the opioid peptides studied in humans with headache*

	Endorphins	Enkephalins	Dynorphins
Precursor	Propiomelanocortin	Proenkephalin	Prodynorphin
Major peptide	β-Endorphin	Met-enkephalin	Dynorphin A
Receptor	μ+δ	δ	κ
Antagonist	Naloxone	Naloxone	Naloxone

modulation. β-Endorphin located within the brain, on the other hand, is closely connected to pain-modulating pathways, especially in the midbrain (8), and is anatomically relatively simple, since almost all cell bodies containing β-endorphin are located in the arcuate nucleus of the hypothalamus (9). It is therefore of considerable interest to establish methods for monitoring the activity of β-endorphin neurons in the brain, and measurement of β-endorphin in the CSF is a tempting choice. Polypeptides are freely interchangable between the extracellular fluid of brain and the CSF, and many β-endorphin-containing nerve terminals are located near the ependyma (10). We have shown that β-endorphin is stable in human CSF (11) and that β-endorphin concentrations in lumbar CSF samples correlate with those in ventricular CSF in certain individuals (12). Finally, it has been suggested that β-endorphin is released from immune cells in inflamed tissue and subsequently binds to opioid receptors on primary sensory neurons (13).

Met-enkephalin is widely distributed both within the central nervous system (CNS) and in the periphery. The adrenal medulla contains large amounts of Met-enkephalin co-stored with catecholamines, and a significant amount of circulating Met-enkephalin may be secreted from that organ, although other sources are equally important. Physiological or pathophysiological roles of circulating Met-enkephalin remain to be established (14). Platelets carry Met-enkephalin in quantities much larger than plasma (partially co-stored with serotonin), and this creates considerable problems for analytical procedures and interpretations, like the problems with serotonin discussed in the chapter by Glover. As would be expected from its wide distribution in the brain and spinal cord, Met-enkephalin is also present in CSF. The more dispersed localization of Met-enkephalin makes it more difficult to relate changes in CSF concentrations of Met-enkephalin to altered activity in a specific subset of neurons than in the case of β-endorphin, for example, but in vivo release of Met-enkephalin to CSF by electrical stimulation of nerve fibers and brain regions has been shown (15,16). Met-enkephalin is also present in immune cells in peripheral tissues and may have a role in peripheral opioid analgesia.

Dynorphin has been less studied than the other peptides. It is present in plasma only in very small quantities, and exact characterization of the peptide fragments present is lacking (14). More work has been done on CSF. Although it is less widely distributed in the CNS than Met-enkephalin, the same considerations about uncertainty of site of secretion goes for dynorphin. Dynorphin has not been found in immune cells.

Some important aspects of measurement in biological fluids are common for the opioid peptides. Since this is the subject of Chapter 2 of this text, it will only be touched on briefly. All opioid peptides are processed from larger precursors by cleavage at dibasic amino acid pairs and may be secreted from cells along with peptide fragments less or more processed. Apart from further cleavage, modification may occur by acetylation of the N terminal, for example, which renders the peptide without opioid activity. As a consequence, it is necessary to characterize the composition of immunoreactive fragments of the peptides in a biological fluid to ensure the specificity of a given assay. Examinations of CSF by antibodies against peptides from all three endorphin families have shown the presence of multiple immunoreactive fragments (11,17,18). Since the processing patterns may vary between compartments, it may be necessary to use different antisera for analysis of different fluids (19). Many peptides are unstable in biological fluids because of the presence of degrading enzymes, which may call for stabilizing additives to the samples. These and other factors may be responsible for some of the differences in results obtained by different groups in the clinical studies referred to in the following discussion.

PLASMA CONCENTRATIONS OF OPIOID PEPTIDES DURING HEADACHE

Following some early studies of opioid activity in plasma using receptor binding assays, the first studies employing more specific radioimmunoassays appeared (20). Unfortunately, the results have not been entirely uniform. Most studies found that patients with migraine have plasma levels of β-endorphin similar to those of control persons (21–24). One group found reduced levels in patients with aura (23). Another study found lower β-endorphin concentrations during attacks than in other patients out of attacks (22), whereas a study in which paired samples were obtained from the same individuals revealed unchanged levels during attack (21). Patients with daily chronic or chronic tension-type headache were reported to have reduced (22,25) or normal (4,23) β-endorphin concentrations, whereas normal β-endorphin concentrations were found in cluster headache and secondary headaches (24).

Plasma levels of Met-enkephalin have been examined by several groups, who met the obstacles of high content of Met-enkephalin in platelets and poor stability of the peptide. Methodological differences are likely to account for some differences in the results, but the major results were that in migraine patients, concentrations of Met-enkephalin were increased in platelets but decreased in plasma. The concentrations increased in both compartments during attack. On the other hand, patients with tension headache revealed decreased levels in platelets and increased levels in plasma (26,27). Plasma Met-enkephalin concentrations increased tenfold during attack in cluster headache (28). Few data are available on dynorphin in plasma. No change in dynorphin immunoreactivity was seen during migraine attacks (29).

Now, what is learned from these examinations of plasma? Probably not much! First, it must be emphasized that the peptides do not cross the blood-brain barrier and do not act directly on central pathways. Second, it still remains to be shown that circulating opioid peptides may influence peripheral pain mechanisms or vascular headache mechanisms. It is possible that the changes from normal described above are results of primary or secondary events during headache, and they may thus serve as markers of more or less specific pathophysiological events during headache.

CEREBROSPINAL FLUID CONCENTRATIONS OF OPIOID PEPTIDES DURING HEADACHE

β-Endorphin has been measured in lumbar CSF in most headache syndromes. Much lower than normal concentrations were found in patients with migraine with interval headache (24). Similar low levels of β-endorphin were found in migraine without aura, whereas patients with symptomatic (post-traumatic and ischemic cerebrovascular) headaches revealed normal concentrations (24). These data received some support in a quite spectacular recent study in which suboccipital CSF was obtained from nine patients during an attack of migraine without aura (30). These patients had a significantly lower mean β-endorphin concentration in suboccipital CSF than 11 patients suffering from epilepsy or neurosis, whereas the mean concentration of 13 patients with migraine without aura outside attack was intermediate, not significantly different from either of the other groups. On the other hand, our study, including 47 patients with chronic tension-type headache without interval migraine, showed almost identical lumbar CSF β-endorphin levels as the control group (4), and the levels were not affected by treatment with sulpiride or paroxetine (31).

It is possible that the low β-endorphin concentrations found by Nappi et al. (24) are related more to migraine than to tension headache. Recently, the same group repeated their study on 15 patients in the same category, finding a smaller but still significant difference from controls (32). However, this time N-acetylated-β-endorphin was also measured. Interestingly, this opioid-inactive derivative of β-endorphin was present in higher concentrations in patients than controls, leading to a clearly lower ratio between N-acetylated-β-endorphin and β-endorphin in migraine with interval chronic tension headache. The authors suggest that inappropriately high biological inactivation of β-endorphin may be a pathogenetic factor in chronic headache of this type, which is supported by the finding of a negative relation between CSF β-endorphin and a headache index (32). The CSF β-endorphin levels in cluster headache patients were not different from those in control persons (33).

Met-enkephalin has not been studied in CSF with specific radioimmunoassays. An early study using a rather nonspecific receptor assay concluded that migraine patients had low Met-enkephalin levels (20). The CSF from 48 patients of the same group with chronic tension-type headache examined for β-endorphin by Bach et al. (4) revealed a higher mean concentration of Met-enkephalin than 48 controls (34). Similar results were obtained in a study on fibromyalgia (35). Significantly reduced levels of Met-enkephalin were found in cluster headache (33).

Dynorphin immunoreactivity was measured in our patients with chronic tension-type headache. We found a slight, but significant, reduction from the control level

(31). Another study found reduced dynorphin concentrations in patients with idiopathic pain syndromes (36). Based on (a) the access of opioid peptides in the brain to opioid receptors involved in modulation of pain (37), and (b) the demonstrated reflection in CSF of opioid peptides released within the brain (15,16,38), it is reasonable to see concentrations of endogenous opioid peptides measured in lumbar CSF as markers of the level of activity of central opioid neuronal systems. The data obtained in patients with primary headaches are not conclusive, but it is fair to say that there may be some headache conditions (migraine with interval headache) in which the endogenous opioid systems are disrupted. Whether this is a primary or secondary event with regard to pathogenesis remains to be established.

CONCENTRATIONS OF OPIOID PEPTIDES IN IMMUNE CELLS DURING HEADACHE

β-Endorphin immunoreactivity has been demonstrated in peripheral blood mononuclear cells, and concentrations of β-endorphin immunoreactivity per cell have been measured in primary headaches, which brings headache into the exciting new field of the interactions between the immune system and the nervous system. Patients with migraine, with or without aura, had reduced β-endorphin levels compared with healthy control persons and patients with episodic tension-type headache (39). The same group found reduced β-endorphin levels in patients with cluster headache during and outside attacks (40). The authors postulate that these changes of β-endorphin content in immune cells are markers of the levels in the brain based on similar changes in CSF concentrations. However, this has not been studied in individual patients, and several discordances weaken this speculation (41).

Met-enkephalin has been measured in neutrophil granulocytes during cluster headaches showing reduced levels during the pain phase and higher than normal levels in pain-free periods (42). The significance of these changes in immune cells is still unclear, but this phenomenon represents an interesting new approach in the study of headache.

NALOXONE IN HEADACHE

To answer the question of whether endogenous opioid peptides are involved in headache, the straightforward thing to do would of course be to administer naloxone. An increased opioid tonus would then show up as an increase in pain, whereas a decreased tonus (which is the primary hypothesis) would not necessarily be recognized. Naloxone did not change pain during migraine attacks (43) or chronic tension-type headache (44) but did reduce the pain tolerance in an ischemic test during migraine attack (45). The latter authors propose that this finding reflects a release of opioids during migraine attack. Facchinetti et al. (46) used the amount of luteinizing hormone (LH) secreted in response to a naloxone injection as a measure of antagonized endogenous opioid inhibition in the hypothalamus. Interestingly, patients with migraine without aura and those with migraine with interval headache showed low LH responses, pointing toward low central opioid activity, which is in good accordance with the β-endorphin findings in CSF made by the same group (24). The unknown dose-response relationships and the opioid receptor multiplicity are factors that make interpretations of naloxone experiments somewhat troublesome.

CONCLUSIONS

The efforts during the last 15 years to confirm the "endorphin theory" of headache have provided us with much new information about endogenous opioid peptides in humans, but it has not been possible to place the peptides in a well-defined and clear pathophysiological role. The involvement of endogenous opioid peptides in the control of headache (as of pain in general) remains uncertain, and it is unlikely that reduced activity of opioid peptides is the primary factor in any form of primary headache. The data presented in this chapter, however, do indicate that primary headaches may exist in which one or more opioid systems are disrupted. New possibilities and perspectives are provided now by advances in molecular biology, for example, by the availability of mice without the μ-receptor (47). Animal models of headache mechanisms should be applied using these mice.

REFERENCES

1. Sicuteri F. Natural opioids in migraine. In: Critchley M, Friedman A, Gorini S, Sicuteri F, eds. *Headache: physiopathological and clinical concepts.* Philadelphia: Lippincott–Raven, 1982:65–74. (*Advances in neurology*; vol 33).
2. Kerdelhue B, Bethea CL, Ling N, Chrétien M, Weiner RI. β-Endorphin concentrations in serum, hypothalamus and central gray of hypophysectomized and mediobasal hypothalamus lesioned rats. *Brain Res* 1982;231:85–91.
3. Schlachter LB, Wardlaw SL, Tindall GT, Frantz AG. Persistence of β-endorphin in human cerebrospinal fluid after hypophysectomy. *J Clin Endocrinol Metab* 1983;57:221–224.
4. Bach FW, Langemark M, Secher NH, Olesen J. Plasma and cerebrospinal fluid β-endorphin during chronic tension-type headache. *Pain* 1992;51:163–168.
5. Foley KM, Kourides IA, Inturrisi CE, et al. β-Endorphin: analgesic and hormonal effects in humans. *Proc Natl Acad Sci USA* 1979;76:5377–5381.
6. Parsons CG, Czlonkowski A, Stein C, Herz A. Peripheral opioid receptors mediating antinociception in inflammation. Activation by endogenous opioids and role of the pituitary-adrenal axis. *Pain* 1990; 41:81–93.
7. Bach FW, Fahrenkrug J, Jensen K, Dahlstrøm G, Ekman R. Plasma β-endorphin during clinical and experimental ischaemic pain. *Scand J Clin Lab Invest* 1987;47:751–758.
8. Pilcher HP, Joseph SA, McDonald JV. Immunocytochemical localization of pro-opiomelanocortin neurons in human brain areas subserving stimulation analgesia. *J Neurosurg* 1988;68:621–629.
9. Bloom F, Battenberg E, Rossier J, Ling N, Guillemin R. Neurons containing beta-endorphin in rat brain exist separately from those containing enkephalin: immunocytochemical studies. *Proc Natl Acad Sci USA* 1978;75:1591–1595.
10. Stengaard-Pedersen K, Larsson L-I. Comparative immunocytochemical localization of putative opioid ligands in the central nervous system. *Histochemistry* 1981;73:89–114.
11. Bach FW, Ekman R, Jensen FM. β-Endorphin-immunoreactive components in human cerebrospinal fluid. *Regul Pept* 1986;16:189–198.

12. Bach FW, Schmidt JF, Faber T. Radioimmunoassay of β-endorphin in ventricular and lumbar cerebrospinal fluid. *Clin Chem* 1992;38:847–852.
13. Stein C, Hassan AHS, Gramsch C, Herz A. Local opioid receptors mediating antinociception in inflammation: endogenous ligands. In: Bond MR, Charlton JE, Woolf CJ, eds. *Proceedings of the VIth World Congress on Pain*. Amsterdam: Elsevier, 1991:83–87. (*Pain research and clinical management*; vol 4).
14. McLoughlin L, Medbak S, Grossman AB. Circulating opioids in man. In: Hertz A, ed. *Opioids II*. Berlin: Springer-Verlag, 1993:673–696. (Born GVR, Cuatrecasas P, Herken H, eds. *Handbook of experimental pharmacology*; vol 104/II).
15. Yaksh TL, Elde R. Factors governing release of methionine enkephalin-like immunoreactivity from mesencephalon and spinal cord of the cat in vivo. *J Neurophysiol* 1981;46:1056–1075.
16. Young RF, Bach FW, van Norman A, Yaksh TL. Release of β-endorphin and methionine-enkephalin into cerebrospinal fluid during deep brain stimulation for chronic pain: effects of stimulation locus and site of sampling. *J Neurosurg* 1993;79:816–825.
17. Nyberg F, Nylander I. Characterization of dynorphin A immunoreactivity in human cerebrospinal fluid. *Regul Pept* 1987;17:159–166.
18. Nyberg F, Nylander I, Terenius L. Enkephalin-containing polypeptide in human cerebrospinal fluid. *Brain Res* 1986;371:278–286.
19. Bach FW. Beta-endorphin-related peptides in human cerebrospinal fluid. In: Genazzani AR, Negri M, eds. *Opioid peptides in biological fluids*. Carnforth: Parthenon, 1989:17–25.
20. Anselmi B, Baldi E, Casacci F, Salmon S. Endogenous opioids in cerebrospinal fluid and blood in idiopathic headache sufferers. *Headache* 1980;20:294–299.
21. Bach FW, Jensen K, Blegvad N, Fenger M, Jordal R, Olesen J. β-Endorphin and ACTH in plasma during attacks of common and classic migraine. *Cephalalgia* 1985;5:177–182.
22. Baldi E, Salmon S, Anselmi B, et al. Intermittent hypoendorphinaemia in migraine attack. *Cephalalgia* 1982;2:77–81.
23. Fettes I, Gawel M, Kuzniak S, Edmeads J. Endorphin levels in headache syndromes. *Headache* 1985;25:37–39.
24. Nappi G, Facchinetti F, Martignoni E, et al. Plasma and CSF endorphin levels in primary and symptomatic headaches. *Headache* 1985;25:141–144.
25. Facchinetti F, Nappi G, Savoldi F, Genazzani AR. Primary headaches: reduced circulating β-lipotropin and β-endorphin levels with impaired reactivity to acupuncture. *Cephalalgia* 1981;1:195–201.
26. Ferrari MD, Odink J, Fršlich M, Portielje JEA, Bruyn GW. Methionine-enkephalin in migraine and tension headache. Differences between classic migraine, common migraine and tension headache, and changes during attacks. *Headache* 1990;30:160–164.
27. Mosnaim AD, Wolf ME, Chevesich J, Callaghan OH, Diamond S. Plasma methionine levels. A biological marker for migraine? *Headache* 1985;25:259–261.
28. Figuerola ML, Vindrola O, Barontini MB, Leston JA. Increase in plasma methionine-enkephalin levels during the pain attack in episodic cluster headache. *Cephalalgia* 1990;10:251–257.
29. Bach FW, Jensen K, Ekman R, Olesen J. Dynorphin-immunoreactivity in plasma during migraine attacks. *Cephalalgia* 1987;7[Suppl 6]:232–233.
30. Vécsei L, Widerlšv E, Ekman R, et al. Suboccipital cerebrospinal fluid and plasma concentrations of somatostatin, neuropeptide Y and beta-endorphin in patients with common migraine. *Neuropeptides* 1992;22:111–116.
31. Bach FW, Langemark M, Ekman R, Rehfeld JF, Schifter S, Olesen J. Effect of sulpiride or paroxetine on cerebrospinal fluid neuropeptide concentrations in patients with chronic tension-type headache. *Neuropeptides* 1994;27:129–136.
32. Facchinetti F, Sances G, Martignoni E, Pagani I, Nappi G, Genazzani AR. Evidence of alpha,N-acetyl β-endorphin in human cerebrospinal fluid. *Brain Res* 1992;586:1–5.
33. Hardebo JE, Ekman R, Eriksson M. Low CSF met-enkephalin levels in cluster headache are elevated by acupuncture. *Headache* 1989;29:494–497.
34. Langemark M, Bach FW, Ekman R, Olesen J. Increased cerebrospinal fluid met-enkephalin-immunoreactivity in patients with chronic-tension-type headache. *Pain* 1993;.63:103–107.
35. Vaerøy H, Nyberg F, Terenius L. No evidence for endorphin deficiency in fibromyalgia following investigation of cerebrospinal fluid (CSF) dynorphin A and Met-enkephalin-Arg6-Phe7. *Pain* 1991;46:139–143.

36. Von Knorring L, Almay BLG, Ekman R, Widerlöv E. Biological markers in chronic pain syndromes. *Nord Psykiatr Tidsskr* 1988;42:139–145.
37. Fields HL, Heinricher MM, Mason P. Neurotransmitters in nociceptive modulatory circuits. *Annu Rev Neurosci* 1991;14:219–245.
38. Bach FW, Yaksh TL. Release of β-endorphin immunoreactivity into ventriculo-cisternal perfusate by lumbar intrathecal capsaicin in the rat. *Brain Res* 1995;701:192–200.
39. Leone ML, Sacerdote P, D'Amico D, Panerai AE, Bussone G. Beta-endorphin concentrations in the peripheral blood mononuclear cells of migraine and tension-type headache patients. *Cephalalgia* 1992;12:155–157.
40. Leone ML, Sacerdote P, D'Amico D, Panerai AE, Bussone G. Beta-endorphin levels are reduced in peripheral blood cells of cluster headache patients. *Cephalalgia* 1993;13:413–416.
41. Bach FW. β-Endorphin and migraine. *Cephalalgia* 1992;12:390.
42. Figuerola ML, Vindrola O, Barontini MB, Leston JA. Changes in neutrofil met-enkephalin containing peptides in episodic cluster headache. *Headache* 1991;31:406–408.
43. Sicuteri F, Boccuni M, Fanciullacci M, Gatto G. Naloxone effectiveness on spontaneous and induced perceptive disorders in migraine. *Headache* 1983;23:179–183.
44. Langemark M. Naloxone in moderate doses does not aggravate chronic tension headache. *Pain* 1989;39:85–93.
45. Steardo L, Barone P, diStasio E, Bonuso S. Headache patients: different responses induced by naloxone during work-test. *Cephalalgia* 1982;2:151–156.
46. Facchinetti F, Martignoni E, Gallai V, et al. Neuroendocrine evaluation of central opiate activity in primary headache disorders. *Pain* 1988;34:29–33.
47. Matthes HWD, Maldonado R, Simonin F, et al. Loss of morphine-induced analgesia, reward effect and withdrawal symptoms in mice lacking the μ-opioid-receptor gene. *Nature* 1996;383:819–823.

Headache Pathogenesis: Monoamines, Neuropeptides, Purines, and Nitric Oxide, edited by J. Olesen and L. Edvinsson.
Lippincott–Raven Publishers, Philadelphia © 1997.

27

Nonopioid Peptides in Migraine and Cluster Headache

Peter J. Goadsby

Institute of Neurology, The National Hospital for Neurology and Neurosurgery, London WC1N 3BG, United Kingdom

Migraine has plagued humans for more than 20 centuries (1), and cluster headache has been recognized for at least 250 years (2). For many years it was held that migraine was a mainly vascular problem (3), but views are shifting (4) as the pathophysiology of migraine becomes better understood. In this review I shall highlight the contribution that the study of nonopioid peptides has made to our understanding of the neurobiology of migraine and cluster headache.

ANATOMY OF THE CRANIOVASCULAR PEPTIDERGIC INNERVATION

To place the data in context, it is important to have some understanding of the neural pathways pertaining to the extrinsic (to the brain) neural innervation of the large cerebral and extracerebral vessels including the pain-producing intracranial venous sinuses. This in part stems from the strong clinical impression that the vessels, or at least their innervation, are in some way involved in the disease (5–7).

Broadly speaking, the innervation of the cerebral circulation is divided into intrinsic and extrinsic neural systems. The intrinsic systems are those that commence within and do not exit the central nervous system, innervating intraparenchymal vessels. Many such systems have been described and are under active investigation (8). Their peptide content is not completely determined; they fall outside the scope of this text and are covered more completely elsewhere (9). The extrinsic system consists of neurons whose pathways ultimately commence in the central nervous system and then exit synapsing outside the central nervous system in ganglia to innervate target vessels. Three systems have been well described: the sympathetic system, the parasympathetic system, and the trigeminal system. Each is defined anatomically and marked by neuropeptides that give clues to their possible normal function and role in pathology.

Sympathetic Nerves

The sympathetic system arises in hypothalamic neurons passing to the intermediolateral cell column of the spinal cord and synapsing before proceeding out to the superior cervical ganglion. Here they again synapse and give rise to the fibers that innervate the vessels. This system is marked by the transmitters or modulator substances noradrenaline and neuropeptide Y (NPY). It is fundamentally a vasoconstrictor pathway (10).

Parasympathetic Nerves

The parasympathetic system arises from cell bodies in the superior salivatory nucleus (11), passing out with fibers of the facial nerve (seventh cranial nerve) (12) and synapsing in the sphenopalatine and otic ganglia (13). In some species there are additional microganglia on the internal carotid artery (14). This system is marked by the neurotransmitters acetylcholine, vasoactive intestinal polypeptide (VIP) (15), peptide histidine isoleucine (methionine) (16), and helospectin-like peptides (17); the ganglia contain nitric oxide synthase (18). This system is physiologically a vasodilator system (19).

Trigeminal Nerve

There is a sensory innervation of the cranial vessels and dura mater from the trigeminal system. The cell bodies are bipolar and located in the trigeminal ganglion. They make functional second-order connections with neurons in the trigeminal nucleus caudalis and dorsal horn neurons at the level of the C1 and C2 cervical spinal cord (20,21). This system is marked by the peptides calcitonin gene-related peptide (CGRP), substance P (SP), and neurokinin A. It is also an essentially vasodilator system in addition to its primary sensory function.

NEUROPEPTIDE CHANGES IN EXPERIMENTAL ANIMALS

Neurogenic Inflammation

In a series of experiments Moskowitz's group have looked at changes in vascular permeability and ultrastructural changes in the dura mater of the rat associated with trigeminal ganglion stimulation (22). It has been demonstrated that trigeminal ganglion stimulation increases vascular permeability in the dura (23) and that there is coincident mast cell degranulation (24). Both these effects are blocked by the potent antimigraine drugs dihydroergotamine and sumatriptan (25). Furthermore, during trigeminal ganglion stimulation, CGRP levels are elevated in the superior sagittal sinus of the rat. This elevation is blocked again by acute-attack antimigraine drugs (26). Recent experimental and clinical data demonstrating that compounds active in the model of plasma extravasation, such as bosentan (27) and RPR100893 (28), are inactive in acute migraine attacks suggest that further aspects of the trigeminovascular system require explanation and exploration (27,29).

Trigeminovascular Studies

Trigeminal ganglion stimulation results in local (cranial) release of both CGRP and SP in the cat and in humans (30). Both CGRP and SP act as markers for trigeminal activation, which can clearly be seen in humans as well as experimental animals. Studies of trigeminal ganglion stimulation are hampered by the fact that the ganglion contains cell bodies of nociceptive neurons as well as those of proprioceptive, light, touch, and other sensory modalities. In short, the trigeminal ganglion has all the sensory modalities of the head and is thus nonspecific in respect to pain. Our studies have therefore turned to the superior sagittal sinus. This structure is pain producing in humans (6,31). It is clear from electrophysiological studies that most of the neurons excited by sinus stimulation are either nociceptive specific or of a wide dynamic range type (including a nociceptive component) (32). Sagittal sinus stimulation increases regional cerebral blood flow more than does trigeminal ganglion stimulation (33) and seems to activate preferentially the cerebral circulation compared with the extracerebral circulation (34). Sinus stimulation leads to the local release of both CGRP and VIP without changes in either SP or NPY (35). Trigeminal ganglion stimulation-evoked release of CGRP can be blocked by sumatriptan and dihydroergotamine (36), while VIP release through a central nervous system reflex is only blocked by centrally acting compounds such as zolmitriptan (37). It is of further interest that the novel, conformationally restricted analog of sumatriptan, which is so potent in the plasma extravasation model (38), is inactive in the blood flow changes seen with sagittal sinus stimulation in the cat (39).

NEUROPEPTIDE CHANGES IN HUMANS DURING HEADACHE

In a study of direct trigeminal ganglion activation in patients being treated for trigeminal neuralgia by thermocoagulation of the ganglion, facial flushing ipsilateral to the side of stimulation was noted. As this flush occurred, blood samples were taken from the external jugular vein and compared with samples taken immediately before coagulation. There was a marked increase of both CGRP and SP in the patients who flushed compared with the control precoagulation levels (30). We have similarly seen cutaneous flushing in a patient with triggerable pain in the trigeminal distribution with CGRP release to levels similar to those reported for trigeminal ganglion stimulation (40). A similar important contribution for facial blood flow has been reported in the rat (41). Furthermore, during subarachnoid hemorrhage, a painful cause of secondary headache, CGRP levels are raised, while CGRP is depleted from human vessels in patients who die (42).

MIGRAINE WITH AURA

Studies of migraine with aura have been conducted in which both cerebrospinal fluid and venous blood have been studied. Venous blood has been studied in the periphery and in the cranial circulation. Opioid peptides are covered elsewhere in this volume and are therefore not further considered. In peripheral blood, VIP and SP levels are not altered during headache (43). The often described premonitory symptoms of altered bladder habit, particularly increased urination, have led to the suggestion that these may reflect hypothalamic disturbance and therefore be a manifestation of an essentially central nervous system disorder (44). Vasopressin levels, however, are unchanged during headache (43). In a study of the cerebral venous outflow it has been shown that CGRP and VIP levels are not altered during headache, although in that study the numbers with headache were small (n = 3), and the baseline levels high with respect to the literature (45). For studies of cranial venous outflow, blood samples were drawn from the cubital fossa and the external jugular vein during headache. Using markers for the sympathetic (NPY), parasympathetic (VIP), and trigeminovascular systems (CGRP, SP), the patients were assessed. There were no changes in the peripheral blood in any of the peptides studied or in NPY, VIP, or SP in the external jugular blood. There were, however, marked increases in CGRP during migraine from control levels of 40 pmol/L to 91 ± 11 pmol/L during headache (46). In two patients with autonomic symptoms, similar to cluster headache patients, there were increases in VIP, but this was not significant for the whole group. These data were confirmed in a further series of patients who had blood sampling during headache and then after administration of sumatriptan. Remarkably, the CGRP levels returned to normal after administration of sumatriptan and successful amelioration of the headache (36). Recently, it has been reported that in addition to CGRP elevation there is elevation of another trigeminal marker peptide, neurokin A (47). The results of these studies are summarized in Table 1.

MIGRAINE WITHOUT AURA

A similar picture emerges for migraine without aura. Plasma levels of SP and VIP are normal both during an attack and interictally (43). Again, as with migraine with aura, plasma vasopressin levels are also unchanged during headache (43). Studies of the cerebrospinal fluid have been limited to demonstrating that there is no change in either SP or somatostatin during headache (48). Again, we have studied patients with migraine without aura during headache by sampling blood from the cubital fossa and external jugular vein (Table 1). As was the case with migraine with aura, substantial increases in CGRP levels were found only in the jugular blood, whereas no changes in substance P, VIP, or NPY were seen in either jugular or peripheral blood (46). Nicolodi and Del Bianco (49) used the relatively novel method of salivary sampling and examined peptide levels in association with migraine without aura. They saw increases in both SP and CGRP along with a reduction in VIP during headache (49).

TABLE 1. Peptide levels during migraine[a]

	Migraine	
Peptide	Aura	No aura
Trigeminal		
Substance P	N	N
CGRP	↑	↑
NKA	↑	↑
PACAP	?	?
Sympathetic		
Neuropeptide Y	N	N
Parasympathetic		
VIP	N	N
PHI(M)	?	?
Helospectin-like	?	?
Opioids		
β-Endorphin	N	N
Met-enkephalin	↑	↑
Others		
ACTH	N	N
Vasopressin	N	N

[a]Levels in plasma
ACTH, adrenocorticotrophin; CGRP, calcitonin gene-related peptide; N indicates the levels were within the normal range for the population studied; NKA, neurokinin A; PACAP, pituitary adenylate cyclase activating peptide; PHI(M), peptide histidine isoleucine [Methionine, PHI(M)]; VIP, vasoactive intestinal polypeptide; ↑, levels above normal; ?, data not available.

The differences in the changes seen with these techniques probably represents the different field of sampling. Whereas the cerebral circulation has a preferentially CGRP-rich trigeminal innervation, the innervation of the salivary glands is not similarly characterized (50). The changes in VIP suggest that some reflex, parasympathetically mediated event is also taking place, but this requires further investigation.

CLUSTER HEADACHE

Plasma levels of SP and somatostatin show only very modest change (51). Cerebrospinal fluid changes have been similar, with only changes in Met-enkephalin being noted reliably (52) (Table 2). Interestingly, both substance P and VIP levels are elevated in the saliva during headache. In a recent study of cluster headache patients during acute attacks it was shown that cranial venous outflow levels of CGRP and VIP are elevated. Furthermore, these are normalized after successful treatment with either oxygen or sumatriptan, whereas they are unaffected by opiate administration (53). It has also been demonstrated that such changes are only seen and triggerable during a cluster bout and not out of the bout (54). These findings indicate activation of the central and peripheral arms of the trigeminovascular reflex and

TABLE 2. *Peptide levels during cluster headache*

Peptide	Cluster headache		
	Plasma	CSF	Saliva
Trigeminal			
Substance P	N	N	↑
CGRP	↑	?	N
Sympathetic			
Neuropeptide Y	N	?	?
Parasympathetic			
VIP	↑	N	↑
Opioids			
β-Endorphin	↑	N	?
Met-enkephalin	↑	↑	?
Others			
Somatostatin	N	N	?

CGRP, calcitonin gene-related peptide; CSF, cerebrospinal fluid; N indicates the levels were within the normal range for the population studied; VIP, vasoactive intestinal polypeptide; ↑, levels above normal; ?, data not available.

underscore the importance of a full description of the physiological mechanisms involved in primary headache syndromes (8).

CONCLUSIONS

The study of neuropeptide levels in migraine and cluster headache has provided a clear link between the clinic and research work. It is essential to the field that markers for disease activity that are robust in humans and in experimental models be identified and explored to understand better the primary headaches. In migraine both with and without aura there are marked changes in cranial levels of CGRP, indicating activation of the trigeminal system. These levels are rendered normal by sumatriptan in association with the headache settling. Similarly, CGRP is released with trigeminal activation in animal studies, an effect that is also inhibited by sumatriptan. In cluster headache there is the trigeminal system (CGRP) and parasympathetic nerve (VIP) activation which is blocked with successful specific treatment. These data tell us that the models employed are at least usefully close to the pathways that are activated in primary vascular headache. They point out compounds of special interest that might act in the trigeminal nucleus; only more clinical data will determine if this interest is appropriate. Whether the animal models will be predictive and will contribute further to our understanding of the disease processes is yet to be seen.

ACKNOWLEDGMENTS

The author acknowledges the valuable collaboration of Lars Edvinsson, with whom all the cited studies have been conducted. The work of the author reported here has been supported by the Wellcome Trust and the Migraine Trust. P.J.G. is a Wellcome Senior Research Fellow.

REFERENCES

1. Lance JW. *Mechanism and management of headache*. 5th ed. London: Butterworth Scientific, 1993.
2. Isler H. Episodic cluster headache from a textbook of 1745: Van Swieten's classic description. *Cephalalgia* 1993;13:172–174.
3. Wolff HG. *Headache and other head pain*. New York: Oxford University Press, 1963.
4. Goadsby PJ, Olesen J. Migraine: diagnosis and treatment in the 1990's. *BMJ* 1996;312:1279–1282.
5. Penfield W. A contribution to the mechanism of intracranial pain. *Proc Assoc Res Nerv Mental Dis* 1934;15:399–415.
6. Feindel W, Penfield W, McNaughton F. The tentorial nerves and localisation of intracranial pain in man. *Neurology* 1960;10:555–563.
7. McNaughton FL, Feindel WH. Innervation of intracranial structures: a reappraisal. In: Rose FC, ed. *Physiological aspects of clinical neurology*. Oxford: Blackwell Scientific Publications, 1977:279–293.
8. Goadsby PJ, Lance JW. Brainstem effects on intra- and extracerebral circulations. Relation to migraine and cluster headache. In: Olesen J, Edvinsson L, eds. *Basic mechanisms of headache*. Amsterdam: Elsevier Science Publishers, 1988:413–427.
9. Edvinsson L, MacKenzie ET, McCulloch J. *Cerebral blood flow and metabolism*. Philadelphia: Lippincott–Raven, 1993.
10. Olesen J, Edvinsson L. *Basic mechanisms of headache*. Amsterdam: Elsevier Science Publishers, BV, 1988.
11. Spencer SE, Sawyer WB, Wada H, Platt KB, Loewy AD. CNS projections to the pterygopalatine parasympathetic preganglionic neurons in the rat: a retrograde transneuronal viral cell body labeling study. *Brain Res* 1990;534:149–169.
12. Chorobski J, Penfield W. Cerebral vasodilator nerves and their pathway from the medulla oblongata. *Arch Neurol Psychiatry* 1932;28:1257–1289.
13. Walters DW, Gillespie SA, Moskowitz M. Cerebrovascular projections from the sphenopalatine and otic ganglia to the middle cerebral artery of the cat. *Stroke* 1986;17:488–494.
14. Gibbins IL, Brayden JE, Bevan JA. Perivascular nerves with immunoreactivity to vasoactive intestinal polypeptide in cephalic arteries of the cat: distribution, possible origins and functional implications. *Neuroscience* 1984;13:1327–1346.
15. Larsson LI, Edvinsson L, Fahrenkrug J, et al. Immunohistochemical localization of a vasodilatory peptide (VIP) in cerebrovascular nerves. *Brain Res* 1976;113:400–404.
16. Edvinsson L, McCulloch J. Distribution and vasomotor effects of peptide HI (PHI) in feline cerebral blood vessels in vitro and in situ. *Regul Peptides* 1985;10:345–356.
17. Uddman R, Goadsby PJ, Jansen I, Edvinsson L. Helospectin-like peptides: immunohistochemical localization and effects on cat pial arteries and on cerebral blood flow. *J Cereb Blood Flow Metab* 1993;13[Suppl 1]:S206.
18. Goadsby PJ, Uddman R, Edvinsson L. Cerebral vasodilatation in the cat involves nitric oxide from parasympathetic nerves. *Brain Res* 1996;707:110–118.
19. Goadsby PJ. Characteristics of facial nerve elicited cerebral vasodilatation determined with laser Doppler flowmetry. *Am J Physiol* 1991;260:R255–R262.
20. Goadsby PJ, Zagami AS. Stimulation of the superior sagittal sinus increases metabolic activity and blood flow in certain regions of the brainstem and upper cervical spinal cord of the cat. *Brain* 1991;114:1001–1011.
21. Kaube H, Keay K, Hoskin KL, Bandler R, Goadsby PJ. Expression of c-fos-like immunoreactivity in the trigeminal nucleus caudalis and high cervical cord following stimulation of the sagittal sinus in the cat. *Brain Res* 1993;629:95–102.
22. Moskowitz MA, Cutrer FM. Sumatriptan: a receptor-targeted treatment for migraine. *Annu Rev Med* 1993;44:145–154.
23. Markowitz S, Saito K, Moskowitz MA. Neurogenically mediated leakage of plasma proteins occurs from blood vessels in dura mater but not brain. *J Neurosci* 1987;7:4129–4136.
24. Dimitriadou V, Buzzi MG, Moskowitz MA, Theoharides TC. Trigeminal sensory fiber stimulation

induces morphological changes reflecting secretion in rat dura mater mast cells. *Neuroscience* 1991; 44:97–112.
25. Buzzi MG, Moskowitz MA. The antimigraine drug, sumatriptan (GR43175), selectively blocks neurogenic plasma extravasation from blood vessels in dura mater. *Br J Pharmacol* 1990;99:202–206.
26. Buzzi MG, Moskowitz MA, Shimizu T, Heath HH. Dihydroergotamine and sumatriptan attenuate levels of CGRP in plasma in rat superior sagittal sinus during electrical stimulation of the trigeminal ganglion. *Neuropharmacology* 1991;30:1193–1200.
27. Brandli P, Loffler B-M, Breu V, Osterwalder R, Maire J-P, Clozel M. Role of endothelin in mediating neurogenic plasma extravasation in rat dura mater. *Pain* 1996;64:315–322.
28. Cutrer FM, Garret C, Moussaoui SM, Moskowitz MA. The non-peptide neurokinin-1 antagonist, RPR 100893, decreases c-fos expression in trigeminal nucleus caudalis following noxious chemical meningeal stimulation. *Neuroscience* 1995;64:741–750.
29. Diener HC. Substance-P antagonist RPR100893-201 is not effective in human migraine attacks. In: Olesen J, Tfelt-Hansen P, eds. *Proceedings of the VIth International Headache Research Symposium*, Copenhagen, 1996.
30. Goadsby PJ, Edvinsson L, Ekman R. Release of vasoactive peptides in the extracerebral circulation of man and the cat during activation of the trigeminovascular system. *Ann Neurol* 1988;23:193–196.
31. McNaughton FL. The innervation of the intracranial blood vessels and the dural sinuses. In: Cobb S, Frantz AM, Penfield W, Riley HA, eds. *The circulation of the brain and spinal cord*. New York: Hafner, 1966:178–200.
32. Goadsby PJ, Hoskin KL. Inhibition of trigeminal neurons by intravenous administration of the serotonin (5HT)-1-D receptor agonist zolmitriptan (311C90): are brain stem sites a therapeutic target in migraine? *Pain* 1996;67:355–359.
33. Lambert GA, Goadsby PJ, Zagami AS, Duckworth JW. Comparative effects of stimulation of the trigeminal ganglion and the superior sagittal sinus on cerebral blood flow and evoked potentials in the cat. *Brain Res* 1988;453:143–149.
34. Goadsby PJ, Hoskin KL, Knight YE, Butler P. Selective activation of the trigeminovascular system by stimulation of the superior sagittal sinus: cerebral vs extracerebral blood flow changes. *J Cereb Blood Flow Metab* 1995;15[Suppl 1]:S164.
35. Zagami AS, Goadsby PJ, Edvinsson L. Stimulation of the superior sagittal sinus in the cat causes release of vasoactive peptides. *Neuropeptides* 1990;16:69–75.
36. Goadsby PJ, Edvinsson L. The trigeminovascular system and migraine: studies characterising cerebrovascular and neuropeptide changes seen in man and cat. *Ann Neurol* 1993;33:48–56.
37. Goadsby PJ, Edvinsson L. Peripheral and central trigeminovascular activation in cat is blocked by the serotonin (5HT)-1D receptor agonist 311C90. *Headache* 1994;34:394–399.
38. Lee WS, Moskowitz MA. Conformationally restricted sumatriptan analogues, CP-122,288 and CP-122,638, exhibit enhanced potency against neurogenic inflammation in dura mater. *Brain Res* 1993; 626:303–305.
39. Goadsby PJ, Hoskin KL, Knight YE, Butler P. Sagittal sinus stimulation selectively increases cerebral blood flow compared to extracerebral blood flow in the anaesthetised cat. *Cephalalgia* 1996;16: 366.
40. Goadsby PJ, Edvinsson L, Ekman R. Cutaneous stimulation leading to facial flushing and release of calcitonin gene-related peptide. *Cephalalgia* 1992;12:53–56.
41. Escott KJ, Beattie DT, Connor HE, Brain SD. Trigeminal ganglion stimulation increases facial skin blood flow in the rat: a major role for calcitonin gene-related peptide. *Brain Res* 1995;669:93–99.
42. Edvinsson L, Juul R, Uddman R. Peptidergic innervation of the cerebral circulation. Role in subarachnoid hemorrhage in man. *Neurosurg Rev* 1990;13:265–272.
43. Blegvad N, Jensen K, Fahrenkrug J, Schaffalitzky de Muckadell OB, Olesen J. Plasma-VIP and substance-P during migraine-attack. *Cephalalgia* 1986;5[Suppl 2]:352–353.
44. Goadsby PJ. The challenge of headache for the nineties. *Cur Opin Neurol* 1994;7:255–282.
45. Friberg L, Olesen J, Olsen TS, Karle A, Ekman R, Fahrenkrug J. Absence of vasoactive peptide release from brain to cerebral circulation during onset of migraine with aura. *Cephalalgia* 1994;14:47–54.
46. Goadsby PJ, Edvinsson L, Ekman R. Vasoactive peptide release in the extracerebral circulation of humans during migraine headache. *Ann Neurol* 1990;28:183–187.
47. Gallai V, Sarchielli P, Floridi A, et al. Vasoactive peptides levels in the plasma of young migraine patients with and without aura assessed both interictally and ictally. *Cephalalgia* 1995;15:384–390.
48. Vecchiet L, Geppetti P, Marchionni A, Spillantini MG, Fanciullacci M, Sicuteri F. Cerebrospinal fluid (methionin^5)-enkephalin, substance P and somatostatin-like immunoreactivities in painful and

pain-less human diseases. In: Sicuteri F, Vecchiet L, Fanciullacci M, eds. *Trends in cluster headache.* Amsterdam: Exerpta Medica, 1987:135–143.
49. Nicolodi M, Del Bianco E. Sensory neuropeptides (substance P, calcitonin gene-related peptide) and vasoactive intestinal polypeptide in human saliva: their pattern in migraine and cluster headache. *Cephalalgia* 1990;10:39–50.
50. O'Connor TP, van der Kooy D. Enrichment of a vasoactive neuropeptide (calcitonin gene related peptide) in trigeminal sensory projection to the intracranial arteries. *J Neurosci* 1988;8:2468–2476.
51. Sicuteri F, Fanciullacci M, Geppetti P, Renzi D, Caleri D, Spillantini MG. Substance P mechanisms in cluster headache: evaluation in plasma and cerebrospinal fluid. *Cephalalgia* 1985;5:143–149.
52. Hardebo JE, Ekman R. Substance P and opioids in cluster headache. In: Sicuteri F, Vecchiet L, Fanciullacci M, eds. *Trends in cluster headache.* Amsterdam: Exerpta Medica, 1987:145–158.
53. Goadsby PJ, Edvinsson L. Human in vivo evidence for trigeminovascular activation in cluster headache. *Brain* 1994;117:427–434.
54. Fanciolacci M, Alessandri M, Figini M, Geppetti P, Michelacci S. Increases in plasma calcitonin gene-related peptide from extracerebral circulation during nitroglycerin-induced cluster headache attack. *Pain* 1995;60:119–123.

28

Increased Plasma Level of Endothelin-1 in Cluster Headache

Linda R. White, *Maurice B. Vincent, †Helene M. G. Arcanjo, †Paulo L. M. Araujo, Lars J. Stovner, and Jan Aasly

*Department of Neurology, University Hospital, N-7006 Trondheim, Norway; *Serviço de Neurologia, Hospital Universitário Clementino Fraga Filho, Rio de Janeiro, Brazil; and †Faculdad de Medicina, Universidade Federal do Rio de Janeiro, 21949-590 Rio de Janeiro, Brazil*

Endothelin 1 (ET 1) is the most powerful vasoconstrictor hitherto found. It is a potent constrictor of cerebral vessels and probably contributes to the control of vessel tone in the cerebral circulation (1). Under normal conditions, a low level of ET-1 can be detected in circulating plasma, but this level has been found to increase in certain pathological conditions, such as stroke (2), subarachnoid hemorrhage (3), and migraine (4,5). In the case of migraine, it is not yet known whether the increase in circulating endothelin is associated with the cerebral vasoconstriction accompanying attacks of migraine with aura, or whether it represents release from damaged endothelial cells. Even in the interictal period, migraineurs were found to have significantly higher endothelin levels than controls (4). However, an increased level of endothelin is not necessarily a factor of all headaches, as no such increase has been found in patients with tension-type headache (4).

This study was carried out to examine the circulating level of ET-1 in cluster headache, which, like migraine, is accompanied by vascular components (6). In contrast with migraine, however, the pain of cluster headache is excruciating. Blood sampling in this study was therefore not carried out during attacks, although all patients sampled were in a cluster headache bout. The results were compared with data obtained from migraineurs outside attack, from patients with chronic low back pain, and from healthy volunteers.

MATERIALS AND METHODS

Peripheral blood was collected from the cubital fossa of cluster headache patients in bout, but outside attack [n = 18; 15 with episodic attacks (12 male, 3 female) and 3 with chronic headache (3 males); mean age, 42 ± 13 years]; migraine patients outside attack (n = 18; 2 male, 16 female; 7 with aura, 11 without aura; mean age, 43 ±

11 years); patients from the ward with chronic low back pain (n = 9; 5 male, 4 female; mean age, 41 ± 19 years); and healthy volunteers (n = 18; 9 male, 9 female; mean age, 41 ± 8 years). All subjects gave informed consent. Headache diagnosis was made according to the classification criteria of the International Headache Society (7). All subjects were pain free, except for the patients with low back pain, all of whom had moderate to severe pain at the time of sampling. These were also the only patients taking drugs (sedative and/or regular analgesic).

The blood was collected from the antecubital vein into ethylenediamine tetraacetic acid vacutainers, which were immediately chilled on ice and centrifuged at 3,000g and 4°C for 20 minutes to obtain platelet-poor plasma. This was stored at –70°C until assayed for ET-1. The assay was carried out using a commercial enzyme immunoassay (R&D Systems Europe, UK) according to the manufacturer's instructions, except that after extraction of 1 mL plasma (1.5 mL acetone/1 M HCl/water, 40:1:5, followed by centrifugation at 1,500g and 4°C for 15 minutes), the supernatant was dried under a stream of nitrogen at 37°C (Techne Dri-block DB-3D sample concentrator), rather than by vacuum concentration. The intra-assay and interassay variations were 7% and 5%, respectively. Cross-reactivity for the assay was reported as 45% for ET-2 (< 20% of the ET-1 level in normal plasma) and 14% for ET-3 ($\approx$50% of the ET-1 level), with negligible cross-reactivity for big ET.

Data are expressed as the mean ± SD. Comparisons between groups were carried out using ANOVA and Newman-Keul's test, $p < 0.05$ being considered significant.

RESULTS

The results for ET-1 concentrations measured in the various samples are shown in Table 1. No difference was found between males (mean = 0.62 ± 0.16 pg mL^{-1}, n = 9) and females (mean = 0.57 ± 0.18 pg mL^{-1}, n = 9) in the control group. Values for all controls lay within the range cited by the manufacturer (0.3 to 0.9 pg mL^{-1}), as did the results obtained from all patients with low back pain and all but one of the migraine patients. The means for these groups were all similar. However, there was much greater variation among results from the cluster headache patients (range, 0.39 to 1.54 pg mL^{-1}), and the mean was statistically greater than the means for the other groups, $p = 0.001$ (Table 1).

TABLE 1. *Endothelin-1 plasma levels in controls, headache patients, and patients with chronic low back pain, as measured by enzyme immunoassay*

Group[a]	No.	Sex	ET-1 (pg · mL^{-1}) (mean±SD)
Control	18	9 M, 9 F	0.59±0.16
Migraine (7 MA, 11 MO)	18	2 M, 16 F	0.59±0.17
Cluster headache	18	15 M, 3 F	0.87±0.37*
Chronic low back pain	9	5 M, 4 F	0.54±0.18

[a]All headache patients were measured outside attack.
*ET-1, endothelin-1; MA, migraine with aura; MO, migraine without aura. Significantly different from all other groups (ANOVA+Newman-Keul's test), $p=0.001$.

DISCUSSION

The results indicate that the circulating level of ET-1 is elevated in cluster headache patients in bout, even outside attack. Previous studies have indicated that interictal migraine patients also have an increased plasma ET, though this result was not confirmed by the present study, in which migraineurs without attack had ET-1 levels similar to those of healthy controls and sufferers of low back pain (4). The reason for this discrepancy is not clear, but it may reflect differences in the assay procedures or slight differences in the specificities for ET isopeptides.

Previous data have shown that there is a substantial increase in circulating ET during the ictal period of migraine, with or without aura (4,5). By contrast, neither episodic nor chronic tension-type headache is associated with such changes in plasma ET-1 (4). It has been suggested that the increase in circulating ET during migraine may be due to changes in vascular tone or hemodynamic alterations, particularly during the initial phase of the attack (4,5). However, the stress of pain itself does not appear to influence the ET-1 level, either in the case of tension-type headache, or in the present results from patients with low back pain (4).

Recent data suggest that neither ET_A nor ET_B receptors are involved in cortical spreading depression, a phenomenon widely believed to underlie the aura of classic migraine (although it has not been implicated in cluster headache) (8). Similarly, a preliminary study has shown the mixed $ET_{A/B}$ antagonist bosentan to be ineffective for the acute treatment of migraine (9). The elevated levels of ET measured during migraine and between cluster headache attacks (this study) are not sufficient to induce vasomotor changes (4). It therefore seems more likely that if ET is involved in the pathophysiology of vascular headaches, it may be through potentiation of other vasoactive transmitter systems implicated in headache pathophysiology, such as 5-hydroxytryptamine or noradrenalin (4,10).

ACKNOWLEDGMENTS

We thank SINTEF-UNIMEDs Forskningsfond for financial support.

REFERENCES

1. Salom JB, Torregrosa, Alborch E. Endothelins and the cerebral circulation. *Cerebrovasc Brain Metab Rev* 1995;7:131–152.
2. Ziv I, Fleminger G, Djadetti MD, Achiron A, Melamed E, Sokolovsky M. Increased plasma endothelin-1 in acute ischemic stroke. *Stroke* 1992;23:1014–1016.
3. Suzuki R, Masaoka H, Hirata Y, Marumo F, Isotani E, Hirakawa K. The role of endothelin-1 in the origin of cerebral vasospasm in patients with aneurysmal subarachnoid hemorrhage. *J Neurosurg* 1992;77:96–100.
4. Gallai V, Sarchielli P, Firenze C, et al. Endothelin-1 in migraine and tension-type headache. *Acta Neurol Scand* 1994;89:47–55.
5. Färkkilä M, Palo J, Saijonmaa O, Fyhrquist F. Raised plasma endothelin during acute migraine attack. *Cephalagia* 1992;12:383–384.
6. Pareja JA, White LR, Sjaastad O. Pathophysiology of headaches with a prominent vascular component. *Pain Res Manage* 1996;1:93–108.

7. Headache Classification Committee of the International Headache Society. Classification and diagnostic criteria for headache disorders, cranial neuralgias and facial pain. *Cephalalgia* 1988;7[Suppl 8]:1–96.
8. Goadsby PJ, Adner M, Edvinsson L. Characterization of endothelin receptors in the cerebral vasculature and their lack of effect on spreading depression. *J Cereb Blood Flow Metab* 1996;16:698–704.
9. May A, Gijsman HJ, Wallnöffer A, Jones R, Diener HC, Ferrari MD. Endothelin antagonist bosentan blocks neurogenic inflammation, but is not effective in aborting migraine attacks. *Pain* 1996;67:375–378.
10. Yang Z, Richard V, von Segesser L, et al. Threshold concentrations of endothelin-1 potentiate contractions to norepinephrine and serotonin in human arteries. A new mechanism of vasospasm? *Circulation* 1990;82:188–195.

29

Plasma Homocysteine Levels in Primary Headache

Stefan Evers, *Hans Georg Koch, and Ingo-Wilhelm Husstedt

*Departments of Neurology and *Pediatrics, University of Münster,
D-48129 Münster, Germany*

Elevation of the amino acid homocysteine has been shown to be a risk factor for vascular diseases such as stroke (1,2) and myocardial infarction (3). Furthermore, hyperhomocysteinemia might be associated with other neurological diseases (e.g., multiple sclerosis) (4). In primary headache, to our knowledge, neither plasma nor cerebral spinal fluid (CSF) homocysteine levels have been examined, although migraine is supposed to be a cerebrovascular risk factor as well, especially in young women (5,6).

Two main mechanisms lead to hyperhomocysteinemia. First, mutations of different genes [e.g., genes for cystathionine-β[beta]-synthase (CBS) or 5'-10'-tetrahydrofolate-reductase] can cause mild hyperhomocysteinemia in the heterozygous state or severe hyperhomocysteinemia or homocystinuria in the homozygous state (7,8). Second, deficiency of vitamin B_{12} or folate can cause mild hyperhomocysteinemia. Physiologically, homocysteine increases with age and is higher in the male gender (9).

We were interested in determining plasma homocysteine levels in different headache types and comparing them with healthy control subjects, to evaluate a possible comorbidity of hyperhomocysteinemia and vascular headache types.

MATERIALS AND METHODS

We enrolled 92 consecutive patients admitted to our headache outpatient clinic and 18 healthy control subjects. Diagnosis was made according to the criteria of the International Headache Society. All patients were free of renal failure and had no history of vascular disease. The patients were headache free on the day of examination, and no medications were allowed on that day and on the day before. The demographic data of the patients and healthy subjects are given in Table 1. All subjects underwent a blood sampling procedure from the cubital vein in the fasting state; 5 mL plasma and 5 mL serum were obtained.

TABLE 1. *Demographic data of the patients and healthy subjects*

	Age (years)	Sex
Migraine without aura (n=45)	42±12	41 F/4 M
Migraine with aura (n=17)	33±11	15 F/2 M
Episodic tension-type headache (n=20)	36±14	17 F/3 M
Episodic cluster headache (n=10)	47±24	2 F/8 M
Healthy control subjects (n=18)	30±8	14 F/4 M

Total (i.e., free and protein-bound) plasma homocysteine levels were measured by high-performance liquid chromatography according to the method described by Araki and Sakoy (10). Serum vitamin B_{12} and folate levels were measured by routine radioimmunoassay methods. All measurements were done twice. Statistical analysis of differences between the different subject groups was performed by Kruskal-Wallis analysis; differences between two subject groups were analyzed by the Mann-Whitney U-test. Correlations were examined by simple regression analysis.

RESULTS

All subject groups did not differ significantly in age or sex distribution except a male preponderance in cluster headache. The plasma homocysteine levels, the vitamin B_{12} levels, and the folate levels are presented in Table 2. There were no significant differences in either headache type compared with healthy controls (Mann-Whitney U-test). However, in migraine with aura, homocysteine levels were significantly higher compared with migraine without aura ($p < 0.05$, Mann-Whitney U-test; controlled over all groups by Kruskal-Wallis analysis).

The rate of mild hyperhomocysteinemia (defined as mean value plus 1 standard deviation of healthy subjects) was 24% in migraine with aura, 4% in migraine without aura, and 17% in healthy subjects. Subgroup analysis of the homocysteine levels

TABLE 2. *Plasma homocysteine levels, serum vitamin B_{12} levels, and serum folate levels in patients and healthy subjects*

	MOA	MWA	CLU	TTH	HC
Homocysteine (µmol/L)	11.7±3.1	17.1±14.1*	15.2±4.4	12.1±2.9	13.1±3.4
Rate of hyperhomo-cysteinemia (%)	4	24	10	—	17
Vitamin B_{12} (pmol/L)	653±383	517±162	456±137	555±147	508±201
Folate (nmol/L)	16.3±4.1	10.7±6.7	10.1±5.3	12.4±4.1	11.7±3.1

*$p < 0.05$ as compounded by MOA.
MOA, migraine without aura; MWA, migraine with aura; CLU, episodic cluster headache; TTH, episodic tension-type headache; HC, healthy controls.

of women with migraine under the age of 35 years revealed no significant differences compared with women without migraine under the age of 35 and with healthy subjects (12.5 ± 2.5 µmol/L, 12.3 ± 3.3 µmol/L, and 13.1 ± 3.4 µmol/L, respectively). In our sample, only a small positive correlation between age and homocysteine levels could be observed ($r = 0.09$; $p < 0.40$). We confirmed the known difference between the male and female gender in homocysteine levels (15.7 ± 11.5 versus 11.7 ± 3.9 µmol/L; $p < 0.03$).

There were no significant differences in vitamin levels among all subject groups. We were unable to detect a significant correlation between vitamin levels and homocysteine. None of the patients with mild hyperhomocysteinemia showed hypovitaminosis (i.e., vitamin B_{12} level < 180 pmol/L or folate < 3 ng/L).

DISCUSSION

We could not detect any difference in plasma homocysteine levels between different primary headache types compared with healthy subjects. However, we observed a significantly increased homocysteine level in migraine with aura compared with migraine without aura that could not be explained by the age or gender distribution in the two groups. The difference could also not be related to hypovitaminosis in migraine with aura. We observed only a trend to lower vitamin levels in those subject groups with higher homocysteine levels. Subclinical hypovitaminosis has been described in patients with chronic pain syndromes, but we could not confirm this finding in our headache patients (11). It also seems unlikely that genetic mechanisms are the cause of our finding because we recently excluded mutations of the CBS gene in cerebrovascular disease associated with hyperhomocysteinemia (12). In fact, the cause of the difference between migraine with and migraine without aura cannot be explained by this study.

Since an association between cerebrovascular events and migraine has been described and attributed to the migraine aura in some studies, it might be that our results reflect a comorbidity of migraine with aura and cerebrovascular risk factors, such as hyperhomocysteinemia (5,13). This hypothesis needs to be confirmed in studies with larger samples. Furthermore, it would be of interest to study whether vitamin B_{12} or folate supplementation can influence the course and symptoms of migraine with aura.

REFERENCES

1. Brattström L, Lindgren A, Israelsson B, et al. Hyperhomocysteinemia in stroke: prevalence, cause, and relationship to type of stroke and stroke risk factors. *Eur J Clin Invest* 1982;22:214–221.
2. Perry IJ, Refsumn H, Morris RW, Ebrahim SB, Ueland PM, Shaper AG. Prospective study of serum total homocysteine concentration and risk of stroke in middle-aged British men. *Lancet* 1995;346:1395–1398.
3. Mayer EL, Jacobsen DW, Robinson K. Homocysteine and coronary atherosclerosis. *J Am Coll Cardiol* 1996;27:517–527.
4. Reynolds EH. Multiple sclerosis and vitamine B12 metabolism. *J Neurol Neurosurg Psychiatry* 1992;55:339–340.

5. Carolei A, Marini C, de Matteis G. History of migraine and risk of cerebral ischaemia in young adults. *Lancet* 1996;347:1503–1506.
6. Tzourio C, Iglesias S, Hubert JB, et al. Migraine and risk of ischaemic stroke: a case-control study. *BMJ* 1993;307:289–292.
7. Mudd SH, Skovby F, Levy HL, et al. The natural history of homocystinuria due to cystathionine-beta-synthase deficiency. *Am J Hum Genet* 1985;37:1–31.
8. Kluijtsmans LA, van den Heuvel LPWJ, Boers GHJ, et al. Molecular genetic analysis in mild hyperhomocysteinemia: a common mutation in the methylenetetrahydrofolate reductase gene is a genetic risk factor of cardiovascular disease. *Am J Hum Genet* 1996;58:35–41.
9. Selhub J, Jacques PF, Weilson PWF, Rush D, Ronnberg IH. Vitamin status and intake as primary determinants of homocyst(e)ine in an elderly population. *JAMA* 1993;270:2693–2698.
10. Araki A, Sakoy Y. Determinants of free and total homocysteine in human plasma by high-performance liquid chromatography with fluorescence detection. *J Chromatogr* 1987;422:42–52.
11. Mader R, Deutsch H, Siebert GK, et al. Vitamin status of inpatients with chronic cephalgia and dysfunction pain syndrome and effects of a vitamin supplementation. *Int J Vitam Nutr Res* 1988;58:436–441.
12. Koch HG, Evers S, Grotemeyer KH, et al. Moderate hyperhomocysteinemia in ischemic stroke. *Ir J Med Sci* 1995;164[Suppl 15]:11.
13. Hernich JB, Horwitz RI. A controlled study of ischaemic stroke risk in migraine patients. *J Clin Epidemiol* 1989;42:773–780.

30

Endothelin-B Receptors in Human Temporal Artery

Linda R. White, *Roar Juul, Guilherme A. Lucas, Knut H. Leseth, Jan Aasly, *Johan Cappelen, and †Lars Edvinsson

*Departments of Neurology and *Neurosurgery, University Hospital, N-7006 Trondheim, Norway; and †Department of Internal Medicine, Lund University Hospital, 22185 Lund, Sweden*

Endothelin (ET), the potent vasoactive peptide produced by endothelial cells, has three isopeptides (ET 1, ET 2, and ET 3) and two receptors (ET_A and ET_B). ET_A receptors are located on smooth muscle cells and are associated with the potent contractile ability of endothelin. ET_B receptors mediate both relaxation and contraction. The ET_B receptor mediating relaxation is predominantly localized on vascular endothelium (1).

Endothelin has been implicated in a number of cerebrovascular disorders, including subarachnoid hemorrhage, cerebral ischemia, and migraine (2). In models of subarachnoid hemorrhage in the dog, endothelin ET_A antagonists have been shown to relieve chronic cerebral vasospasm (3), and recent results have shown that ET-1 is involved in this process through ET_B as well as ET_A receptors (4).

Since ET_B receptors can mediate relaxation as well as contraction, it is important to characterize ET receptor activity in the human cranial vasculature. We have studied ET receptor activity in isolated segments of the human temporal artery, particularly with respect to ET_B receptors.

MATERIALS AND METHODS

Branches of human superficial temporal artery were obtained after various neurosurgical procedures and immediately placed in ice-cold modified Krebs-Ringer buffer solution. Experiments were carried out in organ baths at physiological pH and temperature, and ET_A and ET_B receptors were characterized using in vitro pharmacology (vasomotor response experiments). Isometric tension in the isolated artery segments was monitored using Grass FT03C force-displacement transducers linked to a MacLab analog-digital convertor and continuously analyzed by computer. Segments were tested with buffer in which 60 mM NaCl was replaced by an equivalent amount of KCl. The resulting contraction was considered as 100%, and all ET contractions from basal tension were compared with this value. In experiments in which ET reactions were tested in precontracted arteries, contraction was induced by 10^{-5} M prostaglandin $F_{2\alpha}$, and this was used as 100% for comparison of subsequent reactions. No experiment was carried out more than once on any artery preparation. The presence of an intact endothelium was confirmed by relaxation in the presence of either 10^{-7} M substance P or 10^{-6} M acetylcholine. Antagonists and enzyme inhibitors were added 10 minutes prior to the addition of agonists (ET-1, ET-3, or the specific ET_B agonist IRL 1620). All reagents were added in 50g μl aliquots. Further details of the experimental procedures are available elsewhere (5).

Results are given as the mean ± SE. Statistical analysis was carried out with analysis of variance (ANOVA) and Newman-Keuls test for multiple comparisons, or Student's unpaired t-test as appropriate, values of $p < 0.05$ being considered significant.

RESULTS

Data for ET_A-mediated contractions in human temporal artery are summarized in Table 1. Although the maximum contraction induced by ET-1 and ET-3 was similar, ET-1 was a more potent agonist than ET-3. However, Schild plot analysis showed that the specific ET_A antagonist FR 139317 was a considerably more potent antagonist of contractions induced by ET-3 than ET-1, as shown by the pA_2 values (5). A concentration of 10^{-6} M FR 139317 eliminated ET-3 contraction at concentrations up to 3×10^{-6} M, whereas 10^{-5} M FR 139317 would not block contraction induced by ET-1 at concentrations above 10^{-7} M. Since ET isopeptides are equipotent at ET_B receptors, further studies of ET_B activity were conducted with ET-3 in the presence of 10^{-6} M FR 139317. With 10^{-6} M FR 139317, a marked relaxation was induced by 10^{-6} M ET-3 (Fig. 1a), in contrast to a slight additional contraction in the absence of antagonist (Table 2). A similar relaxation was induced by 10^{-6} M IRL 1620 (Fig. 1b).

The ET-3-induced relaxation was attenuated by the mixed ET_A/ET_B receptor antagonist bosentan, the cyclooxygenase inhibitor indomethacin, and the nitric oxide synthase inhibitor N^G-nitro-L-arginine methyl ester (L-NAME) (Table 2). IRL 1620 did not induce any contraction in arteries at basal tension (not shown).

TABLE 1. *Summary of data obtained for endothelin ET_A activity in human temporal artery[a]*

Agonist	E_{max} (%)	pD_2	pA_2 for FR 139317	No.
ET-1	112±6	7.8±0.2	5.8	7
ET-3	111±5	6.7±0.1	8.3	7

[a]Maximum contraction in response to ET-1 or ET-3, expressed as percent of the contraction induced by 60 mM K^+, and sensitivity expressed as pD_2 (negative logarithm of peptide concentration inducing half-maximum response). The potency of the specific ET_A antagonist FR 139317 is expressed as the pA_2 (negative logarithm of the mean concentration of antagonist eliciting half-maximum effect). Data from Lucas et al. (5).

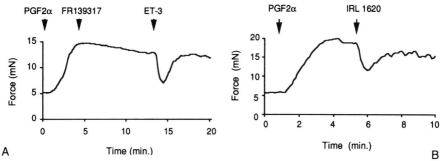

FIG. 1. Typical reaction profiles of ET_B-mediated relaxation in human temporal artery precontracted by 10^{-5} M prostaglandin $F_{2\alpha}$ ($PGF_{2\alpha}$) mediated by **(A)** 10^{-6} M endothelin-3 (ET-3) in the presence of 10^{-6} M FR 139317, or **(B)** 10^{-6} M IRL 1620.

DISCUSSION

It is clear from the data that ET_B, as well as ET_A receptors, are present in human temporal artery. The ET_B receptors appear to mediate only relaxation and probably correspond to the ET_{B1} receptor subtype. They appear to be endothelium dependent, as judged by the results of the pharmacological data with indomethacin and L-NAME, requiring either a product of the cyclooxygenase or nitric oxide synthase pathways.

In the absence of an ET_A antagonist in vitro, ET_B-mediated relaxation is completely masked by strong ET_A-mediated contraction. It is therefore only possible at this time to speculate on the possible physiological role of ET_B-mediated relaxation. However, the presence of ET_B receptors in the human cranial vasculature could have important implications for the field of cerebrovascular disorders, including head-

TABLE 2. *Percentage changes in isometric tension of human temporal artery from a precontraction by 10^{-5} M prostaglandin $F_{2\alpha}$*[a]

Treatment	Reaction	% Change from precontraction (mean±SE)	No.
10^{-6} M ET-3	Contraction	5.8±1.4	8
10^{-6} M ET-3+10^{-6} M FR 139317	Relaxation	49.3±7.4*	8
10^{-6} M ET-3+10^{-5} M bosentan	Relaxation	8.7±1.5	6
10^{-6} M ET-3+10^{-6} M FR 139317+ 10^{-6} M indomethacin	Relaxation	7.0±1.7	6
10^{-6} M ET-3+10^{-6} M FR 139317+ 10^{-4} M L-NAME	Relaxation	3.7±1.2	6

[a]Endothelin-3 (ET-3) alone induced additional contraction, while all other reactions induced relaxations.
*ET-3+FR 139317 was significantly different from all other reactions, at $p < 0.0005$.
Data from Lucas et al. (5).
L-NAME, N^G-nitro-L-arginine methyl ester.

ache. Classic studies by Wolff demonstrated the temporal artery to be dilated during migraine attacks on the headache side, and this dilation is counteracted by ergotamine (6). More recently, the phenomenon has also been shown in cluster headache (7). While it is not yet known precisely which vasoactive substances are involved in these reactions, endothelium-derived factors certainly seem to play a role, probably through a nitric oxide-related mechanism (8). Since ET is elevated in the circulation during migraine, and since it is a potent peptide capable of both contraction and relaxation, it is not unlikely that it plays a role in the pathophysiology of vascular headaches (9).

ACKNOWLEDGMENTS

The authors wish to thank Elin Ødegaard for excellent technical assistance and the Research Council of Norway (project 101464/310). G.A.L. thanks the Brazilian Ministry of Education for a research fellowship (grant 1231/94-4). Bosentan was kindly provided by Dr. Martine Clozel of Hoffmann-La Roche Ltd., Basel, Switzerland.

REFERENCES

1. Bax WA, Saxena PR. The current endothelin receptor classification: time for reconsideration? *Trends Pharmacol Sci* 1994;15:379–386.
2. Cardell LO, Uddman R, Edvinsson L. Endothelins: a role in cerebrovascular disease? *Cephalalgia* 1994;14:259–265.
3. Nirei H, Hamada K, Shoubo M, Sogabe K, Notsu Y, Ono T. An endothelin ET_A receptor antagonist, FR 139317, ameliorates cerebral vasospasm in dog. *Life Sci* 1993;52:1869–1874.
4. Shigeno T, Clozel M, Sakai S, Saito A, Goto K. The effect of bosentan, a new potent endothelin receptor antagonist, on the pathogenesis of cerebral vasospasm. *Neurosurgery* 1995;37:87–91.
5. Lucas GA, White LR, Juul R, Cappelen J, Aasly J, Edvinsson L. Relaxation of human temporal artery by endothelin ET_B receptors. *Peptides* 1996;17:1139–1144.
6. Tunis, MM, Wolff HG. Long term observations of the reactivity of the cranial arteries in subjects with vascular headache of the migraine type. *Arch Neurol Psychiatry* 1953;70:551–557.
7. Iversen HK, Nielsen TH, Krabbe AAE, Tfelt-Hansen P, Olesen J. Temporal artery responses during cluster headache. *Cephalalgia* 1995;15[Suppl 14]:198.
8. Olesen J, Thomsen LL, Lassen LH, Olesen IJ. The nitric oxide hypothesis of migraine and other vascular headaches. *Cephalalgia* 1995;15:94–100.
9. Gallai V, Sarchielli P, Firenze C, et al. Endothelin-1 in migraine and tension-type headache. *Acta Neurol Scand* 1994;89:47–55.

31

Presence of Contractile Endothelin-A and Dilatory Endothelin-B Receptors in Human Cerebral Arteries

Torun Nilsson, Leonor Cantera, Mikael Adner, and *Lars Edvinsson

*Division of Experimental Vascular Research, *Department of Internal Medicine, Lund University Hospital, S-221 85 Lund, Sweden*

The endothelins (ETs) exert their diverse biological actions through at least two classes of receptor subtypes, ET_A and ET_B (1,2). To elucidate which receptor subtype is responsible for endothelin-induced vasomotor responses of human cerebral arteries, we used in vitro pharmacology and reverse transcriptase-polymerase chain reaction (RT-PCR).

MATERIALS AND METHODS

In Vitro Pharmacology

Human cerebral arteries were obtained from patients undergoing surgery for intracranial tumors. The vessel segments were placed in buffer solution aerated with 5% CO_2 and immediately transported to the laboratory for investigation. The protocol was approved by the Human Ethics Committee of Lund University (Sweden).

The vessels were dissected out under a microscope and cut into cylindrical segments (1 to 2 mm long). For continuous recording of the isometric tension, the specimens were mounted in temperature-controlled (37°C) tissue baths, containing an Na^+-Krebs solution, continuously aerated with carbogen gas, giving a physiological pH (3). Vascular effects of agonists were examined by cumulative application of the peptides. The antagonists were added 15 minutes before the agonist. The results are given as percentage of the potassium-induced contraction. To study relaxant activity, the segments were precontracted with 10 nM U46619 (a prostaglandin $F_{2\alpha}$ derivate), causing a contraction that in control experiments remained stable for 45 to 60 minutes. The antagonist was added before U46619. When the precontraction was stable, the agonist was added.

The potency of the agonists was expressed as pEC_{50} values (negative logarithm of the molar concentration of agonist inducing half-maximum response) and the potency of the antagonist as pA_2 values (negative logarithm of the molar concentration of antagonist reducing the effect to half of the original effect).

Reverse Transcriptase-Polymerase Chain Reaction

Total cellular RNA was isolated from human cerebral arterial segments (with intact endothelium or denuded of endothelium) by the method of acid guanidinium thiocyanate/phenol/chloroform extraction (4). The following primers were used:

ET_A forward: 5´-TGGCCTTTTGATCACAATGACTTT-3´
ET_A reverse: 5´-TTTGATGTGGCATTGAGCATACAGGTT-3´
ET_B forward: 5´-ACTGGCCATTTGGAGCTGAGATGT-3´
ET_B reverse: 5´-CTGCATGCCACTTTTCTTTCTCAA-3´

One microgram of total RNA was reverse transcribed using the standard protocol of the GeneAmp RNA PCR kit (Perkin Elmer AB, Sweden). PCR was carried out by using four linked files as follows: file 1, 2 minutes at 95°C for 1 cycle; file 2, 1 minute at 95°C and 1 minute at 60°C for 35 cycles; file 3, 7 minutes at 72°C for 1 cycle; file 4, incubation at 4°C for 5 minutes.

RESULTS

Endothelin-1 induced a concentration-dependent contraction of human cerebral arteries; the pEC_{50} value was 9.4 ± 0.2. The vasoconstriction was significantly antagonized both by bosentan (Ro 47-0203), a combined ET_A and ET_B receptor antagonist (5) (Fig. 1), and FR139317, a selective ET_A receptor antagonist (6) (Fig. 2). The pA_2 values were 7.2 ± 0.4 and 7.4 ± 0.4, respectively.

Sarafotoxin 6c (a selective ET_B agonist) failed to cause contraction of human cerebral arteries. In precontracted vessels, however, sarafotoxin 6c induced relaxation, which was significantly inhibited by bosentan (10 µM) resulting in a pA_2 value of 6.0 ± 0.2 (Fig. 3). Furthermore, mRNA encoding the human ET_A and ET_B receptors was detected in human cerebral arteries both with and without endothelium (Fig. 4).

CONCLUSIONS

The ET-1 induced vasoconstriction of human cerebral arteries is primarily mediated by the ET_A receptor, while the sarafotoxin 6c-induced vasodilation appears to be mediated via the ET_B receptor.

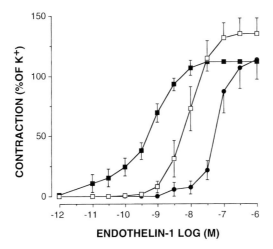

FIG. 1. The contractile responses to ET-1 on human cerebral vessels without (■) and with incremental concentrations of bosentan, 1 µM (□) and 10 µM (●). The results are expressed as percentage of the potassium-induced contraction; each point represents the mean of tested vessel segments from seven patients, with error bars representing SEM.

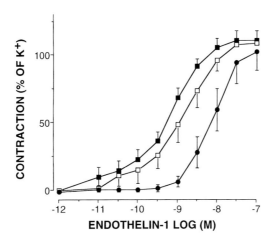

FIG. 2. The contractile responses to ET-1 on human cerebral vessels without (■) and with incremental concentrations of FR139317, 0.1 µM (□) and 1 µM (●). The results are expressed as percentage of the potassium-induced contraction; each point represents the mean of tested vessel segments from seven patients, with error bars representing SEM.

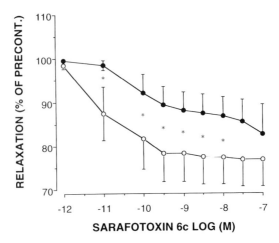

FIG. 3. The dilatory response to sarafotoxin 6c on human cerebral arteries without (○) and with bosentan, 10 µM (●). Results are expressed as percentage of U46619-induced precontraction, and each point is the mean ± SEM of five experiments.

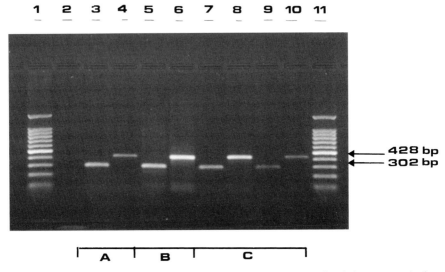

FIG. 4. Detection by RT-PCR of human ET_A and ET_B receptor transcripts in human cerebral arteries from three individuals. The amplified products were of the predicted size for ET_A (302 bp) and ET_B (428 bp) receptors. Lanes 3 and 4: Human cerebral artery from individual A. Lanes 5 and 6: Human cerebral artery from individual B. Lanes 7 and 8: Human cerebral artery from individual C. Lanes 9 and 10: Human cerebral artery from individual C denuded of endothelium. Promega´s 100-bp ladder was run in each of the outside lanes to confirm molecular size of the amplification product (lanes 1 and 11). The absence of contaminants was checked by negative control samples with RNAase-free water (lane 2).

REFERENCES

1. Arai H, Hori S, Aramori I, Ohkubo H, Nakanishi S. Cloning and expressing of a cDNA encoding an endothelin receptor. *Nature* 1990;348:730–732.
2. Saeki T, Ihara M, Fukuroda T, Yamagiwa M, Yano M. [Ala^{1,3,11,15}] Endothelin-1 analogs with ET$_B$ agonistic activity. *Biochem Biophys Res Commun* 1992;179:286–292.
3. Högestätt ED, Andersson K-E, Edvinsson L. Mechanical properties of rat cerebral arteries as studies by a sensitive device for recording of mechanical activity in isolated small blood vessels. *Acta Physiol Scand* 1983;117:49–61.
4. Chomczynski P, Sacchi N. Single-step method of RNA isolation by acid guanidinium thiocyanate-phenol-chloroform extraction. *Anal Biochem* 1987;162:156–159.
5. Sogabe K, Nirei H, Shoubo M, et al. Pharmacological profile of FR139317, a novel, potent endothelin ET$_A$ receptor antagonist. *J Pharmacol Exp Ther* 1993;264:1040–1046.
6. Clozel M, Breu V, Burri K, et al. Pathophysiological role of endothelin revealed by the first orally active endothelin receptor antagonist. *Nature* 1993;365:759–761.

32

Evidence for Calcitonin Gene-Related Peptide-1 Receptors in Human Cranial Arteries

Inger Jansen-Olesen, *Sergio Gulbenkian, †Leonor Cantera, and †Lars Edvinsson

*Department of Biological Sciences, The Royal Danish School of Pharmacy, DK-2100 Copenhagen Ø, Denmark; *Gulbenkian Institute of Science, Oeiras, Portugal 2781;and †Department of Internal Medicine, Lund University Hospital, S-221 85 Lund, Sweden*

The 37-amino acid peptide calcitonin gene-related peptide (CGRP) is one of the most potent vasodilators known today. It is produced in the trigeminal ganglia, from where it is transported to sensory nerve terminals innervating the cranial circulation (1). Electrical stimulation of the trigeminal nerve causes the release of CGRP from sensory nerve endings, which results in cerebral vasodilation (2). Calcitonin gene-related peptide is involved in the pathophysiology of cluster headache and migraine since increased levels of the peptide have been measured during cluster headache attacks (3) as well as during migraine with and without aura (4). Recently, a complementary DNA (cDNA) encoding the human $CGRP_1$ receptor was cloned. This has provided a powerful instrument to study the expression of the receptor in different tissues (5). The aim of the present study was to show the presence of mRNA encoding $CGRP_1$ receptors in the human cranial circulation, to show human α-CGRP binding sites on cranial arteries, and to illustrate the effects of human α-CGRP on cranial arteries.

MATERIALS AND METHODS

For vasomotor experiments and receptor autoradiography, human cerebral, meningeal, and temporal arteries were obtained in conjunction with neurosurgical tumor operations. For second-messenger studies and RNA experiments, tissue was collected at autopsy within 2 to 6 hours post mortem. Specimens were collected in accordance with Swedish legislation and approved by the local ethics committee.

For studies of vasomotor reactivity and second messengers, the vessel specimens were immersed in an ice-cold buffer solution directly after removal, gassed with 5%

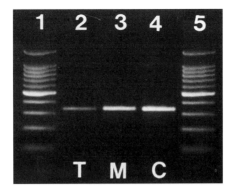

FIG. 1. Gel electrophoresis of RT-PCR reaction products of mRNA fragments corresponding to human $CGRP_1$ (339 bp) receptor transcripts. Lane 2: $CGRP_1$ mRNA in human temporal artery. Lane 3: $CGRP_1$ mRNA human middle meningeal artery. Lane 4: $CGRP_1$ mRNA in human cerebral artery. As a negative control, no amplification product occurred when reverse transcriptase was omitted in the first-strand cDNA reaction (not shown). Promega's 100-bp DNA Ladder (Promega, SDS, Sweden) was run to confirm molecular size of the amplification product (lanes 1 and 5).

CO_2 in O_2, and for the other methods immediately frozen in liquid nitrogen. For further details on the methods for vasomotor response studies in vitro and second-messenger experiments see ref. 6, for reverse transcriptase-polymerase chain reaction (PCR) see ref. 7, and for receptor autoradiography see ref. 8.

RESULTS

Reverse Transcriptase Polymerase Chain Reaction

Agarose gel electrophoresis of the PCR products from human cerebral, meningeal, and temporal arteries demonstrated products of the expected size, corresponding to mRNA encoding $CGRP_1$ receptors (Fig. 1). DNase was successfully used to eliminate any contaminating DNA, since no bands were detected in negative controls in which the reverse transcriptase enzyme was omitted in the first-strand cDNA reaction. The experiments showed expression of mRNAs encoding $CGRP_1$ receptors in cerebral, meningeal, and temporal arteries.

Receptor Autoradiography

The ^{125}I-CGRP binding studies were performed in the human meningeal and temporal arteries in the absence and presence of unlabeled human α-CGRP. Intense binding was observed over the smooth muscle cell layer of both arteries (Fig. 2). In

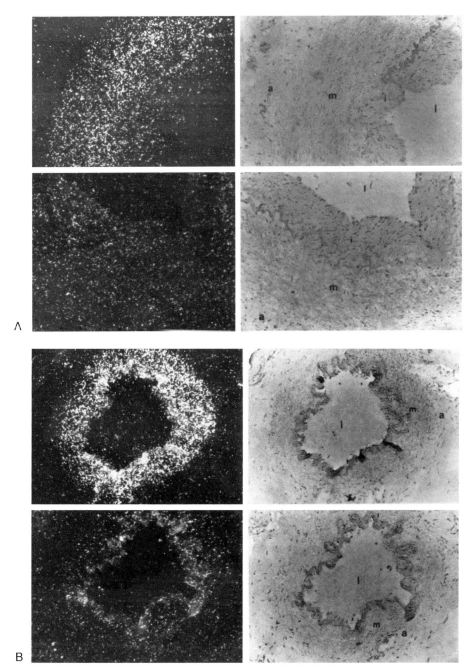

FIG. 2. Autoradiographs illustrating ^{125}I-human α-CGRP binding in the human superficial temporal artery **(A)** and in the middle meningeal artery **(B)** in the absence (*top row*, total binding) or presence (*bottom row*, nonspecific binding) of unlabeled human α-CGRP. Darkfield and brightfield photographs of the same field are shown in the left and right panels, respectively. Notice that silver grains, visible only in the darkfield microscopy, are preferentially accumulated over the smooth muscle medial (*m*) layer. Autoradiographs from nonspecific binding show a small number of silver grains distributed homogenously over the artery wall. *A*, adventitia; *i*, intima; *l*, lumen.

control sections the ^{125}I-CGRP labeling was low and homogeneously distributed over the vessel walls.

Vasomotor Responses In Vitro

Human α-CGRP induced potent relaxations of precontracted human cerebral, middle meningeal, and temporal arteries, measured by I_{max} (maximum relaxant effect) and pIC_{50} (negative logarithm of concentration of agonist that elicit half maximum relaxation) (cerebral—I_{max}: 92 ± 3% of precontraction, pIC_{50}: 9.89 ± 0.25, n = 20; meningeal—I_{max}: 89 ± 5% of precontraction, pIC_{50}: 8.94 ± 0.48, n = 6; temporal—I_{max}: 84 ± 4% of precontraction, pIC_{50}: 9.31 ± 0.31, n = 18). Removal of the endothelium did not significantly change the responses to human α-CGRP with respect to the amount of maximum relaxation or pIC_{50} values.

A single concentration of human α-CGRP$_{8-37}$ (10^{-6} M), given 15 minutes prior to the administration of agonist, induced neither contraction of vessel segments at the resting level of tension nor relaxation of precontracted vessel segments. Human α-CGRP$_{8-37}$ (10^{-6} M) induced a parallel shift toward higher concentrations of human α-CGRP (cerebral—I_{max}: 75 ± 7% of precontraction, pIC_{50}: 9.13 ± 0.42, n = 9; meningeal—I_{max}: 82 ± 5% of precontraction, pIC_{50}: 8.11 ± 0.21, n = 4; temporal—I_{max}: 94 ± 3% of precontraction, pIC_{50}: 8.40 ± 0.27, n = 5).

Capsaicin Experiments

Capsaicin (10^{-15}–10^{-4} M) induced a biphasic relaxation of human cerebral arteries (n = 4). The first phase of the relaxation amounted to 20 ± 4% of precontraction and occurred at capsaicin concentrations up to 10^{-11} M. The maximum relaxant response for the second phase of relaxation was found at capsaicin concentrations between 10^{-5} M and 10^{-4} M, amounting to 91 ± 9%. Pretreatment with 10^{-6} M human α-CGRP$_{8-37}$ significantly inhibited the first phase (I_{max}: 2 ± 2%) but not the second phase (I_{max}: 93 ± 8%) of capsaicin-induced relaxation.

Measurement of Cyclic AMP

The basal formation of cyclic AMP in human cerebral arteries was 235 ± 17 fmol/mg wet weight (n = 4). The adenylyl cyclase activator forskolin given in a concentration of 10^{-6} M induced a production of cyclic AMP in the cerebral vessels, amounting to 2,967 ± 118 fmol/mg wet weight. Human α-CGRP given in a concentration of 10^{-9} M increased the cyclic AMP formation to 48 ± 5% of the production induced by forskolin. When given alone, human α-CGRP$_{8-37}$ (10^{-6} M) only induced a slight (5%) increase in cyclic AMP production. Human α-CGRP$_{8-37}$ (10^{-6} M) totally inhibited the increase in cyclic AMP production induced by 10^{-9} M human α-CGRP (Fig. 3).

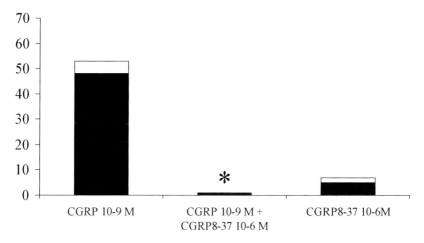

FIG. 3. Increase in cyclic adenosine monophosphate (AMP) levels by 10^{-9} M human α-calcitonin gene-related peptide (CGRP), 10^{-9} M human α-CGRP in the presence of 10^{-6} M $CGRP_{8-37}$, and 10^{-6} M human α-$CGRP_{8-37}$, given in percent relative to the effect induced by 10^{-6} M forskolin in human cerebral arteries. Values are given ± SEM; 4–16 experiments from three to nine patients. *, $p<0.05$.

DISCUSSION

Migraine attacks are associated with intra- and extracranial arterial dilation. The pathophysiology involves CGRP release, which is associated with headache in migraine and cluster headache. We have in previous studies suggested that human α- and β-CGRP acts, at least partly, at two different receptor sites for CGRP in the human cerebral circulation (6). However, there seems to be more mRNA coding for α-CGRP than for β-CGRP in the trigeminal ganglia, and we have therefore in the present investigation studied the effects of human α-CGRP and the receptor upon which this is believed to act (9).

This is the first time that mRNA encoding the $CGRP_1$ receptor and CGRP binding sites has been demonstrated in human cranial vessels, and the findings support the view that this receptor is present in smooth muscle cells. This agrees well with the finding that there is no difference in effect of α-CGRP administered to human cranial arteries with and without endothelium. Antagonist experiments revealed that the $CGRP_1$ receptor antagonist human α-$CGRP_{8-37}$ blocked the responses to human α-CGRP, which further illustrates the existence of this receptor subtype in the human cranial circulation. The blockade of the first phase of the capsaicin-induced relaxation by human α-$CGRP_{8-37}$ suggests that α-CGRP and not β-CGRP is released from sensory nerve endings (6). This result agrees well with studies of the distribution of mRNA for α- and β-CGRP in which the trigeminal ganglion was found to contain tenfold more α-CGRP mRNA than β-CGRP mRNA (9). The increase in cyclic AMP levels induced by human α-CGRP was significantly blocked by $CGRP_{8-37}$. Thus mRNA encoding the $CGRP_1$ receptor is demonstrated for the first time in human cranial vessels and may be coupled to a G protein responsible for the activation of adenylyl cyclase.

REFERENCES

1. Uddman R, Edvinsson L, Ekman R, Kingman T, McCulloch J. Innervation of the feline cerebral vasculature by nerve fibres containing calcitonin gene-related peptide: trigeminal origin and co-existence with substance P. *Neurosci Lett* 1985;62:131–136.
2. Goadsby P, Edvinsson L, Ekman R. Release of vasoactive peptides in the extracerebral circulation of man and the cat during activation of the trigeminovascular system. *Ann Neurol* 1988;23:193–196.
3. Goadsby P, Edvinsson L. Human *in vivo* evidence for trigeminovascular activation in cluster headache: neuropeptide changes and effects of acute attack therapies. *Brain* 1994;117:427–434.
4. Goadsby P, Edvinsson L, Ekman R. Vasoactive peptide release in the extracerebral circulation of humans during migraine headache. *Ann Neurol* 1990;28:183–187.
5. Aiyar N, Rand K, Elshourbagy N, et al. A cDNA encoding the calcitonin gene-related peptide type 1 receptor. *J Biol Chem* 1996;19:11325–11329.
6. Jansen-Olesen I, Mortensen A, Edvinsson L. Calcitonin gene-related peptide is released from capsaicin sensitive nerve fibres and induces vasodilatation of human cerebral arteries concomitant with activation of adenylyl cyclase. *Cephalalgia* 1996;16:310–316.
7. Jansen-Olesen I, Ottosson A, Cantera L, et al. Role of endothelium and nitric oxide for histamine-induced responses in human cranial arteries and detection of mRNA encoding H_1- and H_2-receptors using RT-PCR. *Br J Pharmacol* 1997;121:41–48.
8. Afonso F, Sebastiao AM, Pinho MS, et al. Calcitonin gene-related peptide in the hamster seminal vesicle and coagulating gland. Immunohistochemical, autoradiographical, and pharmacological study. *Peptides* 1996;17:1189–1195.
9. Amara SG, Arriza JI, Leff SE, Swanson LW, Evans RM, Rosenfeld MG. Expression in brain of a messenger RNA encoding a novel neuropeptide homologous to calcitonin gene-related peptide. *Science* 1985;229:1094–1097.

33

Discussion Summary: Involvement of Neuropeptides in Primary Headaches

Lars Edvinsson

Department of Internal Medicine, Lund University Hospital, S-221 85 Lund, Sweden

The first presentation by Flemming Bach on opioid peptides in primary headache raised the question from László Vécsei: "What is the relationship of the co-localization of peptides, turnover, and the synaptic receptor concentration?" This is a good question, for which no one has exact data. Clearly, this is an area that always deserves consideration in evaluating the role of signal substances. However, the levels of the peptides are very low in circulation. β-Endorphin is stable in test tubes, whereas Met-encephalin is rather unstable. Flemming Bach considers that the concentrations in blood or in cerebrospinal fluid (CSF) should mainly be regarded as a reflection of activity in the opioid peptide system.

Mary Heinricher remarked that she was struck by the phrase "central opioid systems." Is there any reason to believe that central opioidergic neurons act in concert so that they actually form a system whose activity could be reflected in CSF? Is it not equally possible that opioidergic neurons comprise a heterogenous population and that only a subset of neurons are involved in pain, particularly in headache?

Flemming Bach agreed with this statement. He would be more cautious in his expression but believes the β-endorphins are connected in some ways and are involved in pain physiology, where they could act in concert, whereas Met-encephalin clearly involves different systems, which probably act separately. Jes Olesen questioned whether pain activation causes opioid system activation. Flemming Bach argued that in experimental animals this may be seen in certain conditions but has never been demonstrated in humans.

The second lecture by Peter Goadsby on plasma and CSF nonopioid peptides in migraine and cluster headache attracted several questions. Salonen questioned whether indomethacin blocks the release of calcitonin gene-related peptide (CGRP) from nerve endings. There is, however, no knowledge concerning this. If not, how would he explain the normalization of CGRP after indomethacin? The concentrations of indomethacin used in the clinic (25 mg, every 8 hr) and in experimental animals attenuate the CO_2 response (hypercapnia response) of the cerebral blood flow. This seems to be a rather unique feature, since other cyclooxygenase inhibitors lack this effect. In the discussion of whether this might be due to a special inhibitory capability of indomethacin, it was suggested that inhibition of nitric oxide synthase is a possibility.

Harri Hirvonen enquired about the time delay for elevation of CGRP. The response was that facial flushing occurs instantaneously after trigeminal stimulation. The CGRP measurements have not been followed exactly on time, but within a few minutes (10 minutes) CGRP levels were already elevated. However, a systematic study would be of importance.

Vivette Glover wondered about the exact role of CGRP. The role of CGRP in the cerebral circulation is clearly not tonic, but it is at present regarded as "nociceptive" for headache problems and also as a protective system in that it acts to antagonize potent vasoconstriction, seen in conjunction with subarachnoid hemorrhage, for example. If primary headaches constitute a group of disorders that can be regarded as cerebrovascular, then the CGRP reflex could be a reaction to counterbalance constriction in spreading depression (for example) by activating the trigeminovascular system.

Merete Bakke raised the question: With so many negative data on substance P (SP) in pain conditions and headache, should we re-evaluate its role in pain mechanisms in general? Clifford Woolf agreed that there is no apparent role for SP in the primary headaches. However, the most interesting aspect is that there seems to be a differential expression between SP and CGRP in the intracranial circulation, which is a fairly unique situation. In other parts of the body there is co-localization of the two peptides, and one can often see plasma extravasation and vasodilation occurring in peripheral tissues as measures of release of both SP and CGRP. Peter Goadsby noted that the anatomical data argue strongly for a differential innervation of CGRP to the intracranial circulation. However, in situations of intense activation of this pathway by stimulation of the trigeminal ganglion, release of SP can be seen. This has not been demonstrated in headache, possibly because the activation is not maximal, as it is during direct trigeminal ganglion stimulation.

Peer Tfelt-Hansen questioned the role of neurokinin A (NKA). Although NKA and SP are formed from the same preprotachychinin and ideally would be released simultaneously, we must await further studies on this peptide during migraine attacks. Also, the use of NK_1 antagonists in migraine therapy might give some clues since they also have affinity for NK_2 receptors, for which NKA has higher affinity. They could thus offer some enlightenment on the usefulness of this type of blocker. Helen Connor noted the lack of efficacy of NK_1 antagonists in migraine (as shown by two independent studies) and questioned the potential usefulness of a CGRP antagonist. Peter Goadsby replied that NK_1 is a good tool for the laboratory, for learning more about migraine pathophysiology and the trigeminovascular system. Whether or not it is a useful antimigraine drug is not easy to determine. Purely on a theoretical basis, CGRP is consistently released in attacks of primary headache, and the idea deserves to be tested.

Linda White was asked by what mechanism she considers endothelin-1 (ET-1) to be released in cluster headache and migraine. She replied that two independent studies (a Finnish one published in 1992 and one by Genari et al. in 1994) demonstrated release of ET-1 during migraine attacks. The mechanism behind the release is difficult to imagine, but it could reflect vasomotor changes, since endothelin can be released by flow, shear stress, and hypoxia. Thus, if there is modulation of vasculature tone in primary headache attacks, ET release from the endothelium could be a reflection of such changes.

Helle Iversen was asked why nitroglycerin (NTG) doesn't release CGRP. Dr. Iversen replied that Moskowitz and colleagues had demonstrated that NTG causes vasodilation in the cerebral circulation via a response that can be completely blocked by a $CGRP_1$ antagonist. They argued that NTG causes release of CGRP, which acts as a vasodilator. Dr. Iversen noted that NTG causes headache and vasodilation of several types of vessels in vivo, with no significant release of CGRP. Thus the mechanism suggested by Wei et al. (1992) does not apply to humans, a finding supported by other laboratory studies.

SECTION VI

Involvement of Nitric Oxide–Cyclic GMP Products in Primary Headache

Headache Pathogenesis: Monoamines, Neuropeptides, Purines, and Nitric Oxide, edited by J. Olesen and L. Edvinsson.
Lippincott–Raven Publishers, Philadelphia © 1997.

34
Nitroxidergic Nerve in Cranial Arteries

Noboru Toda

Department of Pharmacology, Shiga University of Medical Science, Ohtsu/Shiga 520-21, Japan

Nitric oxide (NO) derived from the endothelium and perivascular nerve is an important mediator of vasodilation in intra- and extracranial blood vessels and is also an algogenic substance. Intravenous injections of NO donors, such as nitroglycerin, evokes an attack in migraine patients, in association with cerebral vasodilation (1). Histamine vasodilates human cerebral arteries only when the endothelium is intact, and the response is mediated via histamine H_1 receptor subtypes (2). This amine also induces migraine attacks in patients, and the headache is relieved by treatment with H_1 receptor antagonists (3). These findings led us to speculate that endogenous NO plays an important role in evoking vascular headache in migraineurs (4).

This chapter describes (a) vasodilation mediated by NO derived from perivascular nerves in intracranial and extracerebral arteries, including anterior, middle and posterior cerebral, and basilar arteries; (b) effects of Ca^{2+} channel inhibitors, including flunarizine, on the neurogenic vasodilation; and (c) comparisons of the responsiveness to perivascular nerve stimulation in cerebral and extracranial (retinal central and superficial temporal) arteries obtained from dogs.

ANALYSIS OF MECHANISMS UNDERLYING CEREBRAL VASODILATION INDUCED BY PERIVASCULAR NERVE STIMULATION

Nonadrenergic, noncholinergic nerves responsible for the cerebral arterial relaxation were first found by the use of nicotine, which is known to stimulate neuronal nicotinic receptors located not only in ganglionic cells but also nerve terminals innervating the vascular wall (5). This phenomenon is also observed in the relaxant response to nerve stimulation with electrical pulses (6). Possible involvement of cerebral vasodilator peptides, such as vasoactive intestinal polypeptide, substance P, calcitonin gene-related peptide, and atrial natriuretic peptide, as neurotransmitters is excluded (7). However, the mechanism of neurogenic vasodilation was not clarified until a NO synthase inhibitor was applied to our preparations in 1989.

Figure 1 is a typical tracing of the response to transmural electrical stimulation at

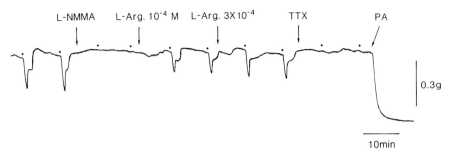

FIG. 1. Abolishment by N^G-monomethyl-L-arginine (L-NMMA) (10^{-4} M) of the relaxant response to transmural electrical stimulation (5 Hz) and restoration of the response by high concentrations of L-arginine (L-Arg.) in a dog middle cerebral arterial strip partially contracted with PGF$_{2\alpha}$. Tetrodotoxin (TTX, 3×10^{-7} M) abolishes neurogenic response; papaverine (PA, 10^{-4} M produces maximal relaxation. From Toda et al. (9).

5 Hz of a canine cerebral arterial strip partially contracted with prostaglandin F$_{2\alpha}$ (PGF$_{2\alpha}$). Treatment with N^G-monomethyl-L-arginine (L-NMMA), a NO synthase inhibitor found by Palmer et al. (8), abolished the relaxation, and L-arginine restored the response (9). The D-enantiomers were without effect. Nicotine-induced relaxations were also abolished by NO synthase inhibitors, such as L-NMMA and N^G-nitro-L-arginine (L-NA), whereas the response to exogenously applied NO, the acidified NaNO$_2$ solution, was unaffected. In superfused, endothelium-denuded cerebral arterial strips, transmural electrical stimulation or nicotine increased the release of NO, measured as NO$_x$, into the superfusate and the content of cyclic guanosine monophosphate (GMP) (10). The effects were abolished by treatment with L-NA. Histochemical study demonstrated the presence of perivascular nerve fibers and bundles containing NO synthase immunoreactivity in the arteries used. On the basis of these findings, we hypothesized that NO acts as a neurotransmitter in the perivascular nerve and produces smooth muscle relaxation via increased production of cyclic GMP (Fig. 2). The nerve is thus called *nitroxidergic* (11).

MODIFICATIONS BY CA^{2+} CHANNEL INHIBITORS OF THE RESPONSE TO NITROXIDERGIC NERVE STIMULATION

Effects of nicardipine (a dihydropyridine-type inhibitor that selectively inhibits the L-type Ca^{2+} channel) and Cd^{2+} (a nonselective Ca^{2+} channel inhibitor) in concentrations sufficient to produce similar magnitudes of attenuation of the contractile response to PGF$_{2\alpha}$ or serotonin were evaluated (12). The response to electrical nerve stimulation or nicotine was not influenced by nicardipine but was markedly inhibited or abolished by Cd^{2+} (Fig. 3), suggesting that the nerve activation permits the influx of Ca^{2+} via non-L-type Ca^{2+} channel into nerve terminals. In addition, ω-conotoxin suppressed the response to electrical stimulation but not to nicotine (13). The N-type channel is involved in the Ca^{2+} influx when the nerve is stimulated by elec-

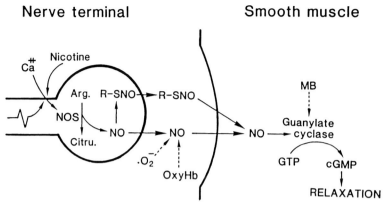

FIG. 2. Schematic presentation of nitroxidergic innervation of cerebral arterial smooth muscle. Arg., L-arginine; Citru., L-citrulline; R-SNO, S-nitroso cysteine; $.O_2^-$ superoxide anion; OxyHb, oxyhemoglobin; MB, methylene blue; GTP, guanosine triphosphate; cGMP, cyclic guanosine monophosphate.

trical pulses, and the non-L, non-N-type channel is responsible for the intracellular introduction of Ca^{2+} by nerve stimulation with nicotine, which does not generate nerve action potentials in isolated blood vessels used.

Flunarizine in concentrations insufficient to produce significant cerebroarterial relaxations attenuated the response to nerve stimulation by electrical pulses and nicotine. Unlike dihydropyridine Ca^{2+} channel inhibitors, flunarizine is reportedly effective in preventing attack in migraine patients, as revealed by double-blind tests (14). Impairment of NO-mediated vasodilator nerve function may participate in the prophylactic action of flunarizine.

EFFECTS OF SUMATRIPTAN

Inhibitory effects of sumatriptan on nerve functions have been recognized. However, the responses to electrical nerve stimulation did not significantly differ in

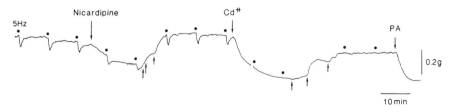

FIG. 3. Modifications by nicardipine and Cd^{2+} of the relaxant response to transmural electrical stimulation (5 Hz) of a dog middle cerebral arterial strip denuded of the endothelium and partially contracted with $PGF_{2\alpha}$. Dot, application of nerve stimulation; upward arrow, supplemental dose of $PGF_{2\alpha}$ applied to restore the arterial tone; PA, 10^{-4} M papaverine. From Toda et al. (12).

cerebral arterial strips contracted with equipotent concentrations of $PGF_{2\alpha}$ and sumatriptan; average values in the relaxation relative to that caused by 10^{-4} M papaverine were $23.5 \pm 4.1\%$ and $28.0 \pm 3.7\%$ (n = 5), respectively. Therefore, prejunctional inhibition by 5-hydroxytryptamine $(5\text{-HT})_{1D}$ receptor stimulation of the neurogenic response is not considered.

Sumatriptan (5×10^{-9} to 10^{-5} M) contracted isolated canine cerebral arteries in a dose-dependent manner. Under prolonged electrical stimulation at 2 Hz that elicited persistent cerebroarterial dilation, sumatriptan in low concentrations (around 10^{-7} M) effectively reversed the effect of nerve stimulation. Physiological antagonism of sumatriptan to endogenous NO-mediated vasodilation is expected to be elicited at the postjunctional site.

COMPARISONS OF THE RESPONSE TO NERVE STIMULATION OF CEREBRAL, RETINAL, AND TEMPORAL ARTERIES

Transmural electrical stimulation and nicotine did not produce contractions of isolated canine cerebral and retinal arteries under resting conditions but relaxed them when partially contracted with $PGF_{2\alpha}$. On the other hand, temporal arteries responded to these stimuli with a contraction that was abolished by α-adrenoceptor blockade. Treatment with L-NA potentiated the contraction elicited by nerve stimulation (15).

Relaxations to nerve stimulation of cerebral arteries contracted with $PGF_{2\alpha}$ were abolished by L-NA, whereas those of retinal arteries were reversed to contractions that were sensitive to α-adrenoceptor antagonists (16). Therefore, adrenergic vasoconstrictor nerve functions are in the order of temporal > retinal >> cerebral arteries.

Under treatment with α-receptor antagonists, temporal arteries responded to nerve stimulation with a relaxation that was abolished by L-NA. L-arginine reversed the response. The rank order of nitroxidergic vasodilator potency is cerebral > retinal > temporal arteries.

These findings may indicate that vasodilation, which is possibly responsible for vascular headache, is elicited by activation of nitroxidergic nerve in cerebral and retinal arteries and that temporal arterial dilation is due to adrenergic nerve suppression in addition to nitroxidergic nerve stimulation.

CONCLUSIONS

Neurogenic vasodilation seen in intracranial and extracerebral arteries and in extracranial arteries, such as the retinal central and superficial temporal arteries, is mediated by NO liberated from perivascular nerves that activates soluble guanylate cyclase in smooth muscle and increases the production of cyclic GMP. The retinal and temporal arterial tone is reciprocally regulated by the nitroxidergic vasodilator and adrenergic vasoconstrictor nerves. The vasodilator nerve function is impaired by flunarizine and physiologically antagonized by sumatriptan. On the basis of the findings presented here, together with those on nitroglycerin action in migraine patients, it is hypothesized that NO, a potent vasodilator and algogenic agent derived from perivascular nerve, is one of the factors involved in migraine and other vascular headaches.

REFERENCES

1. Iversen HK, Olesen J, Tfelt-Hansen P. Intravenous nitroglycerin as an experimental model of vascular headache. Basic characteristics. *Pain* 1989;38:17–24.
2. Toda N. Mechanism underlying responses to histamine of isolated monkey and human cerebral arteries. *Am J Physiol* 1990;258:H311–H317.
3. Krabbe A, Olesen J. Headache provocation by continuous intravenous infusion of histamine. Clinical results and receptor mechanisms. *Pain* 1980;8:253–259.
4. Toda N. Endothelial and neural nitric oxide-induced cerebral artery dilatation. In: Olesen J, Schmidt RF, eds. *Pathophysiological mechanisms of migraine*. New York: VCH Publishers, 1993:37–43.
5. Toda N. Nicotine-induced relaxation in isolated canine cerebral arteries. *J Pharmacol Exp Ther* 1975; 193:374–384.
6. Toda N. Relaxant responses to transmural stimulation and nicotine of dog and monkey cerebral arteries. *Am J Physiol* 1982;243:H145–H153.
7. Toda N, Okamura T. Role of nitric oxide in cerebroarterial relaxation. In: Phillis JW, ed. *The regulation of cerebral blood flow*. London: CRC Press, 1993:233–246.
8. Palmer RMJ, Rees DD, Ashton DS, Moncada S. L-arginine is the physiological precursor for the formation of nitric oxide in endothelium-dependent relaxation. *Biochem Biophys Res Commun* 1988; 153:1251–1256.
9. Toda N, Okamura T. Modification by L-N^G-monomethyl arginine (L-NMMA) of the response to nerve stimulation in isolated dog mesenteric and cerebral arteries. *Jpn J Pharmacol* 1990;52:170–173.
10. Toda N, Okamura T. Nitroxidergic nerve: regulation of vascular tone and blood flow in the brain. *J Hypertens* 1996;14:423–434.
11. Toda N, Okamura T. Regulation by nitroxidergic nerve of arterial tone. *News Physiol Sci* 1992;7: 148–152.
12. Toda N, Okamura T. Different susceptibility of vasodilator nerve, endothelium and smooth muscle functions to Ca^{++} antagonists in cerebral arteries. *J Pharmacol Exp Ther* 1992;261:234–239.
13. Toda N, Uchiyama M, Okamura T. Prejunctional modulation of nitroxidergic nerve function in canine cerebral arteries. *Brain Res* 1995;700:213–218.
14. Toda N, Tfelt-Hansen P. Calcium antagonists. In: Olesen J, Tfelt-Hansen P, Welch MA, eds. *The Headache*. Philadelphia: Lippincott–Raven, 1993:383–390.
15. Toda N, Okamura T. Reciprocal regulation by putatively nitroxidergic and adrenergic nerves of monkey and dog temporal arterial tone. *Am J Physiol* 1991;261:H1740–H1745.
16. Toda N, Kitamura Y, Okamura T. Role of nitroxidergic nerve in dog retinal arterioles in vivo and arteries in vitro. *Am J Physiol* 1994;266:H1985–H1992.

Headache Pathogenesis: Monoamines, Neuropeptides, Purines, and Nitric Oxide, edited by J. Olesen and L. Edvinsson.
Lippincott–Raven Publishers, Philadelphia © 1997.

35

Nitric Oxide Synthase Activation and Inhibition in Migraine

Lisbeth H. Lassen and Jes Olesen

Department of Neurology, Glostrup Hospital, University of Copenhagen, DK-2600 Glostrup, Copenhagen, Denmark

It has long been known that glyceryl trinitrate (GTN) can induce headache in humans. Recently it has been shown that GTN in migraineurs induces an immediate headache during the infusion and a delayed migraine headache with peak headache intensity approximately 5.5 hours after the infusion (1). Glyceryl trinitrate is an *exogenous* direct donor of nitric oxide (NO) (2). Histamine is an *endogenous* donor of nitric oxide via H_1 receptor activation (3). In a double-blind study 20 migraineurs were pretreated with either the H_1 receptor antagonist mepyramine or placebo before histamine infusion. The time course of the histamine-induced headache in placebo-pretreated patients was almost identical with the time course of GTN-induced headache. Patients pretreated with mepyramine experienced very little headache (4) (Fig. 1). After infusion, five of the ten placebo-pretreated patients experienced migraine compared with none of the ten mepyramine-pretreated patients. Furthermore, a decrease in the mean blood velocity in the middle cerebral artery was found in the placebo-pretreated patients during histamine infusion, indicating dilation of this artery; this decrease in blood velocity was significantly attenuated when patients were pretreated with mepyramine (ms. in preparation). In the endothelium of human arteries, NO is formed from L-arginine and molecular oxygen by the enzyme nitric oxide synthase (eNOS). Several substances including histamine stimulate eNOS via receptor activation with subsequent release of endogenous NO (3,5). The common mediator for GTN and histamine-induced migraine is most likely NO, which might cause headache by dilation of cerebral arteries, or via a more direct effect on perivascular nerve endings (6).

Nitric oxide synthase exists in several isoforms. There is one constitutive isoform in endothelial cells, eNOS (7), a different one in neurons, nNOS (8), and there is an inducible isoform represented in macrophages and endothelial cells, iNOS (9). For our studies of inhibition of induced and spontaneous migraine attacks we used the NOS inhibitor, N^G methyl-L-arginine hydrochloride (546C88), kindly provided by Glaxo-Wellcome. 546C88 inhibits both eNOS, nNOS, and iNOS.

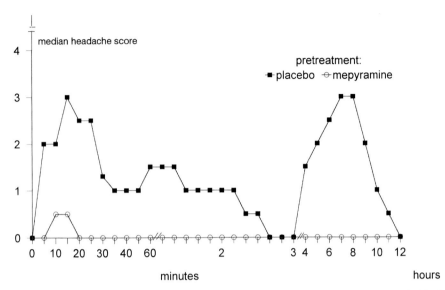

FIG. 1. Time course of the histamine-induced headache, when patients were pretreated with either placebo or mepyramine. The total headache experienced during the 12-hour observation period (summed headache score) was significantly reduced by pretreatment with mepyramine ($p < 0.005$).

A DOSE-RESPONSE STUDY OF 546C88 IN HEALTHY VOLUNTEERS

The objective of the first study was to find the appropriate dose of 546C88 for studies of experimentally induced and spontaneous migraine attacks.

Methods

In a double-blind, placebo-controlled, crossover design six subjects were randomized to receive 546C88 in doses of 0.3, 1, and 3 mg/kg or placebo intravenously over 5 minutes on 4 different study days; in an open study design the same six subjects received 546C88 in the dose of 6 mg/kg intravenously over 15 minutes. The luminal diameter of the radial artery was measured directly with ultrasound (Dermascan C, Denmark), the mean blood velocity in the middle cerebral artery was followed with transcranial Doppler (DWL), and changes in the blood pressure and heart rate were also followed (Tonoprint).

Results

We found no significant difference in blood velocity responses in the middle cerebral artery between the different doses of 546C88 or placebo ($p = 0.27$, MANOVA). Thus inhibition of NOS had no effect on the basal mean blood velocity in the middle cerebral artery. Furthermore, there was no significant difference among the effects of four doses of 546C88 or placebo on the luminal diameters of the radial artery in the first hour after infusion, so inhibition of NOS with 546C88 had no effect on the basal diameter of the radial artery ($p = 0.50$, MANOVA). In the first 60 minutes the mean arterial blood pressure was significantly different from placebo when 3- and 6-mg/kg doses of 546C88 were given. For the 6-mg/kg dose the maximal increase in mean arterial blood pressure was 20% 20 minutes after start of infusion. Decreases in heart rate at doses of 1, 3, and 6 mg/kg were significantly different from placebo. At the 6-mg/kg dose there was a maximal decrease in heart rate of 24% 15 minutes after start of infusion. No subjects reported symptoms related to the drug and (apart from changes in the heart rate and the blood pressure, which were well tolerated and which are known pharmacological effects of the drug) no adverse effects were observed.

Conclusions

On this basis we chose 6 mg/kg of 546C88 given over 15 minutes for further studies of experimentally induced and spontaneous migraine attacks.

EFFECT OF NITRIC OXIDE SYNTHASE INHIBITION ON HISTAMINE-INDUCED HEADACHE

The effect of pretreatment with 546C88 on histamine-induced migraine attacks and arterial dilation was examined next.

Methods

In a double-blind, placebo-controlled, crossover design 12 migraine patients without aura were pretreated with 546C88 at 6 mg/kg or placebo over 15 minutes for 2 days followed by 20 minutes of histamine infusion (0.5 µg/kg/min). Mean blood velocity in the middle cerebral artery and the luminal diameters of the radial and the temporal arteries were measured repeatedly (using the same equipment as described previously). Headache intensity was scored on a verbal scale of 0 to 10: 0, no headache; 1, prepain (a feeling of pressing or throbbing); 5, headache of medium severity; and 10, the worst possible headache (10). Headache intensity and characteristics were scored every 5 minutes during the first 60 minutes and then every hour in the period from 1 to 12 hours after start of histamine infusion.

Results

No patients experienced headache before and immediately after 546C88 or placebo infusion. There was no significant difference between the number of placebo-pretreated patients and 546C88-pretreated patients who experienced head-

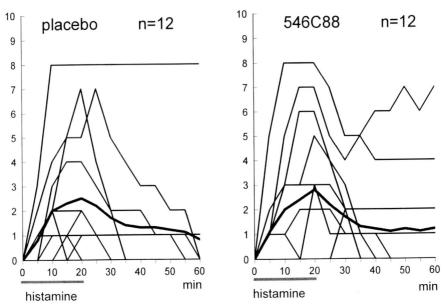

FIG. 2. Histamine-induced headache in the first 60 minutes after start of histamine infusion in placebo- and 546C88-pretreated patients. Bold lines indicate the mean headache score. There was no difference in the sum of headache scores between the placebo- and the 546C88-pretreated group ($p = 0.8$).

ache or migraine either in the first 60 minutes after start of histamine infusion or in the period from 1 to 12 hours after start of histamine infusion (Fisher's exact test).

In the first 60 minutes after start of histamine infusion there was no difference in the sum of headache scores between the placebo- and the 546C88-pretreated patients ($p = 0.80$, Wilcoxon's test) (Fig. 2). Unfortunately, the intensity of the histamine-induced headache in the period from 1 to 12 hours after start of histamine infusion was attenuated by the headache medication that patients were allowed to take in this period. Actually, four of the five 546C88-pretreated patients who developed headache and five of the six placebo-pretreated patients who developed headache took headache medication at different time points in this period. On this ground there was no significant difference in the sum of headache scores in this period ($p = 0.72$, Wilcoxon's test). Confirming results from the dose-response study, 546C88 pretreatment did not affect the baseline mean blood velocity in the middle cerebral artery ($p = 0.99$, Student's t-test for paired data), nor was the magnitude of the histamine-induced decrease in blood velocity affected by 546C88 pretreatment ($p = 0.26$, Student's t-test for paired data). However, an overall multiple analysis of variance (MANOVA) showed a significant difference between the groups, indicating a significant reduction in response in the 546C88-pretreated group in the period 30 to 80 minutes after start of histamine infusion ($p = 0.03$). The 546C88 pretreatment significantly constricted the temporal artery before histamine infusion ($p = 0.002$), but it did not affect the magnitude of the histamine-induced dilation ($p = 0.80$), and, in accordance with the dose-response study, pretreatment with 546C88 did not affect the baseline diameter of the radial artery before histamine infusion ($p = 0.58$), nor was the magnitude of the histamine-induced dilation affected ($p = 0.06$). During basal conditions the temporal artery was more sensitive to NOS inhibition than the radial artery ($p = 0.04$, Student's t-test for paired data).

Conclusions

It was concluded that in the given doses of 546C88 and histamine, NOS inhibition had no effect on the histamine-induced migraine or the magnitude of histamine-induced arterial dilation.

NITRIC OXIDE SYNTHASE INHIBITION: A NEW PRINCIPLE IN THE TREATMENT OF SPONTANEOUS MIGRAINE ATTACKS

Finally the effect of 546C88 as a treatment for *acute migraine* attacks was studied. The primary end point was headache relief, but resolution of nausea, vomiting, and photo- and phonophobia and reduction of clinical disability scores were also studied.

Methods

In a double-blind study 15 patients were randomized to receive 546C88 6 mg/kg over 15 minutes and 3 patients to receive placebo. Furthermore, 11 consecutive, historical placebo controls, who had received placebo intravenously in recent double-blind studies of other drugs for acute migraine attacks, were used in the statistical evaluation. This design was chosen because patient availability did not permit a balanced randomized design in a single center. Candidates for the study were healthy subjects aged between 18 and 50 years with the diagnosis of migraine without aura (11). Patients with a diastolic blood pressure more than 90 mmHg or a heart rate less than 50 bpm were not included. On the study day patients were included provided that their attacks were of moderate or severe intensity, that less than 8 hours had elapsed since start of the actual attack, and that the attack was not already improving. Patients were treated with study medication, followed for 2 hours, and sent home with a headache diary to fill out every 4 hours the following 24 hours. Headache intensity and clinical disability were scored on 4-point verbal scales, and relief was defined as an improvement from grade 3/2 to 1/0 (for explanation see Table 1). Relief of nausea, vomiting, and photo- and phonophobia was defined as improvement from present to absent.

TABLE 1. *Baseline characteristics of the treated migraine attacks*

Characteristic	546C88 (n=15)	Placebo (n=14)
Headache severity		
None (0)	0	0
Mild (1)	0	0
Moderate (2)	9	5
Severe (3)	6	9
Presence of		
Nausea	13	10
Phonophobia	11	12
Photophobia	10	13
Functional disability score		
Normal (0)	0	0
Mild impaired (1)	0	0
Severe impaired (2)	7	4
Bed rest required (3)	8	10

Results

Baseline characteristics of the treated migraine attacks are given in Table 1. There was a significant difference in *headache* relief between the 546C88- and the placebo-treated group after 1 hour ($p < 0.05$, Fisher's exact test). After 2 hours, 10 of 15 patients in the 546C88-treated group experienced *headache* relief compared with 2 of 14 patients in the placebo group ($p < 0.05$, Fisher's exact test) (Table 2).

TABLE 2. *Effect of treatment on various characteristics[a]*

Characteristic (min)	546C88	Placebo	p value[b]
Headache (score 3/2 to 1/0)	(n=15)	(n=14)	
30	5 (33)	1 (7)	
60	8 (53)	1 (7)	<0.05
120	10 (67)	2 (14)	<0.05
Phonophobia (present to absent)	(n=11)	(n=12)	
30	4 (36)	1 (8)	
60	5 (46)	1 (8)	
120	9 (82)	2 (17)	<0.05
Photophobia (present to absent)	(n=10)	(n=13)	
30	4 (40)	0 (0)	
60	6 (60)	0 (0)	<0.05
120	8 (80)	1 (8)	<0.05
Nausea (present to absent)	(n=13)	(n=10)	
30	8 (62)	3 (30)	
60	8 (62)	3 (30)	
120	10 (77)	5 (50)	
Clinical disability (score 3/2 to 1/0)	(n=15)	(n=14)	
30	3 (20)	0 (0)	
60	6 (40)	0 (0)	<0.05
120	8 (53)	2 (14)	

[a] Numbers in parentheses are percentages.
[b] By Fisher's exact test.

There was a significant difference in relief of *photophobia* after 1 hour ($p < 0.05$, Fisher's exact test). After 2 hours, 8 of 10 patients in the 546C88-treated group and 1 of 13 patients in the placebo group experienced relief of *photophobia* ($p < 0.05$). After 2 hours, significantly more patients in the 546C88-treated group than in the placebo-treated group experienced relief of *phonophobia* ($p < 0.05$), but there was no significant difference between the 546C88- and the placebo-treated group in the relief of *nausea*. After 2 hours, 10 of 13 patients in the 546C88 group experienced relief of *nausea*, but this also applied to 5 of the 10 patients in the placebo group ($p = 0.38$).

There was a significant difference between the 546C88- and the placebo-treated groups in the relief of *clinical disability* after 1 hour ($p < 0.05$), but after 2 hours this difference was no longer significant ($p = 0.07$). Apart from changes in blood pressure and heart rate, which were as reported in the dose-response study, the following adverse events were observed among the 546C88-treated patients: one reported a feeling of pressure over the nose, one reported tiredness, and one reported a feeling of tingling in elbows and cold hands.

Conclusions

We conclude that 546C88, a NOS inhibitor, is effective in the treatment of acute migraine attacks and on this basis NOS inhibition is proposed as a new principle in the treatment of migraine attacks. We hope that further experimental and extended clinical trials using more specific NOS inhibitors will elucidate the relative importance of vascular/neurogenic factors in migraine.

ACKNOWLEDGMENTS

Thanks to our colleagues H. K. Iversen, L. L. Thomsen, I. Christiansen, M. Ashina, V. Ulrich, C. Kruuse, and I. Jansen-Olesen, Department of Neurology, Glostrup Hospital, University of Copenhagen, Glostrup, Denmark. The help provided by R. Grover and J. Donaldson, Glaxo-Wellcome Research and Development, Greenford, Middlesex, United Kingdom, is greatly acknowledged.

REFERENCES

1. Thomsen LL, Kruuse C, Iversen HK, Olesen J. A nitric oxide donor (nitroglycerin) triggers genuine migraine attacks. *Eur J Neurol* 1994;1:73–80.
2. Ignarro LJ, Lippton H, Edwards JC, et al. Mechanisms of vascular smooth muscle relaxation by organic nitrates, nitrites, nitroprusside and nitric oxide: evidence for the involvement of S-nitrosothiols as active intermediates. *J Pharmacol Exp Ther* 1981;218:739–749.
3. Toda N. Mechanism underlying responses to histamine of isolated monkey and human cerebral arteries. *Am J Physiol* 1990;258:H311–H317.
4. Lassen LH, Thomsen LL, Olesen J. Histamine induces migraine via H1 receptor activation. Support for the NO-hypothesis of migraine. *NeuroReport* 1995;6:1475–1479.

5. Moncada S, Palmer RMJ, Higgs EA. Nitric oxide: physiology, pathophysiology and pharmacology. *Pharmacol Rev* 1991;43:109–142.
6. Olesen J, Thomsen LL, Lassen LH, Jansen-Olesen I. Nitric oxide hypothesis of migraine and other vascular headaches. *Cephalalgia* 1994;15:94–100.
7. Vane JR, The Croonian lecture. The endothelium: maestro of the blood circulation. *Proc R Soc Lond [Biol]* 1993;343:225–246.
8. Dawson VL, Dawson TM, London ED, Bredt DS, Snyder SH. Nitric oxide mediates glutamate neurotoxicity in primary cortical cultures. *Proc Natl Acad Sci USA* 1991;88:6368–6371.
9. Xie Q, Nathan C. The high-output nitric oxide pathway: role and regulation. *J Leukoc Biol* 1994;56:576–582.
10. Iversen HK, Olesen J, Tfelt-Hansen P. Intravenous nitroglycerin as an experimental model of vascular headache. Basic characteristics. *Pain* 1989:38;17–24.
11. Headache Classification Committee of the International Headache Society. Classification and diagnostic criteria for headache disorders, cranial neuralgias and facial pain. *Cephalalgia* 1988;8[Suppl 7]:1–92.

36

The Nitric Oxide Hypothesis of Migraine and Other Vascular Headaches

Jes Olesen, Lars L. Thomsen, Lisbeth H. Lassen, and
*Inger Jansen-Olesen

*Department of Neurology, Glostrup Hospital, University of Copenhagen,
DK-2600 Glostrup, Copenhagen, Denmark; and *Department of Biological Sciences,
The Royal Danish School of Pharmacy, DK-2100, Copenhagen Ø, Denmark*

Migraine attacks are associated with intra- and extracranial arterial dilation (1–3). This and other findings (4,5) demonstrate that the site of nociception is the perivascular space, where sensory nerve endings are stimulated (4,5). However, the nature of this stimulant remains obscure. Neurogenic inflammation is one possibility (6). This reaction involves the liberation of several neuropeptides, primarily substance P and calcitonin gene-related peptide (CGRP) (7). Unfortunately, neurogenic inflammation has never been shown to occur around cranial blood vessels during migraine attacks, and the concentration of substance P in external and internal jugular venous blood remains normal during migraine attacks (8,9). Also neuropeptide Y and vasoactive intestinal peptide, which are important neuropeptides found in sympathetic and parasympathetic nerve fibers around the intra- and extracranial blood vessels, remain normal in blood from the internal and external jugular veins during migraine attacks (8,9).

The only peptide known to be released during migraine attacks is CGRP. The concentration of this peptide is increased in the external but not in the internal jugular venous blood (8,9). However, CGRP does not cause pain when either infused intravenously or injected into the superficial temporal muscle (10,11). It does not even potentiate pain induced by other substances (11). The spectacular therapeutic effect of 5-hydroxytryptamine (5-HT) receptor agonists in migraine might indicate that 5-HT is involved. However, 5-HT injected intravenously or locally into the superficial temporal muscle does not cause pain (12,13) and it only slightly aggravates bradykinin-induced pain in the temporal muscle (12). It may be concluded that none of the peptides or monoamines examined are likely to cause the nociception responsible for migraine pain.

Nitric oxide (NO) is a much better candidate as the causative molecule in migraine. This small, almost ubiquitous messenger molecule does not interact with a specific receptor but diffuses freely across membranes. It activates intracellular soluble guanylate cyclase, the enzyme catalyzing formation of cyclic guanosine monophosphate (cGMP), which in turn phosphorylates further enzymes. The end result is a decrease of cytosolic calcium (for review, see ref. 14). In vascular smooth muscle, the activation of this so-called NO-cGMP pathway leads to relaxation and vascular dilation. In other tissues it has other effects depending on the type of tissue. Thus cytotoxity, modulation of pain perception, and modulation of transmitter functions in perivascular nonadrenergic, noncholinergic nerves are well-known effects of NO (14). Recent studies of histamine- and glyceryl trinitrate (GTN)-induced headaches, to be discussed below, have prompted us to propose the following hypothesis about the role of the NO-cGMP pathway in migraine and other vascular headaches.

THE NITRIC OXIDE HYPOTHESIS

1. Activation of the NO-cGMP pathway causes migraine attacks in migraineurs, cluster headache attacks in cluster headache sufferers during cluster periods, and nonspecific vascular headaches in others.
2. Drugs that are effective in the treatment of migraine and other vascular headaches, and that are not general analgesics, exert their activity by inhibiting one or more steps in the NO-cGMP pathway or by antagonizing the effects of products of this pathway.
3. Substances that are able to cause an attack of migraine or other vascular headaches do so by stimulating one or more steps in the NO-cGMP pathway or by exerting effects that are agonistic to those of one or more steps in this pathway.

As with all meaningful hypotheses, the present hypothesis is supported by good data, yet cannot be regarded as proved. All parts of the hypothesis have the advantage of being easily testable. In the following discussion, the support for each of the three parts of the hypothesis is discussed separately.

Support for the First Part of the Hypothesis

Histamine and GTN are substances that reliably and dose-dependently produce headache in normal volunteers and migraine sufferers (15–17) (Fig. 1). Several years ago our search for the molecular mechanisms of migraine pain therefore focused on the study of headache induced experimentally by GTN or histamine. By itself, GTN has no known action in the human body but acts via liberation of NO and is thus generally regarded as an NO donor (18–21). It is the most suitable substance for experimental studies of NO-induced headache since it is well tolerated and diffuses freely across membranes due to its lipid solubility. It may thus deliver NO to vascular tissues including those protected by the blood-brain barrier. Histamine also seems to induce headache via NO. In human cerebral blood vessels it stimulates an endothelial H_1 receptor that probably activates nitric oxide synthase (NOS), the enzyme that catalyzes formation of NO from L-arginine (22,23). Histamine thus stimulates the

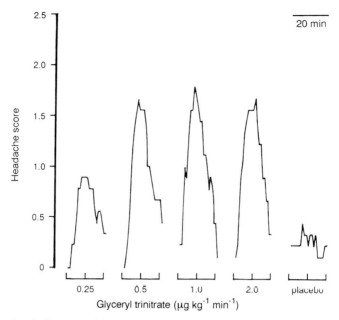

FIG. 1. Mean headache scores (0 to 10 scale) during and after four doses of intravenous glyceryl trinitrate in normal headache-free subjects on day 1 of 2 separate study days. Glyceryl trinitrate was infused for 10 minutes, and during this period a rapid increase in headache was observed. This was followed by a 10-minute washout period, which resulted in a rapid decrease in headache. There was a relatively low day-to-day variation and a ceiling effect at approximately 0.5 µg/kg/min. From Iversen et al. (16).

endogenous formation of NO, whereas GTN delivers NO directly. Most studies supporting a role of NO in migraine pathophysiology have used GTN (24–29). It is therefore important that the following direct studies in humans support the hypothesis that GTN induces headache by liberating NO.

1. The GTN-induced headache in normal controls is very short lived and is therefore unlikely to be caused by metabolites other than NO, since these have a longer half-life (16).
2. Isosorbide mononitrate has a long half-life and is not metabolized to S-nitrosothiols (30). It causes a long-lasting headache and long-lasting arterial dilation in a dose-dependent fashion (17).
3. *N*-acetylcysteine, which augments GTN effects in the heart by increasing the formation of NO or by enhancing the effect of NO itself, also augments the headache response to GTN and prolongs arterial dilation of the superficial temporal artery but not of the radial arteries (25).

It thus seems clear that GTN induces headache via liberation of NO in nonmigraineurs, but how relevant is this for migraine? It has been proposed that only subjects with a family history of migraine develop migraine-like GTN-induced headache (24), but this response does not seem to be an all-or-none phenomenon (16, 27,29). The headache induced in nonmigraineurs varies from being completely absent in a few individuals to being of mild or moderate intensity. It rapidly diminishes after the GTN infusion stops and disappears completely after 10 to 20 minutes. The headache response is dose dependent up to 0.5 µg/kg/min, after which a ceiling effect is observed so that higher doses do not increase headache intensity (16). The headache in nonmigraineurs has some of the features of a migraine attack but differs from migraine by being milder and without nausea or photo- and phonophobia (17). In migraineurs the response is different.

In a recent study comparing 17 headache-free individuals with 17 migraine sufferers, migraineurs developed a significantly stronger headache with more migrainous features than controls (29). The difference between controls and migraineurs became more apparent after the end of the infusion. Thus, none of the control subjects developed significant headache after the initial headache had gone, whereas the migraineurs either had no relief of headache after the infusion or had an initial relief followed by a subsequent worsening. Within 24 hours after infusion 11 migraineurs but no control subjects developed a headache that they labeled as typical migraine. Fourteen of the migraineurs but no control subjects took sumatriptan for the postinfusion headache. However, in this study characteristics of postinfusion headache and accompanying symptoms were not recorded in detail. In another study hourly prospective recordings were made of headache characteristics and accompanying symptoms during 12 hours after infusion of GTN 0.5 µg/kg/min or placebo intravenously for 20 minutes (27) (Fig. 2). The study was done in ten sufferers of migraine without aura using a double-blind placebo-controlled crossover design. Eight

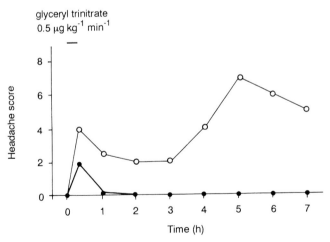

FIG. 2. Comparison of the mean headache scores (0 to 10 scale) in response to glyceryl trinitrate (0.5 µg/kg/min for 20 minutes) in migraineurs (circles) and nonmigraineurs (filled circles). Data from Thomsen et al. (27) and Olesen et al. (29). From Olesen et al. (65).

patients developed headache during the GTN infusion, but only one satisfied the migraine criteria during the infusion. However, eight patients developed a regular migraine attack fulfilling International Headache Society (IHS) criteria after GTN. Peak headache occurred at a mean of 5.5 hours after the infusion. The induced migraine attacks were very similar to the usual migraine attacks of the patients. Thus, five patients, who habitually had unilateral migraine, all developed unilateral attacks after GTN and three patients, who normally had bilateral migraine attacks, all developed bilateral attacks after GTN. The accompanying symptoms experienced after GTN were also similar to patients' usual accompanying symptoms. Only one placebo-treated patient developed a migraine attack.

The next question is where and how NO acts to cause an immediate vascular headache as well as a subsequent migraine attack. The demonstration of numerous endothelial receptors on cerebral arteries has made it clear that cerebral arteries, despite their blood-brain barrier, may be influenced by circulating vasoactive substances such as CGRP, 5-HT, histamine, etc. (31). Although an animal experimental study has shown that GTN dilates cerebral arteries via liberation of CGRP (32), studies of animal and human material both in vitro and in vivo do not support this finding (33,34). It has been suggested that GTN degranulates mast cells and basophils (35). This would liberate histamine around dural blood vessels, where mast cells are abundant, but not around cerebral blood vessels, where they are scarce (36). Theoretically, GTN could therefore induce headache by liberation of histamine. However, pretreatment of patients with the histamine H_1 blocker mepyramine, which is known to prevent histamine-induced headache (15), did not prevent or even reduce GTN-induced headache (26). Nitric oxide from GTN is therefore likely to exert its effect directly on cranial blood vessels and/or perivascular nerves.

Cortical spreading depression, which is presumed to underlie the migraine aura, induces a multiphasic release of NO, characterized by an initial peak or a slow, smaller amplitude second peak when assayed by an NO-selective microelectrode (37). Nitric oxide may therefore be responsible for the pain phase in migraine with aura. Another interesting link to clinical migraine is the marked modulation of NOS caused by the female sex hormones (38). It is important to know which type of cranial blood vessels might be involved. Since no changes occur in cerebral blood flow during attacks of migraine without aura, the arterioles, which control flow, seem to be unaffected (for review, see ref. 39). By contrast, large intracranial arteries seem to be dilated during attacks of migraine with as well as without aura (1,3). Glyceryl trinitrate induces arterial dilation. This has been shown in intracranial arteries using a combination of transcranial Doppler and single-photon emission computed tomography (SPECT) (40,41) and in extracranial arteries by high-frequency ultrasound determination of the superficial temporal artery diameter (17). Glyceryl trinitrate-induced arterial dilation as well as the headache were augmented by *N*-acetylcysteine pretreatment (25). Finally, the dilation of the middle cerebral artery induced by GTN was significantly greater in migraine sufferers than in normal controls (28). The cerebral arteries are, for all these reasons, a likely site of action of GTN-induced headache.

Ekbom (42) gave 1 mg of nitroglycerin sublingually to 28 patients with cluster headache during a cluster period. With a latency of 30 to 50 minutes after administration, all patients developed a typical cluster headache attack (42). Subsequently others have confirmed the provocation of typical cluster headache attacks by nitroglycerin (43,44). Histamine, probably via induction of cerebrovascular endogenous NO formation, as discussed above, also causes cluster headache attacks in sufferers (45). As in migraine, NO triggers attacks only in susceptible individuals and after a surprisingly long latency period. This finding suggests that, in both conditions, NO initiates a slow pathological reaction that eventually leads to the attack.

Meningitis and encephalitis, which cause severe headache, increase the formation of cytokines, which again stimulate macrophage-inducible NOS and production of NO (46). Recently it was shown that migraineurs are more sensitive to endotoxin than nonmigraineurs (47). Endotoxin stimulates the formation of cytokines. Hypoxia is another known cause of vascular headache (48), and, conversely, pure oxygen has been used as an effective treatment for cluster headache (49). Hypoxia augments NO in blood vessels from several species (50,51), and hyperoxia causes a more rapid inactivation of NO and thereby shortens and diminishes its effect (31). Following trauma, headache often occurs with a delay of hours or days (48). There is similar time delay in the development of an inflammatory reaction known to cause an increased formation of NO via inducible NOS (31,52). Thus, the vascular component of post-traumatic headache could easily be caused by endogenous formation of NO. Ischemic cerebrovascular disease is quite often associated with headache of a vascular type and is associated with rapid formation of NO (48). In approximately 10% of cases, headache even occurs before the stroke, the so-called sentinel headache. During platelet aggregation and thrombus formation, a number of substances such as 5-HT, adenosine diphosphate, adenosine triphosphate, platelet activating factor, thrombin, and prostacyclin are released. Several of these substances stimulate the formation of NO in cerebral vascular endothelium (53). Both sentinel headache and headache during stroke could therefore be secondary to thrombus formation and increased vascular concentrations of NO.

Support for the Second Part of the Hypothesis

Our knowledge about the effects of NO on the cranial circulation and perivascular nerves and about the magnitude and importance of spontaneous NO production in human cerebrovascular endothelium is limited. This makes it impossible to analyze fully when and how existing antimigraine drugs interact with the NO-triggered cascade of reactions. However, some observations do suggest an importance of such interactions.

Sumatriptan, the most specific drug for the treatment of migraine attacks, reduces GTN-induced immediate headache and in parallel contracts cerebral and extracerebral arteries (54). In another chapter in this book Rüdinger and Jansen-Olesen report that sumatriptan in arterial homogenates downregulates the activity of NOS. Nitric oxide antagonism may prove to be the most important effect of sumatriptan.

Pure oxygen has been used successfully in the treatment of cluster headache (49) but has not been sufficiently studied in migraine. Nitric oxide is removed from tissues by oxidation to form NO_2^- (nitrite) (31). The action of pure oxygen may thus be explained by its role as an NO scavenger in cerebral arteries.

Calcium antagonists block voltage-dependent Ca^{2+} channels, thereby reducing the concentration of free cytosolic calcium. Since the constitutive NOS in the endothelium is Ca^{2+} dependent (14), calcium antagonists might exert their prophylactic effect in migraine via decreased activity of NOS. Another possibility for non-L-type calcium channels to interact with the NO cascade is described by Professor Toda in Chapter 34 of this volume. Action potentials in nonadrenergic noncholinergic nerves open such channels, and the influx of calcium stimulates the production of NO. Methysergide and pizotifen are nonselective 5-HT antagonists. It has recently been suggested that their effect is via 5-HT_{2B} (previously called 5-HT_{2C} or 5-HT_{1C}) receptor antagonism (55). Activation of this receptor liberates endothelial NO (56). In fact, the 5-HT_{2B} receptor has the highest affinity for 5-HT of any 5-HT receptor and thus may produce NO secondary to only a modest increase in free plasma 5-HT (57). Thus, amine antagonists may well exert their action by reducing endothelial NO production.

Propranolol blocks isoprenaline-induced relaxation of rat thoracic aorta in an endothelium-dependent fashion. The response was also blocked by the NOS inhibitor L-nitroarginine (L-NOARG) (58). Similar observations were made in rabbit aorta (59). The prophylactic effect of β-adrenergic blockers in migraine may thus result from blockade of β-adrenoceptor-induced NO production. Propranolol also antagonizes the 5-HT_{2B} receptor on the endothelium (60). This is another mechanism whereby it may reduce endothelial NO production. In contrast to propranolol, pindolol, which is ineffective in migraine, lacks affinity to the 5-HT_{2C} receptor (56).

Support for the Third Part of the Hypothesis

The only substances that have been reliably shown to cause more headache than placebo in single-dose experiments are GTN, histamine, reserpine, *m*-chlorophenylpiperazine (m-CPP), and, less convincingly, prostacyclin and hypoxia. In this volume Glover reports that fenfluramine is also a reliable inducer of headache and migraine. Alcohol may trigger migraine in some sufferers after a variable period of time. The hangover headache is a complex phenomenon involving a variable proportion of toxic, abstinence, myofacial, and psychological mechanisms. The GTN-induced headache has been described in detail above and the histamine-induced headache in Chapter 35 by Lassen and Olesen. In the following discussion we therefore concentrate on reserpine, m-CPP, prostacyclin, and hypoxia.

Hypoxia is known to induce headache, the best known example being high-altitude headache. However, no formal study of the effects of hypoxia in migraine sufferers is available. Recently Arregui et al. (61) showed that persons living at high altitude had a huge increase in migraine prevalence. Hypoxia increases longevity of NO, whereas pure oxygen acts as a NO scavenger, reducing the lifetime and thereby the effect of NO. Hypoxic vascular headache and hypoxia-induced migraine may thus be due to increased spontaneous NO concentration.

Prostacyclin has been shown in one study to cause a vascular headache in migraineurs (62). Prostacyclin is a vasodilator and may act directly on smooth muscle receptors but, in cerebral vessels protected by the blood-brain barrier, is more likely to act via endothelial receptors by liberating NO (31).

In migraineurs reserpine has been shown to cause a vascular headache with some migrainous features (63). Reserpine depletes not only platelets but also presynaptic nerve terminals of their content of monoamines. The same pertains to fenfluramine, as reported by Glover in Chapter 17 of this volume. Substances released include 5-HT. The 5-HT$_{2B}$ receptor has recently been suggested to play a crucial role in the initiation of migraine attacks (55). The 5-HT caused an endothelium-dependent relaxing response in a number of vessels from different species, and this effect was mediated via the 5-HT$_{2B}$ receptor. The vascular response to 5-HT$_{2B}$ activation, at least in the pig, is primarily a consequence of the release of NO (56). A direct agonist at the 5-HT$_{2B}$ receptor, m-CPP, is therefore likely to cause vascular headache via NO synthesis (55).

It may be concluded that GTN and histamine, which reliably induce vascular headache in nonmigraineurs and migraine in migraineurs, do so by activating the NO-cGMP pathway. Headache induced by other substances such as reserpine, fenfluramine, m-CPP, and prostacyclin, as well as headache induced by hypoxia, has been less well studied regarding both headache characteristics and mechanisms. For each substance there is, however, at least one known mechanism whereby the NO-cGMP pathway is stimulated. Whether this is the only or the major mechanism of the headache-inducing ability remains to be shown.

As more substances with headache-inducing properties become known, it will rapidly become clear whether our hypothesis can explain all experimental vascular headaches or whether other mechanisms must be implied as well.

CALCIUM CHANNELS AND THE NITRIC OXIDE-CYCLIC GUANOSINE MONOPHOSPHATE PATHWAYS

Constitutive NOS (enzyme NOS and nerve NOS) are calcium-calmodulin sensitive. An overload of intracellular calcium in neurons and endothelial cells activates NOS. Also, calcium channels in perivascular nerve terminals are crucial for signal transduction in NOS-containing nerves. These factors may be of importance in relating the newly cloned gene for familial hemiplegic migraine to migraine pathophysiology in general and to NO mechanisms in particular (64).

REFERENCES

1. Friberg L, Olesen J, Iversen HK, Sperling B. Migraine pain associated with middle cerebral artery dilatation: reversal by sumatriptan. *Lancet* 1991;338:13–17.

2. Iversen HK, Nielsen TH, Olesen J, Tfelt-Hansen P. Arterial responses during migraine headache. *Lancet* 1990;336:837–839.
3. Thomsen LL, Iversen HK, Olesen J. Cerebral blood flow velocities are reduced during unilateral attacks of unilateral migraine without aura. *Cephalalgia* 1995;15:109–116.
4. Blau JN, Dexter SL. The site of pain origin during migraine attacks. *Cephalalgia* 1981;1:143–147.
5. Drummond PD, Lance JW. Extracranial vascular changes and source of pain in migraine headache. *Ann Neurol* 1983:13:32–37.
6. Moskowitz MA. Neurogenic inflammation in the pathophysiology and treatment of migraine. *Neurology* 1993;43[Suppl 3]:S16–S20.
7. Buzzi G, Moskowitz M. The antimigraine drug sumatriptan (GR43175) selectively blocks neurogenic plasma extravasation from blood vessels in dura mater. *Br J Pharmacol* 1990;99:202–206.
8. Goadsby PJ, Edvinsson L, Ekman R. Vasoactive peptide release in the extracerebral circulation of humans during migraine headache. *Ann Neurol* 1990;28:183–187.
9. Friberg L, Olesen J, Skyhøj Olsen T, Karle A, Ekman R, Fahrenkrug J. Absence of vasoactive peptide release from brain to cerebral circulation during onset of migraine with aura. *Cephalalgia* 1994; 14:47–54.
10. Shekar YC, Anand IS, Sarma R, Ferrari R, Wahi PL, Poole-Wilson PA. Effect of prolonged infusion of human alpha calcitonin gene-related peptide on hemodynamics, renal bloodflow and hormone levels in congestive heart failure. *Am J Cardiol* 1991;67:732–736.
11. Pedersen-Bjerregård U, Nielse LB, Jensen K, Edvinsson L, Jansen I, Olesen J. Calcitonin gene-related peptide, neurokinin A and substance P: effects on nociception and neurogenic inflammation in human skin and temporal muscle. *Peptides* 1991;12:333–337.
12. Jensen K, Tuxen C, Pedersen-Bjerregård U, Jansen I, Edvinsson L, Olesen J. Pain and tenderness in human temporal muscle induced by bradykinin and 5-hydroxytryptamine. *Peptides* 1990,11.1127–1132.
13. Roberts MHT. 5-Hydroxytryptamine in nociception and antinociception. In: Olesen J and Saxena PR, eds. *5-HT mechanisms of primary headaches*. Philadelphia: Lippincott–Raven, 1992:69–76.
14. Moncada S, Palmer RMJ, Higgs EA. Nitric oxide: physiology, pathophysiology and pharmacology. *Pharmacol Rev* 1991;43:109–141.
15. Krabbe AE, Olesen J. Headache provocation by continuous intravenous infusion of histamine. Clinical results and receptor mechanisms. *Pain* 1980;8:253–259.
16. Iversen HK, Olesen J, Tfelt-Hansen P. Intravenous nitroglycerin as an experimental model of vascular headache. Basic characteristics. *Pain* 1989;38:17–24.
17. Iversen HK, Nielsen TH, Garre K, Tfelt-Hansen P, Olesen J. Dose-dependent headache response and dilatation of limb and extracranial arteries after three doses of 5-isosorbide-mononitrate. *Eur J Clin Pharmacol* 1992;42:31–35.
18. Ignarro LJ, Lipton H, Edwards JC, et al. Mechanisms of vascular smooth muscle relaxation by organic nitrates, nitrites, nitroprusside and nitric oxide: evidence for the involvement of S-nitrosothiols as active intermediates. *J Pharmacol Exp Ther* 1981;218:739–749.
19. Feelisch M, Noack EA. Correlation between nitric oxide formation during degradation of organic nitrates and activation of guanylate cyclase. *Eur J Pharmacol* 1987;139:19–30.
20. Gruetter CA, Kadowitz PJ, Ignarro LJ. Methylene blue inhibits coronary arterial relaxation and guanylate cyclase activation by nitroglycerin, sodium nitrate and amyl nitrate. *Can J Physiol Pharmacol* 1981;59:150–156.
21. Harrison DG, Bates JN. The nitrovasodilators—new ideas about old drugs. *Circulation* 1993;87: 1461–1467.
22. Ottosen ALP, Jansen I, Langemark M, Olesen J, Edvinsson L. Histamine receptors in the isolated human middle meningeal artery. A comparison with cerebral and temporal arteries. *Cephalalgia* 1991; 11:183–188.
23. Toda N. Mechanism underlying responses to histamine of isolated monkey and human cerebral arteries. *Am J Physiol* 1993;258:H311–H317.
24. Sicuteri F, Del Bene E, Poggioni M, Bonazzi A. Unmasking latent dysnociception in healthy subjects. *Headache* 1987;27:180–185.
25. Iversen HK. N-acetylcysteine enhances nitroglycerin-induced headache and cranial arterial responses. *Clin Pharmacol Ther* 1992;52:125–133.
26. Iversen HK, Olesen J. Nitroglycerin-induced headache is not dependent on histamine release. Support for a direct nociceptive action of nitric oxide. *Cephalalgia* 1994;14:437–442.
27. Thomsen LL, Kruuse C, Iversen HK, Olesen J. A nitric oxide donor (nitroglycerin) triggers genuine migraine attacks. *Eur J Neurol* 1994;1:73–80.

28. Thomsen LL, Iversen HK, Brinck TA, Olesen J. Arterial supersensitivity to nitric oxide (nitroglycerin) in migraine sufferers. *Cephalalgia* 1993;13:395–399.
29. Olesen J, Iversen HK, Thomsen LL. Nitric oxide supersensitivity. A possible molecular mechanism of migraine pain. *NeuroReport* 1993;4:1027–1030.
30. Abshagen U, Betzien G, Endele R, Kaufmann B. Pharmacokinetics of intravenous and oral isosorbide-5-mononitrate. *Eur J Clin Pharmacol* 1981;20:269–275.
31. Lüscher TF, Vanhoutte PM. *The endothelium: modulator of cardiovascular functions.* Boston: Chemical Rubber Company Press, 1990:1–228.
32. Wei EP, Moskowitz MA, Boccalini P, Kontos HA. Calcitonin gene related peptide mediates nitroglycerin and sodium nitroprusside induced vasodilation in feline cerebral arterioles. *Circ Res* 1992; 70:1313–1319.
33. Jansen-Olesen I, Iversen HK, Olesen J, Edvinsson L. The effect of nitroglycerin on sensory neuropeptides in isolated guinea pig basilar arteries. In: Moncada S, Feelish M, Busse R, Higgs EA, eds. *Biology of nitric oxide.* vol 3. *Physiology and clinical aspects.* London: Portland Press 1994;368–372.
34. Iversen HK, Jansen I, Edvinsson L, Olesen J. Calcitonin gene-related peptide levels during nitroglycerin-induced headache. *Cephalalgia* 1993;13[Suppl 13]:185.
35. Rozniecki JJ, Kuzminska B, Prusinski A. The possible mechanism of nitroglycerin induced cluster headache attack—a proposed explanation. *Cephalalgia* 1989;9[Suppl 10]:80–81.
36. Edvinsson L, Cervos-Navarro J, Larsson LI, Owman CH, Ronnberg AL. Regional distribution of mast cells containing histamine, dopamine, or 5-hydroxytryptamine in the mammalian brain. *Neurology* 1977;27:878–883.
37. Read SJ, Smith MI, Hunter AJ, Parsons AA. Measurement of NO release using a selective microelectrode following repeated waves of cortical spreading depression. *Br J Pharmacol* 1996;118: 79(abst).
38. Weiner CP, Lizasoain I, Baylis SA, Knowles RG, Charles IG, Moncada S. Induction of calcium-dependent nitric oxide synthase by sex hormones. In: Moncada S, Freelisch M, Basse R, Higgs EA, eds. *The biology of nitric oxide.* vol 3. *Physiological and clinical aspects.* London: Portland Press, 1994:368–372.
39. Olesen J. Cerebral and extracranial circulatory disturbances in migraine: pathophysiological implications. *Cerebrovasc Brain Metab Rev* 1991;3:1–28.
40. Dahl A, Russell D, Nyberg-Hansen R, Rootwell K. Effect of nitroglycerin on cerebral circulation measured by transcranial Doppler and SPECT. *Stroke* 1989;20:1733–1736.
41. Iversen HK, Holm S, Friberg L. Intracranial hemodynamics during intravenous nitroglycerin infusion. *Cephalalgia* 1989;9[Suppl 10]:84–85.
42. Ekbom K. Nitroglycerin as a provocative agent in cluster headache. *Arch Neurol* 1968;19:487–493.
43. Hannerz J, Hellstrøm G, Klum T, Wahlgren NG. Cluster headache and dynamite headadache: blood flow velocities in the middle cerebral artery. *Cephalalgia* 1990;10:31–38.
44. Dahl A, Russell D, Nyberg-Hansen R, Rootwelt K. Cluster headache: transcranial Doppler ultrasound and rCBF studies. *Cephalagia* 1990;10:87–94.
45. Horton BT. Histaminic cephalgia: differential diagnosis and treatment. *Proc Mayo Clin* 1956;31: 325–333.
46. Hibbs JB, Faintor RR, Vavrin Z, et al. Nitric oxide: a cytotoxic activated macrophage effector molecule. *Biochem Biophys Res Commun* 1988;157:87–94.
47. Sicuteri F, Nicolodi M. Nitric oxide action in the mechanisms of fever-induced migraine pain. In: *Abstracts 7th World Congress on Pain.* Paris: IASP Publications, 1993:13.
48. Malinski T, Bailey F, Zhang ZG, Chopp M. NO measurements by a phorphyrinic microsensor in rat brain after transient middle cerebral artery occlusion. *J Cereb Blood Flow Metab* 1993;3:355–358.
49. Kudrow L. Response of cluster headache attacks to oxygen inhalation. *Headache* 1981;21:1–14.
50. Park KH, Rubin LE, Gross SS, Levi R. Nitric oxide is a mediator of hypoxic coronary vasodilatation. Relation to adenosine and cyclooxygenase-derived metabolits. *Circ Res* 1992;71:992–1001.
51. Iwamoto J, Yoshinaga M, Yang SP, Krasney E, Krasney J. Methylene blue inhibits hypoxic cerebral vasodilatation in awake sheep. *J Appl Physiol* 1992;73:2226–2232.
52. Nussler AK, Billiar TR. Inflammation, imunoregulation and inducible nitric oxide synthase. *J Leukoc Biol* 1993;54:171–178.
53. Vanhoutte PM. Platelet-derived serotonin, the endothelium, and cardiovascular disesase. *J Cardiovasc Pharmacol* 1991;17[Suppl 5]:S6–S12.
54. Iversen HK, Olesen J. Headache induced by a nitric oxide donor (nitroglycerin) responds to sumatriptan: A human model for development of migraine drugs. *Cephalalgia* 1996;16:416–418.

55. Fozard JR, Kalkman HO. 5-Hydroxytryptamine (5-HT) and the initiation of migraine: new perspectives. *Naunyn Schmiedebergs Arch Pharmacol* 1994;350:225–229.
56. Glusa E, Richter M. Endothelium-dependent relaxation of porcine pulmonary arteries via 5-HT$_{1c}$-like receptors. *Naunyn Schmiedebergs Arch Pharmacol* 1993;347:471–477.
57. Martin GR. Vascular receptors for 5-hydroxytryptamine distribution, function and classification. *Pharmacol Ther* 1994;62:283–324.
58. Gray DW, Marshall I. Novel signal transduction pathway mediating endothelium-dependent beta-adrenoceptor vasorelaxation in rat thoracic aorta. *Br J Pharmacol* 1992;107:684–690.
59. Aikawa J, Akatsuka N. Vascular smooth muscle relaxation by endothelium-dependent beta 1-adrenergic action. *Comp Biochem Physiol* 1990;97:311–315.
60. Martin GR, Browning C, Giles M. Further characterisation of an atypical 5-HT receptor mediating endothelium-dependent vasorelaxation. *Br J Pharmacol* 1993;110:137.
61. Arregui A, Carera J, Leon-Velarde F, Paredes S, Viscarra D, Arbaiza D. High prevalence of migraine in high-altitude population. *Neurology* 1991;41:1668–1669.
62. Peatfield RC, Gawel MJ, Rose FC. The effect of infused prostacyclin in migraine and cluster headache. *Headache* 1981;21:190–195
63. Lance JW. 5-Hydroxytryptamine and its role in migraine. *Eur Neurol* 1991;31:279–281.
64. Ophoff R, Terwindt G, Vergouwe MN, et al. Familial hemiplegic migraine and episodic ataxia type-2 are caused by mutations in the Ca^{++} channel gene CACNL 1A4.
65. Olesen J, Thompsen LL, Fressen H. Nitric oxide is a key molecule in migraine and other vascular headaches. *TIPS* 1994;5:149–153.

37

Normal Radial Artery Dilation during Reactive Hyperemia in Migraine without Aura

Lars L. Thomsen, Dorthe Daugaard, Helle K. Iversen, and Jes Olesen

Department of Neurology, Glostrup Hospital, University of Copenhagen, DK-2600 Glostrup, Copenhagen, Denmark

Nitric oxide (NO) seems to be involved in the mechanisms of migraine pain (1,2). Several well-known effects of the NO-activated cascade of reactions may be implicated. The NO-mediated dilation of large arteries is one possibility. Thus, dilation of cranial arteries has been reported during spontaneous migraine headache (3,4). Furthermore, NO-induced large cerebral artery dilation seems to be more pronounced in migraineurs than in controls (2). The NO-induced large-artery dilation may be caused by NO released from endothelial cells. This release is triggered by increased friction against the vessel wall (shear stress) (for review, see ref. 5). This happens when the velocity of blood in an artery increases. Blood velocity increases during reactive hyperemia, which causes endothelium-dependent dilation of large arteries (6). The aim of the present study was to evaluate whether disturbances in these endothelial mechanisms are involved in the pathophysiology of migraine.

MATERIALS AND METHODS

Twelve female sufferers of migraine without aura were studied outside of a migraine attack and had been headache free for at least 3 days prior to the examination (7). Twelve healthy subjects matched for age and sex were included for comparison. None of the participants were on migraine prophylaxis or any other daily medication. The design was randomized and single blind, the investigators being blind to the diagnostic group. Before and during induction of reactive hyperemia, radial luminal artery diameter and blood flow velocity were measured with two different ultrasound scanners. One investigator measured the luminal diameter of the left radial artery with a high-resolution ultrasound unit (Dermascan C, Cortex Technology, Hadsund, Denmark; 20 MHz probe, bandwidth 15 MHz, resolution in the axial direction 0.05 mm) (8). These measurements were performed proximal to the distal volar wrist crease, where maximal pulsations of the artery were felt by palpation. Radial arterial blood velocity (V_{mean}) was measured distal to the Dermascan probe by a second investigator using a pulsed Doppler device (Multi-dop X Software TCD-7, DWL, Elektronische Systeme, Sipplingen, Germany; 8 MHz probe).

No medication, coffee, tea, alcohol, or tobacco was allowed 12 hours prior to the examination (sumatriptan 24 hours, ergotamine 48 hours). After arrival in the laboratory the participant was placed in the supine position and remained in this position throughout the study period. Baseline values of diameter and blood velocity in the radial artery were measured after a 30-minute rest. An upper arm arterial occlusion cuff was then inflated to 300 mmHg for 4 minutes (6). After release of arterial occlusion, the radial arterial diameter and blood flow velocity were measured simultaneously every 20 seconds for the first 3 minutes, and then every minute for the next 12 minutes.

RESULTS

Baseline values of arterial diameters [2.41 ± 0.12 mm (mean $\pm$ SEM) in migraineurs and 2.17 ± 0.12 mm in healthy subjects] and blood velocity (7.4 ± 1.3 cm/sec in migraineurs and 9.1 ± 1.8 cm/sec in healthy subjects) did not differ between groups ($p = 0.18$ diameter; $p = 0.44$, blood velocity, by Student's t-test). Radial artery diameter and radial artery blood velocity changes are shown in Figs. 1 and 2.

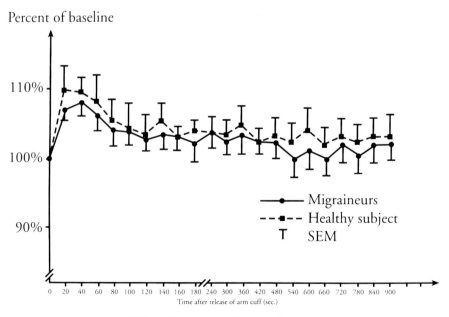

FIG. 1. Radial artery diameter changes.

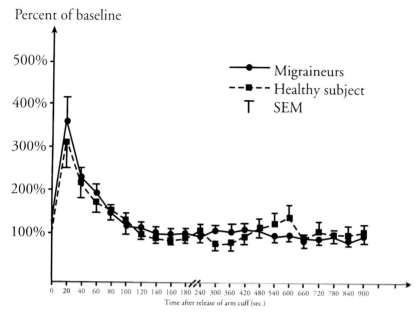

FIG. 2. Radial artery blood velocity changes.

The diameter increased significantly during the first 60 seconds after release of the upper arm arterial occlusion cuff in both groups ($p = 0.0019$, migraineurs; $p = 0.0022$, healthy subjects, MANOVA; $p < 0.05$, multiple range test). No significant group differences were detected in these responses. Thus, the peak response was 111 ± 2% of baseline in migraineurs and 112 ± 3% of baseline in the healthy control group ($p = 0.79$, by Student's t-test). Also the time to peak diameter change was not statistically different between groups (47 ± 9 seconds in migraineurs and 47 ± 13 seconds in healthy subjects; $p = 1.0$, by Student's t-test). The sum of diameter changes during the first 3 minutes (940 ± 16% in migraineurs and 950 ± 23% in healthy subjects) and in the total 15-minute observation period (2,145 ± 40% in migraineurs and 2,185 ± 50% in healthy subjects) did not differ between groups ($p = 0.74$, $p = 0.54$, respectively, by Student's t-test).

The blood velocity increased significantly during the first 40 seconds after release of the upper arm arterial occlusion cuff in both groups ($p < 0.0001$, migraineurs; $p < 0.0001$, healthy subjects, MANOVA; $p < 0.05$ multiple range test). No significant group differences were detected in these responses ($p > 0.05$, by Student's t-test).

DISCUSSION

The present study supports previous human studies showing that the diameter of large peripheral arteries increases in response to reactive hyperemia (6,9,10). Anderson and Mark (9) ruled out that large-artery dilation in response to hyperemia is caused by either (a) changes in local arterial distending pressure, (b) systemic changes in blood pressure, (c) systemic release of ischemic metabolites, or (d) axon reflexes (9). An effect of prostacycline has also been ruled out (10). Rather, the induced large-artery dilation is dependent on the integrity of vascular endothelium and is mediated via release of NO (6,10). Thus, by focusing on large-artery diameter changes in response to reactive hyperemia, the method seems suitable for the detection of dysfunction in stimulated velocity-mediated endothelium-derived NO release.

Nitric oxide seems to be involved in the pathophysiology of migraine pain (1), and hypersensitivity to NO in large arteries has been suggested (2). This could theoretically be explained by increased release of endothelium-derived NO in response to several well-known liberators of NO. On the other hand, arterial hypersensitivity to NO in migraine was found during NO challenge with the NO donor glyceryl trinitrate, which delivers NO directly and endothelium *in*dependently to vascular smooth muscle. Since the molecular target of NO in vascular smooth muscle cells, soluble guanylate cyclase, is upregulated in case of removed endothelium (11), a hypofunction in endothelium-derived NO synthesis/release in migraineurs provides a more likely theoretical explanation for the reported arterial hypersensitivity to NO in migraineurs. The present data do not provide support for this hypothesis. Thus, the comparison of arterial diameter changes revealed no group differences. It remains to be settled whether the same is true in extra- and intracranial arteries.

ACKNOWLEDGMENTS

We appreciate the skillful assistance of laboratory technician Kirsten Enghave and thank the Danish Headache Society, the Foundation for Research in Neurology, the University of Copenhagen, the Danish Foundation for Advancement of Medical Science, and the Henry and Karla Hansen Foundation for financial support.

REFERENCES

1. Olesen J, Iversen HK, Thomsen LL. Nitric oxide supersensitivity. A possible molecular mechanism of migraine pain. *Neuroreport* 1993;4:1027–1030.
2. Thomsen LL, Iversen HK, Brinck TA, Olesen J. Arterial supersensitivity to nitric oxide (nitroglycerin) in migraine sufferers. *Cephalalgia* 1993;13:395–399.
3. Iversen HK, Nielsen TH, Olesen J, Tfelt-Hansen P. Arterial responses during migraine headache. *Lancet* 1990;336:837–839.
4. Friberg L, Olesen J, Iversen HK, Sperling B. Migraine pain associated with middle cerebral artery dilatation: reversal by sumatriptan. *Lancet* 1991;338:13–17.
5. Moncada S, Palmer RMJ, Higgs EA. Nitric oxide: physiology, pathophysiology and pharmacology. *Pharmacol Rev* 1991;43:109–141.
6. Celermajer DS, Sorensen KE, Gooch VM, et al. Non-invasive detection of endothelial dysfunction in children and adults at risk of artherosclerosis. *Lancet* 1992;340:1111–1115.
7. Headache Classification Committee of the International Headache Society. Classification and diagnostic criteria for headache disorders, cranial neuralgias and facial pain. *Cephalalgia,* 1988;8[Suppl 7]:1–96.

8. Nielsen TH, Iversen HK, Tfelt-Hansen P, Olesen J. Small arteries can be accurately studied in-vivo, using high frequency ultrasound. *Ultrasound Med Biol* 1993;19:717–725.
9. Anderson EA, Mark AL. Flow-mediated and reflex changes in large peripheral artery tone in humans. *Circulation* 1989;79:93–100.
10. Joannides R, Haefeli WE, Linder L, et al. Nitric oxide is responsible for flow-dependent dilatation of human peripheral conduit arteries in vivo. *Circulation* 1995;91:1314–1319.
11. Moncada S, Rees DD, Schulz R, Palmer RMJ. Development and mechanism of a specific supersensitivity to nitrovasodilators after inhibition of vascular nitric oxide synthesis in vivo. *Proc Natl Acad Sci USA* 1991;88:2166–2170.

38

Effect of the Nitric Oxide Donor Glyceryl Trinitrate on Nociceptive Thresholds in Humans

Lars L. Thomsen, *Jannick Brennum, Helle K. Iversen, and Jes Olesen

*Department of Neurology, Glostrup Hospital, University of Copenhagen, DK-2600 Glostrup, Copenhagen, Denmark; and *Department of Neurosurgery, Rigshospitalet, DK-2100 Copenhagen, Denmark*

Animal studies suggest that the messenger molecule nitric oxide (NO) plays a role in central and peripheral modulation of nociception (for review, see ref. 1). Most animal studies suggest that NO is involved in centrally induced hyperalgesia, a state of enhanced sensitivity at the spinal level to peripherally applied noxious stimuli. In the periphery, however, NO seems to have antinociceptive effects in rats (2). In humans the role of NO in nociceptive modulation is largely unknown. The aim of the present study was to examine the influence of intravenous infusion of the NO donor glyceryl trinitrate (GTN) on the perception of noxious stimulations in humans and thereby indirectly to examine whether NO modulates human nociception.

MATERIALS AND METHODS

On 2 different days separated by at least a week, 12 healthy subjects (6 female and 6 male; mean age, 24 years; range, 20 to 29 years) received either a staircase i.v. infusion of GTN in four different doses (0.015, 0.25, 1.0, and 2.0 µg/kg/min) for 20 minutes each dose, or placebo (isotonic saline) in a randomized double-blind crossover design. Before and during the infusion, pressure pain detection (and tolerance) thresholds were determined by algometry (Somomedic AD, Sweden) (3,4). The following threshold definitions were presented to the subjects: pressure pain detection threshold—the lowest pressure that evokes a sensation of pain, i.e., the pressure at which sensation changes from one of pressure alone to a combination of pressure and pain; pressure pain tolerance thresholds—the maximal pressure tolerated by the subject. Interpretation of "painful" was left to the subject, who was instructed to apply the same interpretation throughout the study.

The subject was placed in the supine position and remained in this position throughout the study period. During the subsequent 30-minute resting period, pressure pain detection and pressure pain tolerance training were performed on the second left finger. Then baseline determinations of pressure pain detection (and tolerance threshold) were performed in three different regions, the dorsum of the second right finger (middle phalanx) and in two neighboring right-sided temporal locations with and without interposed myofacial tissue (M. temporalis) (4). Then GTN or placebo was infused through a cannula inserted into a right cubital vein. Pressure pain detection (and tolerance) thresholds were determined at steady state (between 15 and 20 minutes of infusion) on each dose. Throughout the study, headache, which is known to occur during GTN infusion, was scored on a 0 to 10 numerical verbal scale (0, no headache; 5, moderate headache; 10, worst possible headache) every 5 minutes as previously described (5).

RESULTS

Changes in pressure pain detection (and tolerance) thresholds on each of the four doses of GTN and placebo are shown in Tables 1 and 2. A biphasic response was seen regarding the GTN minus placebo differences in pressure pain detection (and

TABLE 1. *Pain detection thresholds in percent of baseline[a]*

Region (μg/kg/min)	GTN	Placebo	GTN minus placebo
Finger			
Baseline	100	100	0
0.015	115 (98–168)	115 (80–151)	−2 (−39–59)
0.25	104 (86–169)	125 (76–164)	−19 (−50–60)
1.00	117 (96–186)	122 (81–184)	−9 (−67–59)
2.00	121 (74–186)	134 (59–156)	−20 (−57–86)
p value	0.005	0.0002	0.11
Cranial region			
Without myofascial tissue			
Baseline	100	100	0
0.015	101 (72–130)	109 (71–158)	−1 (−56–30)
0.25	107 (73–128)	111 (86–170)	−20 (−61–36)
1.00	91 (69–136)	112 (77–164)	−23 (−60–34)
2.00	101 (73–139)	118 (82–139)	−13 (−48–52)
p value	0.93	0.06	0.36
With myofascial tissue			
Baseline	100	100	0
0.015	116 (100–144)	100 (80–134)	+20 (−28–34)
0.25	101 (67–141)	115 (85–138)	−6 (−44–16)
1.00	89 (76–192)	126 (88–171)	−26 (−49–33)
2.00	101 (81–188)	129 (92–173)	−25 (−69–21)
p value	0.03	0.0003	0.003

[a] Data are medians, with ranges in parentheses.
p value, probability that pain detection thresholds differ between doses (by Friedman's test).
GTN, glyceryl trinitrate.
From Thomsen et al. (12).

TABLE 2. *Pain tolerance thresholds in percent of baseline*[a]

Region (µg/kg/min)	GTN	Placebo	GTN minus placebo
Finger			
Baseline	100	100	0
0.015	117 (98–141)	112 (73–150)	+4 (−31–58)
0.25	115 (85–156)	109 (64–157)	+2 (−39–69)
1.00	129 (96–162)	118 (73–155)	+6 (−14–58)
2.0	116 (94–162)	124 (59–149)	−16 (−25–70)
p value	0.002	0.003	0.11
Cranial region			
Without myofascial tissue			
Baseline	100	100	0
0.015	101 (86–136)	100 (71–162)	+1 (−33–55)
0.25	104 (77–154)	95 (77–174)	0 (−67–68)
1.00	103 (77–128)	99 (73–164)	+1 (−51–46)
2.00	96 (57–113)	97 (74–196)	−9 (−99–39)
p value	0.14	0.56	0.44
With myofascial tissue			
Baseline	100	100	0
0.015	109 (79–129)	100 (87–121)	+9 (−42–22)
0.25	100 (77–116)	103 (77–120)	−3 (−24–29)
1.00	100 (62–135)	112 (82–149)	−15 (−61–18)
2.00	88 (76–146)	120 (89–161)	−26 (−79–22)
p value	0.01	0.002	0.002

[a]Data are medians, with ranges in parentheses. *p* value, probability that pain detection thresholds differ between doses (by Friedman's test).
GTN, glyceryl trinitrate.
From Thomsen et al. (12)

tolerance) thresholds when stimulations were applied in the temporal region with interposed myofascial tissue ($p = 0.003$, detection threshold; $p = 0.002$, tolerance threshold, Friedman's test). Relative to placebo GTN increased thresholds at the low GTN dose (0.015 µg/kg/min), and relative to placebo GTN decreased thresholds at the three higher GTN doses. Regarding GTN minus placebo responses in the two other stimulated regions, no significant changes were found (Tables 1 and 2).

No subjects had headache at baseline. All subjects complained of headache during GTN infusion, whereas only one experienced headache on the placebo day. The peak and summed nitroglycerin-induced headache scores on each GTN dose increased with increasing doses ($p < 0.0001$ and $p < 0.0001$, respectively, Friedman's test, Statgraphic 2.6).

DISCUSSION

The role of NO in central modulation of nociception in humans is unknown. Theoretically, systemic administration of the clinically well-tolerated NO donor GTN combined with pressure pain algometry could provide some answers. Thus, GTN is a lipophilic compound that easily penetrates the blood-brain barrier and may be demonstrated in the central nervous system (6). It is most likely converted to NO in astrocytes (7). Furthermore, central hyperexitability is reflected by mechanical rather than thermal hyperalgesia in humans (8). The results are, however, difficult to interpret in terms of a central hyperalgesic effect of NO in humans. Thus, relative to placebo, GTN altered pressure pain thresholds only in the temporal region with interposed myofascial tissue. Furthermore, this response was biphasic and consisted of an increase in thresholds at low GTN doses and a decrease at high GTN doses. The biphasic response may be explained by previously described opposite effects of activation of the L-arginine-NO-cyclic guanosine monophosphate pathway peripherally and centrally; peripherally, NO downregulates nociceptors (2), and centrally, NO facilitates pain transmission (1). High GTN doses may have caused high enough NO concentrations in the central nervous system to outbalance peripheral antinociceptive effects. A decrease in thresholds induced by high doses of GTN was, however, only observed in one (temporal with interposed myofacial tissue) of three stimulated regions, and other mechanisms may therefore be more likely.

Convergens of noxious stimuli from blood vessels and myofascial tissue provide a possible explanation of our results. Trigeminal afferents from the cephalic extra- and intracranial arteries terminate on central, wide, dynamic range neurons in the trigiminal nucleus caudalis (9). The same second-order neurons are also activated by electrical stimulation of different extracranial tissues (10). Noxious vascular input from cranial arteries dilated by GTN may cause depolarization just below the firing level of nucleus caudalis neurons, and it may then only take a modest additional input from pressure on extracranial tissues to fire the neuron and cause pain. In that case myofascial noxious stimulation must produce greater effects on central, wide, dynamic neurons than cutaneous noxious stimulation. This has previously been described in animals (11).

ACKNOWLEDGMENTS

This study was supported financially by the University of Copenhagen, the Danish Foundation for the Advancement of Medical Science, the Foundation for Research in Neurology, and the Danish Headache Society.

REFERENCES

1. Meller ST, Gebhart GF. Nitric oxide (NO) and nociceptive processing in the spinal cord. *Pain* 1993; 52:127–136.
2. Ferreira SH. The role of interleukins and nitric oxide in the mediation of inflammatory pain and its control by peripheral analgesics. *Drugs* 1993;46[Suppl 1]:1–9.
3. Jensen K, Andersen HØ, Olesen J, Lindblom U. Pressure pain threshold in human temporal region. Evaluation of a new pressure algometer. *Pain* 1986;25:313–323.
4. Petersen KL, Brennum J, Olesen J. Evaluation of pericranial myofascial nociception by pressure algometry reproducibility and factors of variation. *Cephalalgia* 1992;12:33–37.
5. Iversen HK, Olesen J, Tfelt-Hansen P. Intravenous nitroglycerin as an experimental model of vascular headache. Basic characteristics. *Pain* 1989;38:17–24.
6. Torfgård K, Ahlner J, Axelsson KL, Norlander B, Bertler Å. Tissue distribution of glyceryl trinitrate and the effect on cGMP levels in rat. *Pharmacol Toxicol* 1989;64:369–372.

7. Salvemini D, Mollace V, Pistelli A, Änggård E, Vane J. Cultured astrocytoma cells generate a nitric oxide like factor from endogenous L-arginine and glyceryl trinitrate: effect of *E. coli* lipopolysaccharide. *Br J Pharmacol* 1992;106:931–936.
8. Dahl JB, Brennum J, Arendt-Nielsen L, Jensen TS, Kehlet H. The effect of pre- versus postinjury infiltration with lidocaine on thermal and mechanical hyperalgesia after heat injury to the skin. *Pain* 1993;53:43–51.
9. Davis KD, Dostrovsky JO. Responses of feline trigeminal spinal tract nucleus neurons to stimulation of the middle meningeal artery and sagittal sinus. *J Neurophysiol* 1988;59:648–666.
10. Sessle BJ, Hu JW, Amano N, Zhong G. Convergence of cutaneous, tooth pulp, viceral, neck and muscle afferents onto nociceptive and non-nociceptive neurons in trigeminal subnucleus caudalis (medullary dorsal horn) and its implications for referred pain. *Pain* 1986;27:219–235.
11. Woolf CJ, Wall PD. Relative effectiveness of C primary afferent fibers of different origins in evoking a prolonged facilitation of the flexor reflex in the rat. *J. Neurosci* 1986;6:1433–1442.
12. Thomsen LL, Brennun J, Iversen HK, Olesen J. Effect of a nitric oxide donor (glyceryl trinitrate) on nociceptive thresholds in man. *Cephalagia* 1996;16:169–174.

39

Nitric Oxide as the Final Mediator of Headaches Induced by Central and Peripheral Serotoninergic Mechanisms

Richard Peatfield, *N. Jarrett, F. Ahmed, and *Vivette A. S. Glover

*Princess Margaret Migraine Clinic, Charing Cross Hospital, London W6 8RF, United Kingdom; and *Department of Pediatrics, Queen Charlotte's Hospital, London W6 0XG, United Kingdom*

Although infused serotonin [5-hydroxytryptamine (5-HT)] will lessen established migrainous headache (1), presumably by acting on the same 5-HT_{1D} receptors as sumatriptan, it has been recognized for many years that agents releasing 5-HT from stores, such as reserpine or fenfluramine, can trigger headaches after a delay of 2 to 3 hours (2). It remains uncertain whether these stores are central (within the brain), peripheral (in the cerebral or extracranial blood vessels, platelets, gut, or elsewhere), or both. Our experimental studies with fenfluramine (3), presented elsewhere at this meeting, have found that migraine and tension headache patients are very likely to develop a headache within 2 to 3 hours of fenfluramine challenge, whereas control subjects are not. Both cortisol and prolactin are released by fenfluramine, which suggests that the drug is certainly having an action within the brain.

The trazodone metabolite m-CPP (*m*-chlorophenylpiperazine) was first shown to induce headache in migrainous subjects by Brewerton and colleagues (4) in 1988. This drug has no serotonin-releasing properties but is particularly active at $5\text{-HT}_{2B/2C}$ receptors—the 5-HT_{2C} receptor is found only on the choroid plexus, while the 5-HT_{2B} receptor is found in blood vessels, which suggests it may be the more relevant (5,6). A dose of m-CPP will cause prolactin and cortisol release within 2 to 3 hours, but the headache is delayed for 5 to 8 hours (7).

About 12% of migraine clinic patients say that headaches can be precipitated by red wine in social quantities; a high proportion but by no means all of these patients are also sensitive to cheese and/or chocolate (8). In experimental studies we have shown that red wine can induce headache in selected susceptible subjects, but that there is no effect on prolactin or cortisol (9). This finding suggests that the effect is largely if not exclusively peripheral.

Red wine will release serotonin from preloaded platelets in vitro and is also a $5\text{-HT}_{1A, 1D, 2B/2C}$ ligand. The experiment reported by Jarman et al. (10), in which

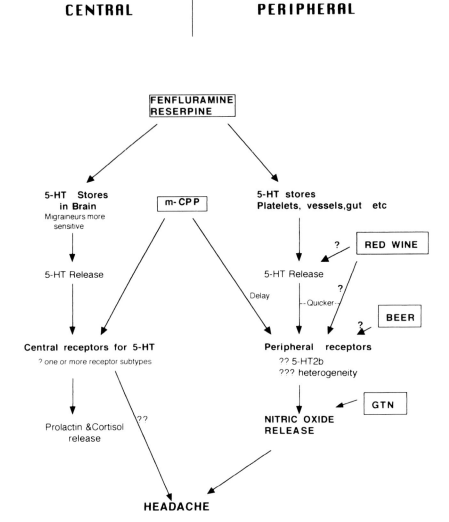

FIG. 1. Summary diagram of the hypothesis in the text. 5-HT, 5-hydroxytryptamine; m-CPP, m-chlorophenylpiperazine.

platelets taken from red wine-sensitive or -nonsensitive migrainous subjects reacted similarly when exposed to red wine in vitro, suggests that the direct pharmacological effect may be more important than serotonin release. Serotonin release, perhaps from nerve endings rather than platelets, could still be an important mechanism, particularly if the inhibitory effect of red wine on the serotonin-metabolizing enzyme phenolsulphotransferase in the gut may cause more potent ligands to enter the circulation from wine than from beer (11).

Central serotoninergic receptor stimulation may be responsible not only for the endocrine effects but also for the headache-producing effect of fenfluramine and m-CPP. We feel that the lack of endocrine effects when headache is induced by red wine is evidence that its effects are peripheral. The nature of the vulnerability in only a minority of the migraine clinic population is obscure, although it may relate either to serotonin release from nerve endings (although not platelets) or to a heterogeneity within one or more serotonin receptors on peripheral structures. The fact that headache induced by fenfluramine or red wine occurs faster than that induced by m-CPP (although the endocrine effects of m-CPP are speedy) is also unexplained.

We know that stimulation of the 5-HT_{2B} receptor can lead to nitric oxide release (12), and Olesen et al.'s (13) experiments with glyceryl trinitrate suggests that this can produce headache in most migrainous subjects. Chabriat et al. (14), in a positron emission tomography scan study, have shown no difference in the 5-HT_{2C} receptor distribution in the human brain, and genetic studies appear to have excluded the 5-HT_{2A} and 5-HT_{2C} receptors (15,16). We speculate that sensitive migraine patients' 5-HT_{2B} receptors may show a greater affinity for the ligand in foods and drinks and are thus more likely to induce headache. Figure 1 summarizes the hypothesis in the text.

REFERENCES

1. Kimball RW, Friedman AP, Vallejo E. Effect of serotonin in migraine patients. *Neurology* 1960; 10:107–111.
2. Del Bene E, Ansalmi B, Del Biano PL, et al. Fenfluramine headache: a biochemical and monoamine receptorial human study. In: Sicuteri F, ed. *Headache: new vistas*. Florence: Biomedical Press, 1977: 101–109.
3. Glover V, Ahmed F, Hussein F, et al. Central 5-hydroxytryptamine supersensitivity in migraine. In: Sandler M, Ferrari M, Harnett S, eds. *Migraine: pharmacology and genetics*. Chapman & Hall, 1996: 117–126.
4. Brewerton TD, Murphy DL, Mueller EA, Jimerson DC. Induction of migrainelike headaches by the serotonin agonist *m*-chlorophenylpiperazine. *Clin Pharmacol Ther* 1988;43:605–609.
5. Fozard JR, Kalkman HO. 5-Hydroxytryptamine and the initiation of migraine: new perspectives. *Naunyn Schmiedebergs Arch Pharmacol* 1994;350:225–229.
6. Schmuck K, Ullmer C, Kalkman HO, et al. Activation of meningeal 5-HT_{2B} receptors: an early step in the generation of migraine headache? *Eur J Neurosci* 1996;8:959–967.
7. Mueller EA, Murphy DL, Sunderland T. Further studies of the putative serotonin agonist, m-chlorophenylpiperazine: evidence for a serotonin receptor mediated mechanism of action in humans. *Psychopharmacology* 1986;89:388–391.
8. Peatfield RC. Relationship between food, wine, and beer-precipitated migrainous headaches. *Headache* 1995;35:355–357.
9. Peatfield RC, Jarrett N, Glover V. The pharmacology of food and drink. In: Sandler M, Ferrari M, Harnett S, eds. *Migraine: pharmacology and genetics*. Chapman & Hall, 1996:127–131.
10. Jarman J, Pattichis K, Peatfield R, et al. Red wine-induced release of [^{14}C]5-hydroxytryptamine from platelets of migraine patients and controls. *Cephalagia* 1996;16:41–43.
11. Littlewood JT, Glover V, Sandler M. Red wine contains a potent inhibitor of phenosulphotransferase. *Br J Clin Pharmacol* 1985;19:275–278.
12. Glusa E, Richter M. Endothelium-dependent relaxation of porcine pulmonary arteries via 5-HT_{1C}-like receptors. *Naunyn Schmiedebergs Arch Pharmacol* 1993;347:471–477.
13. Olesen J, Thomsen LL, Iversen H. Nitric oxide is a key molecule in migraine and other vascular headaches. *Trends Pharmacol Sci* 1994;15:149–153.

14. Chabriat H, Tehindrazanarivelo A, Vera P, et al. 5HT$_2$ receptors in cerebral cortex of migraineurs studied using PET and ^{18}F-fluorosetoperone. *Cephalalgia* 1995;15:104–108.
15. Buchwalder A, Welch SK, Peroutka SJ. Exclusion of 5-HT$_{2A}$ and 5-HT$_{2C}$ receptor genes as candidate genes for migraine. *Headache* 1996;36:254–258.
16. Nyholt DR, Curtain RP, Gaffney PT, et al. Migraine association and linkage analyses of the human 5HT$_{2A}$ receptor gene. *Cephalalgia* 1996;16:463–467.

40

Spreading Depression Evokes a Quantity of Release of Cortical Nitric Oxide Not Correlated to a Change in Pial Artery Diameter or Regional Pial Cerebral Blood Flux

Simon J. Read, M. I. Smith, and A. A. Parsons

Department of Neuroscience, SmithKline Beecham Pharmaceuticals, Harlow, Essex, CM19 5AW, United Kingdom

Cortical spreading depression (SD) is implicated in the pathophysiology of migraine, cerebral trauma, and cerebral ischemia. Typically, SD is characterized by increased cortical and subcortical neuronal metabolism, a change in local ionic environment, release of neurotransmitters into the interstitium, and arterial dilation. This is followed by prolonged suppression of neuronal metabolism (represented as a depression of electroencephalographic activity) and a decrease in regional cerebral blood flow.

It has previously been demonstrated that SD induces a multiphasic release of nitric oxide (NO), characterized as an initial peak followed by a slow, smaller amplitude second peak, which then returns to a basal plateau when assayed by an NO-selective microelectrode (1). In this study, the increases in local concentrations of NO following SD induction reached a mean peak of approximately 0.85 μM, which was of a similar order of magnitude to that observed in cerebral ischemia studies (2). The aim of the present analysis was to pool data from several studies to assess whether this initial peak of NO release was directly correlated to the associated vasomotor effect of SD in the pial vasculature.

MATERIALS AND METHODS

Anesthesia was induced in male cats (3 to 4.2 kg) using 5% halothane and maintained with α-chloralose (100 mg·kg^{-1} i.v.). Recordings of cortical direct current (d.c.) potential regional laser Doppler blood flux (rCBF$_{ldf}$) and NO release were

TABLE 1. Correlation between SD-induced NO release and percentage changes in $rCBF_{ldf}$ and pial artery diameter as determined by the method of least squares analysis[a]

NO	$rCBF_{ldf}$		Pial artery diameter	
	r	p value	r	p value
Saline (n=12)	−0.32	0.32	−0.02	0.94
Glyceryl trinitrate (n=12)	0.47	0.1	−0.21	0.50
β-Cyclodextrin (n=16)	0.17	0.51	Not determined	

[a] r, Pearson product moment linear correlation coefficient. A significance level of $p < 0.05$ was adopted throughout.
NO, nitric oxide; $rCBF_{ldf}$, regional laser Doppler blood flux; SD, spreading depression.

made from the suprasylvian gyrus of the left parietal cortex, as previously described (1). Pial artery diameter measurements were made using a videomicroscope and videomicroscaler (For-a IV, Cameron Comm., Glasgow). Spreading depression was evoked using a 30-mg KCl pellet placed onto the exposed cortex. Analysis was performed on three treatment groups: saline-infused animals (0.1 ml·kg^{-1}·min^{-1} i.v.), glyceryl trinitrate-infused animals (0.25 µg·kg^{-1}·min^{-1} i.v.) or 10% β-cyclodextrin-pretreated animals (2 ml·kg^{-1} i.v.). Relationships among variables were determined by the method of least squares analysis to fit a linear model to the data, and the Pearson product moment linear correlation coefficient was calculated. A significance level of $p < 0.05$ was adopted throughout.

RESULTS

Examining the relationship between local NO concentration and percentage changes in $rCBF_{ldf}$ and pial artery diameter in all treatment groups, no significant linear correlation was observed between variables (least squares analysis, $p > 0.05$) (Table 1, Fig. 1). There was no statistical difference in d.c. depolarization amplitudes (data not shown) (ANOVA, post hoc Dunnett's t-test, $p > 0.05$).

DISCUSSION

This study demonstrates that SD induces an increase in cortical NO release that is not linearly correlated to changes in $rCBF_{ldf}$ or changes in pial artery diameter. There are several possible explanations: (a) the involvement of more than one mediator, e.g., calcitonin gene-related peptide (3); and (b) NO release during SD is supramaximal for further expression as $rCBF_{ldf}$ and pial artery diameter changes. This supramaximal release of NO is particularly interesting as it could then represent a potential mechanism of sensitization of nociceptive afferents in migraine or it could be involved in neuronal injury in cerebral ischemia or cerebral trauma.

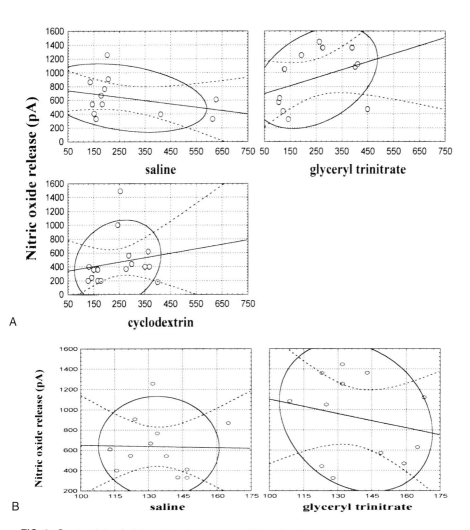

FIG. 1. Scatterplots of nitric oxide release versus **(A)** regional cerebral blood flux (rCBF$_{ldf}$) (percentage change from baseline) and **(B)** pial artery diameter (percentage change from baseline) by treatment. Data are represented with confidence ellipses (80% confidence interval), (X,Y) linear regression best fit (solid line), and 95% confidence intervals (dotted line). No significant correlation was found between variables in all treatments (see Table 1 for correlation coefficients).

REFERENCES

1. Read SJ, Smith MI, Hunter AJ, Parsons AA. Measurement of NO release using a selective microelectrode following repeated waves of cortical spreading depression. *Br J Pharmacol* 1996;118:79P(abst).
2. Malinski T, Bailey F, Zhang ZG, Chopp M. NO measurement by a porphyrinic microsensor in rat brain after transient middle cerebral artery occlusion. *J Cereb Blood Flow Metab* 1993;13:355–358.
3. Wahl M, Schilling L, Parsons AA, Kaumann A. Involvement of CGRP and NO in the pial artery dilatation elicited by cortical spreading depression. *Brain Res* 1994;637:204–210.

41

Nitric Oxide Synthesis in Nitric Oxide Donor Migraine

Paolo Martelletti, *Simona D'Alò, †Giuseppe Stirparo, ‡Cristina Rinaldi, *Maria Grazia Cifone, and Mario Giacovazzo

*Departments of Clinical Medicine and ‡Experimental Medicine and Pathology, University "La Sapienza," I-00161 Rome, Italy; and †Institute of Biomedical Technologies, National Council of Research, I-00161 Rome, Italy; and *Department of Experimental Medicine, University of L'Aquila, I-67100 L'Aquila, Italy*

A definitive and precise demonstration of large intracranial vessel involvement in the origin of migraine pain, already assumed 50 years ago by Ray and Wolff (1), was performed recently by Friberg et al. (2). Using the combined technique of transcranial Doppler/single-photon emission computed tomography, they demonstrated distension of the intracranial vessels during migraine attack.

There is growing interest in nitric oxide (NO) as a causative molecule of migraine pain (3). Lassen recently demonstrated that NO formation in the endothelium of cerebral arteries is a potential initiator of migraine attack (4). Sumatriptan, a potent vasoconstrictor of cerebral vessels via 5-hydroxytryptamine $(5-HT)_{1D}$ receptors, relieved both spontaneous migraine attacks (5) and those induced by the administration of NO donors (6).

It is likely that NO (exogenous and/or endogenous) is the key to these molecular changes during migraine attack, and therefore we pursued the "nitroxide hypothesis" to investigate the pathophysiology of migraine pain.

MATERIALS AND METHODS

Patient Population

This preliminary study was conducted in 13 migraine patients without aura (MWA) (7 males and 6 females; mean age, 36.5 years ± 5.1), randomly recruited among the outpatients of the University "La Sapienza" Headache Center and diagnosed according to the 1988 International Headache Society (IHS) criteria. All subjects gave informed consent and were tested while recumbent in bed at a time when they had been asymptomatic and had not taken any medication for at least 10 days.

Experimental Study Design

Peripheral venous blood (5 ml) was obtained from each subject at two time points: immediately before (baseline, T0) sublingual administration of 5 mg of isosorbide dinitrate (ID), an analog of nitroglycerin, acting as NO donor, and at 1 hour after administration (T1). The T1 time point was chosen on the basis of the clinical observation that both ID-induced and spontaneous headache start about 30 to 35 minutes after baseline and that the headache progressively worsens and usually reaches its maximum peak at the first hour after onset (T1) (3). Plasma samples were then stored at –70°C until assay.

Measurement of Nitric Oxide Synthesis

Synthesis of NO was measured as nitrite accumulation (7,8). Since NO is a highly labile molecule, its direct measurements are difficult. One product of the L-arginine-dependent NO pathway is nitrite. Nitrite is freely permeable to the plasma membrane of cells and easily detected by spectrophotometric analysis of serum samples. Nitrite concentrations were quantified by a colorimetric assay based on the Griess reaction (9). Briefly, 100 µl of serum was mixed with an equal volume of Griess reagent in a U-well microtiter plate and incubated at room temperature for 10 minutes. The OD was measured at 550 nm using a micro-ELISA reader (Easy Reader EAR 400, Kontron Analytic) using $NaNo_3$ as a standard and Dulbecco's medium supplemented with 10% fetal calf serum as a blank.

Statistical Procedure

The SAS system was used for statistical analysis of data. Paired-comparisons t-test and the NPAR1WAY procedure were used to reveal differences between pre-treatment and post-treatment values. The data were reported as means ± SD. Values of p (for a confidence interval of 95%) less than 0.05 were set as the significance level for hypothesis testing.

RESULTS

Experimental headache was induced in all cases. Ten of 13 MWA patients (77%) stated that the headache attack induced by ID was analogous to their spontaneous migraine attack. The attacks were generally shorter, less intense, and had fewer accompanying symptoms, but they fulfilled IHS criteria for an MWA attack. In MWA patients, the crises lasted from 5 to 15 hours.

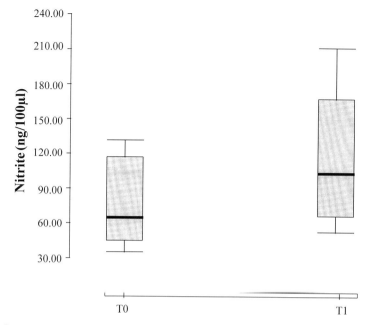

FIG. 1. Box plot illustrating the comparative values (post-treatment minus pretreatment) at different times (T0, basal values; T1, 1 hour) of serum nitrite accumulation in experimental (isosorbide dinitrate 5 mg) migraine. The bars represent the median and the range values plus (upper part from median) 75% of percentiles with the maximum deviation and minus (lower part from median) 25% of percentiles with the minimun deviation. Confidence interval at 95%, 5.1–74.6; mean difference, 39.8 (T1 – T0); $p < 0.05$; Prob > t, 0.0280 (paired-comparisons t-test). T0 versus T1, F 4.42, Pr > F 0.04 (NPAR1WAY).

Nitrite Accumulation

The mean values of serum nitrite as a NO-oxidized derivative were markedly increased in the patients studied during the NO donor-induced migraine attack. Figure 1 illustrates this response, which was significantly increased at T1 compared with the patients' own basal values (t-test = $p < 0.05$, Prob > t 0.0280; NPAR1WAY = F value 4.42, Prob > F 0.04).

DISCUSSION

We have shown that pain crises induced in migraine patients by administering the NO donor were able to induce strong NO production as detected by accumulation of NO-oxidized derivatives.

NO has been proved to play an important role in both central and peripheral nervous systems. NO synthase has been detected in all areas of the human brain, suggesting that NO plays a role in neurotransmission as well as either nociceptive or antinociceptive responses depending on the tissue level (10). In addition, NO seems to be involved in the regulation of cerebral circulation (11). It is still not clear how exogenous NO could play role in the local regulation of blood flow to brain, as is the case of NO donor migraine. However, a metabolic mechanism necessary to convert organic nitrates, such as ID, to a biologically active forms exists, mainly in the vasculature (11). Mounting evidence suggests that not only exogenously added NO but also enzymatically generated NO inhibits the activity of NOS (12). In our case the sharp increase of nitrite levels—a more stable and detectable NO metabolite—that we observed during NO donor migraine attack could be consistent with a very strong activation of NOS during the pain phase and only partially with the hypothesis of a downstream product of the administered NO donor.

This study has attempted to characterize the pathophysiological approach to experimental NO donor migraine, since this is currently quite contentious. The reliability of the NO donor headache model is demonstrated by the similar response to sumatriptan shared by NO donor headache induced either in migrainous patients (5) or in healthy subjects (6).

In summary, NO donor migraine seems to represent an ideal experimental model for the study of the multifactorial mechanisms that lie at the origin of vascular headaches, such as migraine (13). If the predominant pathway of migraine machinery is via NO, the study of this remarkable molecule appears to be the direction in which we are heading.

REFERENCES

1. Ray BS, Wolff HG. Experimental studies on headache. Pain sensitive structures of the head and their significance in headache. *Arch Surg* 1940;41:813–856.
2. Friberg L, Olesen J, Jverson HK, Sperling B. Migraine pain associated with middle cerebral artery dilation: reversal by sumatriptan. *Lancet* 1991;338:13–17.
3. Olesen J, Thomsen LL, Lassen LH, Olesen IJ. The nitric oxide hypothesis of migraine and other vascular headaches. *Cephalalgia* 1995;15:94–100.
4. Lassen LH, Ashina M, Christiansen I, Ulrich V, Olesen J. Nitric oxide synthase in migraine. *Lancet* 1997;349:401–402.
5. Martelletti P, Stirparo G, Rinaldi C, Giacovazzo M. Upregulated expression of peripheral serotonergic receptor in migraine and cluster headache by sumatriptan. *Int J Clin Pharmacol Res* 1994;14:165–175.
6. Iversen HK, Olesen J. Headache induced by a nitric oxide donor (nitroglycerin) responds to sumatriptan. A human model for development of migraine drugs. *Cephalalgia* 1996;16:412–418.
7. Cifone MG, Festuccia C, Cironi L, et al. Induction of the nitric oxide-synthesizing pathway in fresh and interleukin-2 cultured rat natural killer cells. *Cell Immunol* 1994;157:181–194.
8. De Maria R, Cifone MG, Trotta R, et al. Triggering of human monocyte activation through CD69, a member of the natural killer cell gene complex family of signal transducing receptors. *Exp Med* 1994;180:1999–2004.
9. Cifone MG, Cironi L, Meccia A, et al. Role of nitric oxide in cell-mediated tumor cytotoxicity. *Adv Neuroimmunol* 1995;5:443–461.
10. Holthusen H, Arndt JO. Nitric oxide evokes pain at nociceptors of the paravascular tissue and veins in humans. *J Physiol* 1995;487:253–258.
11. Mizutani T, Layon J. Clinical applications of nitric oxide. *Chest* 1996;110:506–524.
12. Griscavage JM, Hobbs AJ, Ignarro LJ. Negative modulation of nitric oxide synthase by nitric oxide and nitroso compounds. *Adv Pharmacol* 1995;34:215–234.
13. Olesen J, Thomsen LL, Iversen H. Nitric oxide is a key molecule in migraine and other vascular headaches. *Trends Pharmacol Sci* 1994;15:149–153.

42

Endothelium-Dependent Mechanics of Nitric Oxide Donor Migraine

Paolo Martelletti and Mario Giacovazzo

Department of Clinical Medicine, University "La Sapienza," I-00161 Rome, Italy

The idea of vascular involvement in migraine is not new. Such a theory was proposed at the end of 1930s by Graham and Wolff (1), who stated that migraine is the result of a stimulation of the sensitive nerves of the large arteries and of meningeal circulation. More recently, the demonstration that the dura mater has a sensitive innervation that transmits information to the vascular bed of the central nervous system (CNS) through the fifth pair of the cranial nerves also supports this notion (2).

MIGRAINE PATHOPHYSIOLOGY AND NITRIC OXIDE

The integrated neurovascular hypothesis for migraine is based on the model of trigeminal-induced plasma extravasation demonstrated in animals and theoretically applied to humans (3). Stimulation of the trigeminal ganglion leading to sterile inflammation in the dura mater of animals is blocked by pretreatment with the 5-hydroxytryptamine $(5-HT)_{1D}$ agonist sumatriptan, thus confirming the serotonergic-mediated mechanisms in the onset of pain in migraine (3). The remarkable importance of the serotonergic receptor system in migraine was underlined by an experimental neuroimmunological model for studying 5-HT receptor expression in humans with migraine (4).

Nitric oxide (NO) is a short-lived radical that has been identified in recent years as a pleiotropic mediator; it is an important mediator of blood vessel relaxation. Nitric oxide is a biologically active compound produced by the vascular endothelium that may interfere with the ability of polymorphonuclear leukocytes to adhere to the vascular endothelium (5). It inhibits leukocyte-endothelial cell interactions, thereby preventing adherence and infiltration of neutrophils into the vessel wall. This phenomenon may be caused by a direct effect of NO on expression of glycoprotein adhesion molecules mediating endothelial cell-leukocyte interactions.

The influence of NO on endothelial activation was recently suggested by in vitro experiments on human endothelial cells showing that NO can reduce cytokine-induced expression of a number of pathophysiological effector molecules characteristic of endothelial activation; NO inhibits the expression of vascular cell adhesion molecule 1 (VCAM-1), E-selectin, and intercellular adhesion molecule 1 (ICAM-1), as well as the secretion of interleukin (IL)-8 and IL-6 in endothelial cell cultures stimulated by IL-1, IL-4, and tumor necrosis factor (6).

We have previously demonstrated an increase in the proinflammatory cytokine IL-1β during the painful period of another form of vascular headache, the cluster headache (7). We thus attempted to identify the role of cell adhesion molecules in NO-derived head vascular pain. Adhesion of peripheral blood cells to the endothelium is a critical step for transendothelial migration toward sites of inflammation. Cell adhesion is achieved through the interaction of cellular adhesion molecules, expressed by endothelial cells with their counterpart ligand expressed by leukocytes.

CELL ADHESION MOLECULES AND EXPERIMENTAL NITRIC OXIDE DONOR MIGRAINE

We have recently shown that pain crises induced in migraine without aura (MWA) patients by administering a NO donor can reduce the monocyte expression of ICAM-1 and its soluble isoform (sICAM-1), as well as serum IL-4 (8). Interestingly, we observed that ICAM-1, sICAM-1, and IL-4 were also significantly lower during spontaneous MWA attacks in a selected subgroup of the MWA patients studied. There was no change with respect to IL-1 receptor expression values. Two control groups (healthy subjects and episodic tension headache patients) tested with the same experimental procedure showed no changes in ICAM-1 and IL-1 receptor (R) expression, nor in the values of sICAM-1 and IL-4 (8).

Our data suggest a specific action of NO, released by isosorbide dinitrate (ID), on cerebral vessel walls and consequently on the onset of head pain. The headache crises caused by NO donor administration were similar to spontaneous migraine attacks, and therefore we can assume that endogenous NO may play a role in migraine pain. At sites of hypothesized "neurogenic inflammation," several cell types, such as vascular smooth muscle cells, monocytes, endothelial cells, and neurons, could have the capacity to generate a high concentration of inducible NO, at levels comparable with the amount of NO released by NO donor in our study (9). Such local generation of large amounts of NO could provide homeostatic regulation of leukocyte adhesion within the cerebral vessel wall. Exogenous as well as endogenous sources of NO can limit the degree of endothelial activation. In addition to its vasodilatory effect, NO inhibits leukocyte transvascular migration, blocking the postulated neurogenic perivascular "sterile inflammation" (3). Since ICAM-1 is upregulated following activation during inflammatory responses, it has been suggested that adhesion molecules could mediate the leukocyte extravasation into the perivascular cerebral tissue (9). The transendothelial migration is a response to inflammatory stimuli, produced or displayed by endothelium. On the basis of our results, leukocyte transmigration seems not to occur in the case of migraine (Fig. 1).

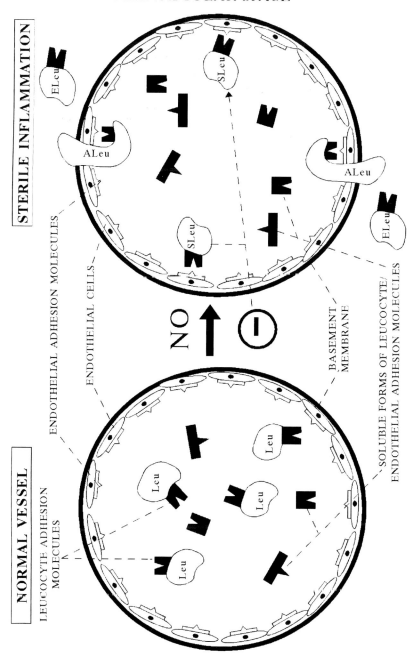

FIG. 1. Inhibitory effect of nitric oxide (NO) donor on the interactions between eukocytes and endothelial surface of cerebral vessels (rolling along and samping the endothelial surface, attachment, and migration into the tissue) during the proposed sterile inflammation phase of migraine. Leu, leukocyte; ALeu, activated leukocyte; SLeu, sampling leukocyte; ELeu, extravasated leukocyte.

PROPOSED MACHINERY OF NITRIC OXIDE/ENDOTHELIAL INTERACTIONS IN MIGRAINE

A possible explanation of these results could be that the increase in NO (exogenous, endogenous?) may induce an IL-4 inhibition through a feedback mechanism, which in turn downregulates ICAM-1 expression and sICAM-1 (Fig. 2). This mechanism seems to be IL-1 independent. This downregulation observed in MWA patients and not in the two control groups could be due to a described supersensitivity to exogenous NO that is present in migraine sufferers (10).

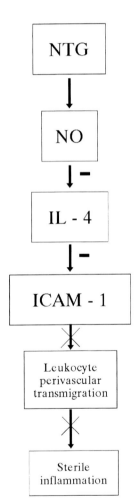

FIG. 2. Proposed mechanics of nitric oxide (NO) donor inhibitory effect on sterile inflammation hypothesis in migraine via interleukin-4 (IL-4)/intercellular adhesion molecule 1 (ICAM-1) sequence. NTG, nitroglycerin.

We do not have sufficient data to claim rejection of the "sterile inflammation hypothesis" in migraine, and at this time it is difficult to draw a valid conclusion. However, NO seems to activate a common final pathway of the old/new hypotheses of vascular involvement in this disease (1,11). Considering that vascular NO synthase is mainly localized in the endothelium of cerebral vessels, the downregulation of ICAM-1, sICAM, and IL-4 that we observed may be much greater at the cerebral endothelium level than that measured in the CD14-positive peripheral cells and in the plasma (12).

This hypothesis for the endothelial mechanisms leading to the vascular disturbances that occur during migraine attack (spontaneous and NO donor-induced) could be coupled with recent data stating that release of NO (spontaneous and NO donor-induced) provides a common final pathway for several substances that trigger migraine pain (4,11).

All the mechanisms described above may be relevant for headache, and activation by a NO donor of the NO cascade could act as a nonspecific trigger factor rather than a downstream product. Further work is now required to assess the in vivo relevance of the NO precursor L-arginine and the metabolites nitrate and nitrite with respect to migraine pain.

REFERENCES

1. Graham JR, Wolff HG. Mechanisms of migraine headache and action of ergotamine tartrate. *Arch Neurol Psychiatry* 1938;39:737–763.
2. Nichols III FT, Mawad M, Mohor JP, Stein B, Hilal S, Michelsen WJ. Focal headache during balloon inflation in the internal carotid and middle cerebral arteries. *Stroke* 1990;21:555–559.
3. Moskowitz MA, McFarlane R. Neurovascular and molecular mechanisms in migraine headaches. *Cerebrovasc Brain Metab Rev* 1993;5:159–177.
4. Martelletti P. Serotonin, its receptors and the mechanisms of migraine: a transforming ancient union. *J Serotonin Res* 1995;1:59–66.
5. Kubes P, Suzuki M, Granger DN. Nitric oxide: an endogenous modulator leukocyte adhesion. *Proc Natl Acad Sci USA* 1991;88:4651–4655.
6. De Caterina R, Libby P, Peng H. Nitric oxide decreases cytokine-induced endothelial activation. *J Clin Invest* 1995;96:60–68.
7. Martelletti P, Granata M, Giacovazzo M. Serum interleukin-1 beta is increased in cluster headache. *Cephalalgia* 1993;13:343–345.
8. Martelletti P, Stirparo G, Morrone S, Giacovazzo M, Rinaldi C. Inhibition of intercellular adhesion molecule-1 (ICAM-1), soluble ICAM-1 and of interleukin-4 by nitric oxide expression in migraine patients. *J Mol Med* 1996;75:1–6.
9. Borgerding RA, Murphy S. Expression of inducible nitric oxide synthase in cerebral endothelial cells is regulated by cytokine activated astrocytes. *J Neurochem* 1995;65:1342–1347.
10. Thomsen LL, Iversen KI, Brinck TA, Olesen J. Arterial supersensitivity to nitric oxide (nitroglycerin) in migraine sufferers. *Cephalalgia* 1993;13:395–399.
11. Lassen LH, Thomsen LL, Olesen J. Histamine induces migraine via the H_1-receptor. Support for the NO hypothesis of migraine. *Neuroreport* 1995;6:1475–1479.
12. Fostermann U, Pollock JS, Schmidt HHHV, Heller M, Murad F. Calmodulin-dependent endothelium-derived relaxing factor/nitric oxide synthase activity is present in the particulate and cytosolic fractions of bovine aortic endothelial cells. *Proc Natl Acad Sci USA* 1991;88:1788–1792.

43

5-Hydroxytryptamine$_1$ Agonists Inhibit the Activity of Constitutive Nitric Oxide Synthase in Guinea Pig Cerebral Vessels

Bertel Rüdinger and Inger Jansen-Olesen

Department of Biological Sciences, The Royal Danish School of Pharmacy, DK-2100 Copenhagen Ø, Denmark

Nitric oxide (NO) is formed from L-arginine during its conversion to L-citrullin, a reaction that is facilitated by the enzyme nitric oxide synthase (NOS). There are at least three types of NOS: neuronal-, endothelial-, and macrophage-type enzyme (1). The neuronal and endothelial enzymes are constitutive (c), whereas the macrophage enzyme is inducible (i). The release of NO onto the smooth muscle cell results in the formation of cyclic guanosine monophosphate through guanylyl cyclase, mediating vasodilation via a decrease in the intracellular Ca^{2+} concentration and/or reduction of Ca^{2+} sensitivity of the contractile proteins (2).

Infusion of the NO donor glyceryl trinitrate (GTN) causes a delayed migraine attack in migraineurs (3), and NO has been suggested to be a causative molecule in migraine pain (4). Sumatriptan, the most specific drug for the treatment of migraine attacks, reduces GTN-induced headache (5). Recently, Lassen and Olesen found that the NOS inhibitor N^G-monomethyl-L-arginine (L-NMMA) had a significant antimigraine effect (see Ch. 35, this volume). This finding inspired us to examine the effect of sumatriptan on cNOS activity in isolated guinea pig cerebral vessels in vitro.

MATERIALS AND METHODS

The activity of NOS in guinea pig cerebral vessels was quantified by monitoring the conversion of L-[^{3}H]arginine to L-[^{3}H]citrulline, as previously described (6). Thirty guinea pigs were exsanguinated under barbiturate anesthesia. The brains were removed, and cerebral blood vessels were dissected under a dissection microscope, immediately frozen on dry ice, and stored at –80°C. The arteries were homogenized in HEPES-HCl buffer (100-mg arteries/320-μl buffer) containing sucrose (0.11 g/ml), dithiothreitol (0.15 mg/ml), leupeptin (0.01 mg/ml), and pepstatin A (0.01 mg/ml). The homogenate was divided into five portions; two served as controls, and

3×10^{-7} M sumatriptan, naratriptan, or sumatriptan + 10^{-6} M methiothepin was added to each of the three other portions. All tubes were incubated for 15 minutes at 37°C and then centrifuged for 15 minutes at 10.000g at 0°C. Supernatant (25 µl) was then distributed in tubes with 100 µl of incubation buffer, and supernatant from one of the control groups was incubated with and without N^G-nitro-L-arginine methyl ester (L-NAME) 10^{-4} M or sumatriptan 3×10^{-7} M for 30 minutes at 37°C. The incubation was then terminated by the addition of 1 ml ice-cold (4°C) stopbuffer to each tube.

Tritiated L-citrullin was recovered by running the reaction mixture through a 1-ml Dowex-50 WX-8 column (Na^+ form). The levels of L-$[2,3-^3H]$citrulline in the eluent were determined by a liquid scintillation counter.

RESULTS

The addition of 10^{-4} M L-NAME to the supernatant of homogenized guinea pig basilar arteries significantly ($p < 0.001$) inhibited cNOS activity by 68%. The addition of 3×10^{-7} M sumatriptan to the supernatant had no inhibitory effect on cNOS activity. However, if sumatriptan was added to the homogenate and incubated for 15 minutes before centrifugation, a significant ($p < 0.001$) inhibition of cNOS activity by 48% was observed (Fig. 1).

The addition of 10^{-4} M L-NAME to the supernatant of homogenized arteries from guinea pig cortex significantly ($p < 0.001$) inhibited cNOS activity by 67%. The addition of 3×10^{-7} M sumatriptan or 3×10^{-7} M naratriptan to the homogenate significantly ($p < 0.001$) inhibited cNOS activity by 28% and 20%, respectively (Fig. 2). Methiothepin given in a concentration of 10^{-6} M totally blocked the decrease in cNOS activity obtained with sumatriptan (Fig. 3).

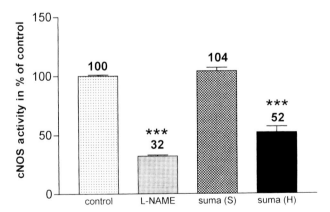

FIG. 1. Effect of N^G-nitro-L-arginine methyl ester (L-NAME; 10^{-4} M) given to the supernatant and sumatriptan (suma) (3×10^{-7} M) given to supernatant (S) or homogenate (H) on constitutive nitric oxide synthase (cNOS) activity in basilar arteries from guinea pig. Values are given as means ± SEM; number of measurements is 6 to 20 on 30 animals. Statistical evaluation was performed by Student's t-test; ***, $p < 0.001$ compared with control values.

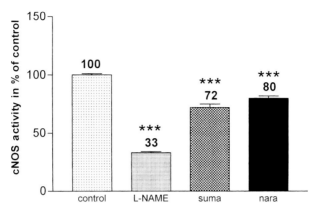

FIG. 2. Effect of N^G-nitro-L-arginine methyl ester (L-NAME; 10^{-4} M) given to the supernatant, sumatriptan (suma) (3×10^{-7} M) and naratriptan (nara) (3×10^{-7} M) given to homogenate on constitutive nitric oxide synthase (cNOS) activity in cortex arteries from guinea pig. Values are given as means ± SEM; number of measurements is 6 to 20 on 30 animals. Statistical evaluation was performed by Student's t-test; ***, $p < 0.001$ compared with control values.

DISCUSSION

In the present study we have shown for the first time that the 5-hydroxytryptamine $(5\text{-HT})_{1D,B,F}$ agonists sumatriptan and naratriptan, used in the acute treatment of migraine, are able to reduce the activity of cNOS in guinea pig cerebral vessels. This finding is important, as NO has been suggested to be a causative molecule in mi-

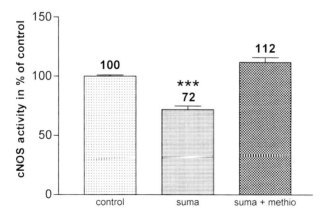

FIG. 3. Effect of sumatriptan (suma) (3×10^{-7} M) in the absence and presence of the 5-HT$_1$ antagonist methiothepin (methio) (10^{-6} M) given to homogenate on constitutive nitric oxide synthase (cNOS) activity in cortex arteries from guinea pig. Values are given as means ± SEM; number of measurements is 6 to 20 on 30 animals. Statistical evaluation was performed by Student's t-test; ***, $p < 0.001$ compared with control values.

graine pain, a hypothesis supported by the recent finding that injection of L-NMMA during a migraine attack significantly aborted the acute migraine attack (4) (see Ch. 35, *this volume*). We found no reduction in NOS activity when the 5-HT$_{1D,B,F}$ agonists were added to the supernatant in which NOS was dissolved. The L-NAME, which acts directly on the enzyme, had a clear NOS-inhibiting effect when administered to the supernatant. Thus, the mode of action on NOS by the 5-HT$_{1D,B,F}$ agonists and NOS inhibitors is different. When sumatriptan or naratriptan was added to brain vessel homogenates in which the vascular cell membranes were present, we observed a significant decrease in cNOS activity that was reversed by simultaneous addition of the nonselective 5-HT$_1$ antagonist methiothepin.

The mechanism by which the 5-HT$_{1D,B,F}$ agonists inhibit cNOS activity is an interesting question. In 1992 it was shown that neuronal and endothelial NOS were phosphorylated by cyclic AMP-dependent protein kinase (PKA), proteinkinase C (PKC), or calcium/calmodulin-dependent protein kinase (CaM-K). Phosphorylation by PKC was the most rapid, whereas CaM-K and PKA phosphorylated NOS more slowly. In our experiments, the cerebral vessel membranes were incubated with sumatriptan for 15 minutes before centrifugation. During this time NOS will be maximally phosphorylated by PKC but only to 30% by CaM-K or PKA (7). Activation of 5-HT$_{1D}$ receptors is known to inhibit forskolin-stimulated adenylyl cyclase activity in calf substantia nigra (8), Chinese hamster ovary cells (9), and intact murine fibroblasts transfected with the 5-HT$_{1D}$ and 5-HT$_{1B}$ receptor genes (10). The action of sumatriptan on adenylyl cyclase in guinea pig cerebral blood vessels should in that case lead to a decrease in PKA activity. Thus decreased phosphorylation of NOS would occur. It has been shown that 5-HT activates phospholipase C in rabbit basilar artery (11). This activation produces two distinct second messengers, inositol triphosphate (IP$_3$), which elevates cytosolic free calcium [Ca^{2+}]$_i$, and diacylglycerol (DAG), which elevates PKC formation. However, this effect has been shown to be mediated by activation of 5-HT$_2$ or 5-HT$_{1C}$ receptors (12,13). Only in one study, performed on 5-HT$_{1F}$-transfected NIH-3T3 and LM (tk-) fibroblasts, did the activation of 5-HT$_{1F}$ receptors induce stimulation of IP$_3$ and a rapid increase of [Ca^{2+}]$_i$ in the LM (tk-) cells but not the NIH-3T3 cells (14). Another possibility for 5-HT$_{1D,B,F}$-induced activation of PKC is the sumatriptan-stimulated release of NO through the activation of a 5-HT$_1$-like receptor located in the endothelium (15–17). Agonists that release endothelial NO activate phospholipase C and therefore also the production of IP$_3$ and DAG (18).

In conclusion, several possible modes of sumatriptan-induced inhibition on NOS activity exist. At present it is not possible for us to explain which of these mechanisms is the most important.

REFERENCES

1. Förstermann U, Schmidt HHHW, Pollock JS, et al. Isoforms of nitric oxide synthase. Characterization and purification from different cell types. *Biochem Pharmacol* 1991;42:1849–1857.

2. Karaki H. Ca^{2+} localization and sensitivity in vascular smooth muscle. *Trends Pharmacol Sci* 1989; 10:320–324.
3. Thomsen LL, Kruuse C, Iversen HK, Olesen J. A nitric oxide donor (nitroglycerin) triggers genuine migraine attacks. *Eur J Neurol* 1994;1:73–80.
4. Olesen J, Thomsen LL, Lassen LH, Olesen IJ. The nitric oxide hypothesis of migraine and other vascular headaches. *Cephalalgia* 1995;15:94–100.
5. Iversen HK, Olesen J. The effect of sumatriptan on nitroglycerin (NTG)-induced headache and vascular responses. *Cephalalgia* 1993;13[Suppl 13]:186.
6. Bredt DS, Snyder SH. Nitric oxide mediates glutamate-linked enhancement of cGMP levels in the cerebellum. *Proc Natl Acad Sci USA* 1989;86:9030–9033.
7. Bredt DS, Ferris CD, Snyder SH. Nitric oxide synthase regulatory sites: phosphorylation by cyclic AMP-dependent protein kinase, protein kinase C and calcium/calmodulin protein kinase; identification of flavin and calmodulin binding sites. *J Biol Chem* 1992;267:10976–10981.
8. Schoeffter P, Hoyer D. How selective is GR 43175? Interaction with functional 5-HT$_{1A}$ and 5-HT$_{1B}$, 5-HT$_{1C}$ and 5-HT$_{1D}$ receptors. *Naunyn Schmeidebergs Arch Pharmacol* 1989;340:135–138.
9. Dickenson JM, Hill SJ. Coupling of an endogenous 5-HT$_{1B}$-like receptor to increases in intracellularcalcium through a pertussis toxin-sensitive mechanism in CHO-K1 cells. *Br J Pharmacol* 1995; 116:2889–2896.
10. Zgombick JM, Borden LA, Cochran TL, Kucharewics SA, Weinshank RL, Branchek TA. Dual coupling of cloned human 5-hydroxytryptamine 10 alpha and 5-hydroxytryptamine 10 beta receptors stably expressed in murine fibroblasts: Inhibition of adenylate cyclase and elevation of intracellular calcium concentrations via pertussis toxin-sensitive G protein(s). *Mol Pharmacol* 1993;44:575–582.
11. Clark AH, Garland CJ. 5-Hydroxytryptamine-stimulated accumulation of 1,2-diacylglycerol in the rabbit basilar artery: a role for protein kinase C in smooth muscle contraction. *Br J Pharmacol* 1991; 102:415–421.
12. Berta P, Seguin J, Vidal N, Haitech J, Mathieu MN, Chevillard C. Influence of Ca^{2+} on 5-HT$_2$- and alpha$_1$-induced arterial contraction and phosphoinositide metabolism. *Eur J Pharmacol* 1986;132: 253–257.
13. Zhang L, Hu XQ. Serotonin stimulates rapid increase of inositol 1,4,5-triphosphate in ovine uterine artery: correlation with contractile state. *J Pharmacol Exp Ther* 1995;275:576–583.
14. Adham N, Borden LA, Schechter LE, et al. Cell specific coupling of the cloned human 5-HT$_{1F}$ receptor to multiple signal transduction pathways. *Naunyn Schmeidebergs Arch Pharmacol* 1993;348: 566–575.
15. Sweeney G, Templeton A, Clayton RA, et al. Contractile responses to sumatriptan in isolated bovine pulmonary artery rings: relationship to tone and cyclic nucleotide levels. *J Cardiovasc Pharmacol* 1995;26:751–760.
16. Whiting MV, Cambridge D. Canine renovascular responses to sumatriptan and 5-carboxamidotryptamine: modulation through endothelial 5-HT$_1$-like receptors and endogenous nitric oxide. *Br J Pharmacol* 1995;114:969–974.
17. Yildiz O, Tuncer M. Comparison of the effect of endothelium on the response to sumatriptan in rabbit isolated iliac, mesenteric and carotid arteries. *Arch Int Pharmacodyn Ther* 1994;328:200–212.
18. Hirata K, Kuroda R, Sakoda T, et al. Inhibition of endothelial nitric oxide synthase activity by protein kinase C. *Hypertension* 1995;25:180–185.

44
Discussion Summary: Involvement of Nitric Oxide-Cyclic GMP Pathway Products in Primary Headaches

Jes Olesen

Department of Neurology, Glostrup Hospital, University of Copenhagen, DK-2600 Glostrup, Copenhagen, Denmark

The first part of the discussion focused on nitroxidergic nerves. The first question was about co-localization with other neurotransmitters in these nerves, and it was confirmed that other neurotransmitters probably exist in addition to nitric oxide (NO). The relation of these nerves to existing migraine therapies was emphasized. Flunarizine is effective in migraine prophylaxis and inhibits the release of NO from nitroxidergic nerves. There seems to be no solid evidence, however, that flunarizine exerts this effect via N-type calcium channels, and it is also uncertain whether the concentrations used in the isolated artery experiments of Professor Toda were actually equal to concentrations normally obtained in humans during prophylactic treatment. The effect of verapamil in cluster headache cannot be explained on the basis of an action on nitroxidergic nerves, since L-channel blockers seem to have no effect on these nerves. It was stressed that the effect of verapamil in cluster headache has not been substantiated by controlled double-blind trials.

Turning to the studies of nitric oxide synthase (NOS) activation and NOS inhibition in human patients with migraine, Dr. Lassen was asked why N^G-monomethyl-L-arginine (L-NMMA) did not have an effect on nausea in migraine patients. In nausea, he responded, there was such a high placebo effect that the drug effect in the small study group was not significant. In the studies of histamine-induced migraine, L-NMMA reduced the diameter of the temporal artery by approximately 15%. However, in this model L-NMMA had no effect on the headache, indicating that the headache is not from the extracranial territory.

A question also arose of whether unspecific cranial vasoconstriction could perhaps explain the treatment effect of L-NMMA in migraine attacks. This is considered unlikely, since ongoing studies have shown no change in blood velocity in the middle cerebral artery and no change in regional cerebral blood flow. The increased blood pressure after L-NMMA would be likely to increase, not to decrease, the headache of migraineurs. This was shown more than 50 years ago in studies of experimental histamine-induced headache when histamine was given as a single injection. When in these studies the concomitant drop in blood pressure was prevented, the headaches induced were worse than when blood pressure was allowed to fall. The interesting question of the various molecular species of NO such as NO• and NO+ was raised, but no information is available to allow any conclusions about their relative roles.

The study of L-NMMA in acute migraine utilized in part historical controls and was not a straightforward double-blind randomized trial. Dr. Lassen explained that the study had been extremely difficult to do, partly because it was difficult to get the substance and partly because it was not financially supported and therefore had to be done in a single center. It would simply not have been possible within a reasonable time frame to obtain enough patients treated in-hospital for acute migraine to allow a straightforward randomized double-blind controlled design.

The question also arose of why histamine-induced headache and migraine did not respond to L-NMMA when spontaneous migraine attacks did. The most likely explanation is that L-NMMA does not cross the blood-brain barrier, and therefore it cannot act on the endothelial NOS inside the cells. Thus, L-NMMA had no effect on histamine-induced arterial dilation. By contrast, the H_1 blocker mepyramine is able to abolish both arterial dilation and the immediate and delayed headache. It may also be that L-NMMA, in addition to having poorer penetration, is simply a weak NOS inhibitor in the big arteries. Finally, it was asked if an aura could be produced by an NO donor. This has not been observed, and it is not even known whether patients who have migraine with aura respond with migraine attacks or whether they behave like nonmigraineurs in this experimental model.

In discussing the NO hypothesis of Olesen et al., it was first asked why NO may cause pain in migraine. There are several possible explanations. One is the vasodilation induced by NO. This is not likely to be the whole explanation, especially not in the delayed migraine. It may perhaps explain the immediate headache during nitroglycerin infusion, since this is fairly marked. Another possibility is the sensitization of perivascular sensory nerves, perhaps even a slightly toxic effect on these nerves. Professor Pat Humphrey had previously done studies showing that NO may sensitize various nerve terminals, but he found that the concentrations needed were higher than those normally encountered around blood vessels. He was therefore skeptical about the possibility that NO can exert a direct nociceptive action on sensory nerve terminals.

This brought up the intriguing fact that after a NO challenge induced by nitroglycerin or histamine it often takes up to several hours before patients develop genuine migraine attack. The normal regulation in situations of an increase of transmitter is counterregulation or desensitization, but Dr. Andrew Parsons had data showing that a brief infusion of nitroglycerin may induce not only an immediate peak of NO in the cerebral cortex but also a delayed and protracted increase in NO. Thus there seems to be some sort of feedforward system, and this might explain precisely the delayed headache although even the delayed and larger response would still not be enough to equal the concentrations used in the experiments by Professor Humphrey. Dr. Parsons had also shown in his poster that cortical spreading depression would induce a rather marked NO release, a response that came very quickly and therefore had to be the result of activation of constitutive NOS, either neural NOS or endothelial NOS. It was suggested that Peter Goadsby, in his interesting model of superior sagittal sinus stimulation, could investigate which concentrations of free NO are necessary to irritate sensory nerve endings. It was also suggested that NO is able to activate inducible cyclooxygenase, and Dr. Costa from Italy reported that they were in the process of finishing a study in which pretreatment with indomethacin seems to be able to prevent the delayed migraine in the nitroglycerin model.

One possibility for NO-induced headache could be a direct action on central nociceptive pathways mediated via the N-methyl-D-aspartate receptor. It is well known that NO facilitates transmission across this receptor. However, a poster presentation by Dr. Thomsen et al. had shown no marked changes in pressure pain threshold in the head or outside the head after nitroglycerin infusion. The intriguing thing is that nitroglycerin diffuses easily across the blood-brain barrier and therefore should be able to deliver very large quantities of NO to neural tissues. It is uncertain, however, whether the enzymes necessary for conversion of nitroglycerin to NO are present in brain parenchyma. Mary Heinricher pointed to another possibility, derived from her observation that NO stimulates both on and off cells in the ventral medial medulla. The lack of effect could thus be due to an equal effect on pain-facilitatory and pain-inhibitory mechanisms.

The posters by Paolo Martelletti indicated that during both spontaneous and nitroglycerin-induced migraine attacks the intercellular adhesion molecule and cytokines were downregulated. It is, therefore, unlikely that NO causes migraine pain via activation of inflammatory mechanisms. The results also indicated that inflammation as a cause of spontaneous migraine pain is unlikely.

It is not clear how the migraine aura induces pain, and it is especially difficult to understand why there is a free interval between the aura and the headache. This may perhaps relate to the above-mentioned slow second phase of NO production after nitroglycerin, or it may be due to some other mechanism.

Finally, the second-messenger mechanisms of migraine were discussed. Could it be that cyclic AMP is just as important as cyclic guanosine monophosphate (GMP)? Dr. Olesen explained that all known models that readily produce vascular headache and/or migraine seem to stimulate cyclic GMP and not cyclic AMP. However, good studies of drugs that exclusively activate cyclic AMP are lacking. One such compound is calcitonin gene-related peptide. In past studies this messenger molecule has not been noted to induce headache when given intravenously, but these studies had different aims, and headache may therefore have been overlooked. Prospective studies in migraineurs with this or other compounds stimulating cyclic AMP are needed.

Lastly it was discussed whether there could be a relation between a mechanism of action of sumatriptan and the NO/cGMP pathway. In the poster of Rüdinger and

Jansen-Olesen, it was shown that sumatriptan in homogenized cerebral blood vessels from guinea pig reduces NOS activity. Since other 5-hydroxytryptamine$_{1D}$ receptor agonists also exert this action, it was considered highly unlikely that it could be a direct inhibition of the enzyme. It was expected that the inhibition could be mediated via a sumatriptan effect on cellular elements, resulting secondarily in NOS inhibition. The interesting possibility that this mechanism may wholly or partly explain the therapeutic efficacy of sumatriptan clearly deserves further study.

Subject Index

A
A23187, 62, 63, 68
Acetylcholine (ACh)
  activation of eNOS, 74
  in cerebral arteries, 37–38
  endothelium-dependent dilation and, 68
  vasodilatory activity of, 61, 74
N-Acetylcysteine, 257
Acetylsalicylic acid, cortical spreading depression and, 120
ACh. *See* Acetylcholine
Adenosine, 75
Adenosine diphosphate (ADP), 68
Adenosine receptors, in cluster headache, 150–151
Adenosine triphosphate (ATP)
  activation of cutaneous afferent neurons, 111–116
  endothelium-dependent contraction and, 68
ADP (adenosine diphosphate), 68
Adrenaline, cerebrovascular adrenoceptors and, 25
α-Adrenoceptor agonists, for benign intracranial hypertension, 73
α-Adrenoceptor blockers, 30
α-Adrenoceptor variability, on human omental vessels, 177–179
Amino acids
  in cluster headaches, 149–150
  excitatory
    serotonin receptor agonists and, 155
    valproate and, 156
  inhibitory, serotonin receptor agonists and, 155
  in tension-type headache, 146–147, 149
γ-Aminobutyric acid (GABA)
  in migraine, 139, 140
  valproate and, 155–156
Amygdala, pain modulation and, 103
Angiotensin, 68
Angiotensin II, 62
Animals, experimental
  cerebral arteries, NOS inhibition by 5–HT$_1$ agonists, 297–300
  monkey, sensory nerve fibers in, 52–55
  neuropeptide changes in, 202–203
  rats. *See* Rat
Anticonvulsant drugs
  for migraine prophylaxis, 96, 157
  valproate. *See* Valproate
Antidepressant drugs, for tension-type headache, 146, 148

Antimigraine drugs
  amine/amino acid levels and, 157–158
  anticonvulsants as, 157
L-Arginine, 41
Arginine-vasopressin (AVP), 63, 125–126, 127
Aspartate, in tension-type headache, 149
Aspartic acid
  in migraine, 147
  in migraineurs, 139, 140
  in tension-type headache, 147
ATP. *See* Adenosine triphosphate
Atropine, 61
Aura. *See also* Migraine, with aura
  time lapse between headache, 118
Autoregulation, cerebral, 30
AVP (arginine-vasopressin), 63, 125–126, 127

B
Basilar artery, 3
Blood pressure changes, headaches and, 17
Bosentan, 213
Bradykinin, 62, 81, 82
Brain
  damage
    migraines from, 7
    protection against, sympathetic nerves and, 30, 31
  forebrain, RVM pain-modulating circuits and, 103–104
  PAG-RVM system, 99–101
  rostral ventromedial medulla. *See* Rostral ventromedial medulla

C
Calcitonin gene-related peptide (CGRP)
  in cluster headache, 205–206
  cortical spreading depression and, 121
  cranial sensory innervation and, 48–49
  elevation, time delay for, 236
  expression, 94
  histamine release in dura mater and, 167–171
  in human cerebral arteries, 55–56
  individual response variability, 175
  indomethacin and, 235
  localization, 167
  in migraine, 203, 255
    with aura, 204
    without aura, 204–205

307

Calcitonin gene-related peptide (CGRP) (contd.)
  nitroglycerin and, 255
  pial artery response and, 188
  in rat sensory nerve fibers, 50–52
  release, 237, 255
  substance P and, 74–75
  superior cervical ganglionectomy and, 24
  vasodilation and, 117
Calcitonin gene-related peptide-1 receptors (CGRP$_1$), in cranial arteries, 229–234
Calcium
  extracellular depletion, cerebral arteries and, 26
  intracellular, central sensitization and, 91
Calcium antagonists, 26, 261
Calcium/calmodulin-dependent protein kinase (CaM-K), 300
Calcium channel inhibitors, nitroxidergic nerve stimulation and, 242–243
Calcium channels, nitric oxide-guanosine monophosphate pathway and, 262
CaM-K (calcium/calmodulin-dependent protein kinase), 300
Cannabinoids, for idiopathic headache, 107–109
Capsaicin
  central sensitization and, 133
  cerebral artery relaxation, 232
  histamine release in dura mater and, 168
  loss of SP immunoreactivity, 48
Catecholamines
  in cluster headaches, 149–150
  endothelial PGD$_2$ and, 63
  in migraine, 140, 141
  in tension-type headache, 146–147, 149
CCK, 102–103
Cell adhesion molecules, nitric oxide donor migraine and, 292–293, 294, 295
Central sensitization
  generation, 133–134
  headache and, 94–96
  mechanisms, 91–93
  nitric oxide and, 82
  termination, 134
Cerebral arteries
  acetylcholine in, 37–38
  blood flow velocity in migraine, 5–6
  cyclic AMP formation in, 232–233
  dilation, 267
    acetylcholine and, 61
    induced by perivascular nerve stimulation, 241–242
    migraine pain and, 80
    by reactive oxygen species, 67
  endothelin$_A$ receptors in, 223–226
  endothelin$_B$ receptors in, 223–226
  extracellular calcium depletion, 26
  middle, 3, 52–55

  nitric oxide synthase inhibition, by 5-HT$_1$ agonists, 297–300
  relaxation, capsaicin-induced, 232
  stimulation, vs. retinal and temporal artery stimulation, 244
  vascular receptors, variability of, 173–176
Cerebral blood volume, 29
Cerebral circulation
  adrenergic innervation, 22
  innervation
    extrinsic system, 201
    intrinsic system, 201
  NOS-immunoreactive nerve fibers, 41
  NPY-containing perivascular nerves in, 23
  peptidergic receptors and, 25–26
  regulation, 21
  in situ microcirculatory responses, 27–28
  sympathetic neural control, 28
    autoregulation and, 30–31
    species differences in, 28–29
    in vivo experiments on, 29
  ultrastructure, 24–25
Cerebral edema, formation, 30
Cerebral infarction, 3
Cerebral regional blood flow, spreading depression-induced NO release and, 283–285
Cerebrospinal fluid (CSF)
  endogenous opioid peptides in, during headache, 196–197
  production, 31, 32
Cerebrovascular adrenoceptors, 25
Cerebrovascular hypertrophy, 31
C fibers, 117
C-fos expression
  induced
    by cortical spreading depression, 119
    by trigeminal nerve electrical stimulation, 119
  in trigeminal nucleus caudalis, 119–120
CGRP. See Calcitonin gene-related peptide
m-Chlorophenylpiperazine (m-CPP)
  fos expression in trigeminal nucleus caudalis, 161–164
  headache induced by, 143, 161, 181–185
    experimental method for, 181–182
    mechanism for, 262
    prolactin levels in, 187, 279
  protein extravasation in rat dura, 161, 163
  receptor/enzyme binding, 164
Choroid plexus, 25, 31–33
Clonidine, 25
Cluster headache
  adenosine receptors in, 150–151
  amino acids in, 149–150
  catecholamines in, 149–150
  cerebral serotoninergic system in, 181–185
  classification, 148
  endothelin-1 in, 211–213

histamine in, 148
induced by *m*-chlorophenylpiperazine, 181–185
neuropeptides in, 205–206
oxygen therapy for, 261
provocation, by nitroglycerin, 259–260
serotonin in, 148
Cortical spreading depression (CSD)
c-fos expression and, 95
characteristics, 283
definition of, 117
elicitation, experimental
c-fos and, 119
method of, 118
endothelin receptors in, 213
glyceryl trinitrate-induced headache and, 259
migraine and, 120–121
neurogenic inflammation and, 117–118
regional cerebral blood flow and, 117
Corticotropin releasing hormone (CRH), 126, 127
Cortisol, in *m*-chlorophenylpiperazine-induced headache, 182–185, 187
m-CPP. *See m*-Chlorophenylpiperazine
Cranial arteries
$CGRP_1$ receptors in, 229–234
dilation, 267
neurotransmitters, 73–76
nitroxidergic nerve stimulation, 244–245
Ca^{2+} channel inhibitors and, 242–243
mechanisms, 241–242
sumatriptan and, 243–244
vs. other nerve stimulation responses, 244
pain sensitivity, 3–4
serotonin injection and, 6, 7
sumatriptan injection and, 6
Craniovascular peptidergic innervation, anatomy, 201
CRH (corticotropin releasing hormone), 126, 127
CSD. *See* Cortical spreading depression
CSF. *See* Cerebrospinal fluid
Cutaneous afferent neurons, ATP activation of, 111–116
Cyclic adenosine monophosphate (cyclic AMP), 232–233, 305
Cyclic guanosine monophosphate (cyclic GMP), 242, 305
Cyclooxygenase products, 62–63, 68
Cytochrome P450 enzymes, 75
Cytochrome P450 epoxides, 66–67
Cytochrome P450 monooxygenase products, 68
Cytokines, 260

D

Dibenamine, 25
Dihydroergotamine
blockage of trigeminal ganglion stimulation, 203

for cerebral edema, 73
cortical spreading depression and, 120
for migraine prophylaxis, 96
Dihydrophenylacetic acid (DOPAC), 154
Dopamine
in tension-type headaches, 146–147
valproate and, 156
Dopamine-β-hydroxylase, 124–125, 127, 149
Doppler ultrasound, transcranial, 5–6
Drugs. *See also specific drugs*
dosage variability
cerebral artery vascular receptors and, 173–176, 188
omental α-adrenoreceptors and, 177–179, 188
prophylactic, 155–157
Dura mater, histamine release in, 167–171
Dynorphin
B, 49
CSF concentrations, during migraine, 196–197
distribution, 194

E

EDCFs (endothelium-derived contracting factors), 63, 68
EDHF (endothelium-derived hyperpolarizing factor), 66–68, 76
EETs (epoxyeicosatrienoic acids), 66–67, 76
Encephalitis, 260
β-Endorphin
in cluster headache, 205–206
distribution, 193–194
during migraine, 235
in cerebrospinal fluid, 196
in immune cells, 197
in plasma, 195
Endothelin, 75, 219
$Endothelin_A$ receptors, in cerebral arteries, 223–226
$Endothelin_B$ receptors
in cerebral arteries, 223–226
in human temporal artery, 219–222
Endothelin-1 (ET-1)
in cerebrovascular disorders, 219
in cluster headache, 211–213, 236–237
endothelium contraction and, 68
Endothelin receptors, in cortical spreading depression, 213
Endothelium, vasoconstrictor agents, 75
Endothelium-derived contracting factors (EDCFs), 63, 68
Endothelium-derived hyperpolarizing factor (EDHF), 66–68, 76
Endothelium-derived relaxing factors (EDRFs), 63–66. *See also* Nitric oxide
Enzyme nitric oxide synthase (eNOS), 247

Epinephrine
  in cluster headaches, 149
  in tension-type headaches, 146–147
Epoxyeicosatrienoic acids (EETs), 66–67, 76
Ergotamine, 5, 177
ET-1. See Endothelin-1

F

Female sex hormones, 259
Fenfluramine-induced headache
  characteristics of, 143
  prolactin release and, 187
  serotoninergic receptor stimulation and, 279, 280, 281
  serotonin release and, 142
FK88 inhibition, of SP-induced histamine release, 168, 169, 170
Flunarizine, 243, 303
Flupirtine, in tension-type headache, 149
Flushing, facial, 203
Fluvoxamine, for tension-type headache, 146, 148
Forebrain, RVM pain-modulating circuits and, 103–104
Fos expression
  in rat brain, 123–128
  in trigeminal nucleus caudalis, m-chlorophenylpiperazine and, 161–164

G

GABA. See γ-Aminobutyric acid
Gabapentin, 157
GAP-43 (growth-associated protein-43), 94
Glutamate
  in migraine, 139, 140
  release from peripheral nerve terminals, 75
  in tension-type headache, 147, 149
Glutamic acid
  in migraine, 139, 140, 147
  in tension-type headache, 147
Glyburide, 67
Glyceryl trinitrate-induced headache
  characteristics of, 257–258
  exogenous nitric oxide donation and, 247
  mechanisms, 259
  in migraineurs vs. nonmigraineurs, 258–259
  nitric oxide donation and, 256–257
  nociceptive thresholds in humans and, 273–276
  temporal relationships in, 80, 247
Glycine
  in cluster headache, 149–150
  in migraine, 140
  in tension-type headache, 149
Growth-associated protein-43 (GAP-43), 94
GTN. See Glyceryl trinitrate

GTN-induced headache. See Glyceryl trinitrate-induced headache
Guinea pig cerebral arteries, NOS inhibition by $5-HT_1$ agonists, 297–300

H

Headaches. See specific types of headaches
Heliospectin
  I, 40–41
  II, 40–41
  vascular relaxation, 74
Hemorrhage hypotension, 31
5–HIAA (5–hydroxyindoleacetic acid), 141–142, 154
High-performance liquid chromatography radioimmunoassay (HPLC-RIA), of neuropeptides, 12
Histamine
  in cluster headache, 148, 150
  as endogenous nitric oxide donor, 247
  endothelium-dependent contraction and, 68
  pial artery response and, 188
  release, in dura mater, 167–171, 188
Histamine-induced headache
  L-NMMA and, 304
  nitric oxide formation and, 256–257
  nitric oxide synthase inhibition and, 249–251
  time course, 248
Homocysteine, in primary headache, 215–217
5–HT receptors. See Serotonin receptors
Hydrogen peroxide
  cerebral arteriolar dilation and, 67
  endothelium-dependent contraction and, 68
6–Hydroxydopamine, 23
5–Hydroxyindoleacetic acid (5–HIAA), 141–142, 154
5–Hydroxytryptamine. See Serotonin
5–Hydroxytryptophan, for migraine prevention, 142
Hyperhomocysteinemia, 215
Hypoxia
  cerebral arterial dilations during, 67–68
  vascular headache and, 260, 261–262

I

ICAM-1 (intracellular adhesion molecule-1), 292–293, 294, 295
ICP (intracranial pressure), 31
Immune-competent cells
  opioid peptides in, during headache, 197
  in pain generation, 81–82
Indomethacin, calcitonin gene-related peptide and, 235
Inducible nitric oxide synthase (iNOS), 247
Inflammation, neurogenic
  cortical spreading depression and, 120–121
  in headache pathogenesis, 169, 171

nerve growth factor up-regulation and, 93–94
neuropeptides in, 202–203, 255
substance P expression after, 94, 95
iNOS (inducible nitric oxide synthase), 247
Interindividual variability, of vascular receptors, 173–176, 188
Internal carotid artery
  ipsilateral frontal pain and, 3
  neurotransmitters in, 55–56
Intracellular adhesion molecule-1 (ICAM-1), 292–293, 294, 295
Intracranial hypertension, benign, 73
Intracranial pressure (ICP), 31
Isosorbide mononitrate, 257

K
Kallidin, 81
Kinins, 81

L
Lamotrigine, 157
LC132 opioid receptor, 103
LH (luteinizing hormone), 197–198
Lignocaine, cortical spreading depression and, 120
Locus ceruleus, 7–8
Luteinizing hormone (LH), 197–198
LY83583, 67
Lypoxygenase products, 68

M
MALDI-TOF MS (matrix-assisted laser desorption/ionization time-of-flight mass spectrometry), 12–14, 18
Mass spectrometry (MS), 12
Mast cells, histamine-containing, 167–168, 188
Matrix-assisted laser desorption/ionization time-of-flight mass spectrometry (MALDI-TOF MS), 12–14, 18
Meningeal artery, ipsilateral retro-orbital pain and, 3
Meningitis, 260
Messenger molecules. *See* Neurotransmitters
Met-enkephalin
  in cluster headache, 205–206
  distribution, 193, 194
  during headache
    in cerebrospinal fluid, 196
    in immune cells, 197
    in plasma, 195
  during migraine, 235
N-Methyl-*D*-aspartate receptor (NMDA receptor), 134
Methysergide, 261
Mianserine, for tension-type headache, 146, 148
Miconazole, 66, 76

Middle cerebral artery
  frontal pain and, 3
  of monkey, 52–55
  retro-orbital pain and, 3
Migraine. *See also* Migraineurs
  with aura
    neuropeptide changes in, 204
    prevalence of, 117
    prodromal phase. *See* Cortical spreading depression
  blood flow velocity changes, 5–6
  clinical observations, 4–5
  cortical spreading depression and, 120–121
  as hypoendorphin syndrome, 193
  induced. *See specific types of induced migraine headaches*
  neuropeptide changes in, 204–205
  nitric oxide donor. *See* Nitric oxide donor migraine
  pathophysiology
    blood vessels in, 17
    central factors in, 6–8
    central sensitization and, 95
    extracranial vasodilation and, 5
    model of, 17
    neurogenic theory of, 117
    nitric oxide and, 270, 291–292
    nitric oxide hypothesis of. *See* Nitric oxide hypothesis
    second-messenger mechanisms, 305
    trigeminal afferent activity and, 79–80
    vascular theory of, 3, 117
  prevalence, 117
  reactive hyperemia, radial artery dilation in, 267–270
  transcranial Doppler studies, 5–6
  triggers, 7, 140, 142, 143
Migraineurs
  aminobutyric acid levels in, 139, 140
  aspartic acid levels in, 139, 140
  with cannabinoid addiction, symptom variations and, 107–109
  glutamate levels of, 139, 140
  glutamic acid levels in, 139, 140
  glyceryl trinitrate-induced headache in, 258–259
Monkey, sensory nerve fibers in, 52–55
Myofascial pain syndrome, 95, 133

N
NADPH-diaphorase, 126–127
Naloxone, 100, 197–198
L-NAME, 298
Naratriptan, 297–300
Nausea
  L-NMMA and, 303
  NOS inhibitor 546C88 for, 251–253

Nerve growth factor (NGF)
  characteristics, 83
  hyperalgesia and, 84
  as inflammatory mediator, 83–84
  neuronal development and, 83
  nociceptive activity, 84–86
  in pain processing, 131–133
  trkA receptor and, 93–94
  upregulation, 85
  vascular headache and, 86
Nerve terminals, ultrastructure, 24, 25
Neural-endothelial modulation, 68
Neural plasticity
  pain and, 89–90
  types of
    central sensitization, 91–93
    chemical-induced transcription-dependent, 93–94
    peripheral sensitization, 90–91
Neurogenic inflammation. *See* Inflammation, neurogenic
Neurokinin A (NKA)
  characteristics, 48
  in human cerebral arteries, 55–56
  in migraine, 236
Neurokinin $_1$ receptor antagonist (FK88), 168, 169, 170
Neuron nitric oxide synthase (nNOS), 247
Neuropeptides. *See also specific neuropeptides*
  changes
    in experimental animals, 202–203
    in humans during headache, 203
  in cluster headache, 205–206
  functions, 11
  in migraine
    with aura, 204, 206
    without aura, 204–205, 206
  in neurogenic inflammation, 255
  in primary headaches, 235–237
  radioimmunoassay, 11–12
Neuropeptide Y (NPY)
  in cerebrospinal fluid, from depressed patients, 13
  in cluster headache, 205–206
  co-localization
    with noradrenaline, 22–23
    with vasoactive intestinal peptide, 38–39
  gene expression, 23–24
  interaction, with noradrenaline, 26, 27
  in migraine
    with aura, 204
    without aura, 204–205
  receptors, 25–26
  release, 28
  structure, 23
  in tension-type headache, 146, 149
  vasoconstriction, 73–74
Neurotensin, 102–103

Neurotransmitters. *See also specific neurotransmitters*
  in cranial blood vessels, 73–76
  in cranial parasympathetic nervous system
    acetylcholine. *See* Acetylcholine
    heliospectin-like peptides, 40–41
    nitric oxide, 41–43
    pituitary adenylate cyclase-activating peptide, 39–40
    vasoactive intestinal peptide, 38–39
  in cranial sympathetic nervous system
    neuropeptide Y. *See* Neuropeptide Y
    noradrenaline. *See* Noradrenaline
  in pain processing, 131–135
  in parasympathetic nervous system, 41–43, 74
  in sensory nerve fibers, 50
    around cerebral vessels, 47–49
    of human, 55–56
    of monkey, 52–55
    of rat, 50–52
NGF. *See* Nerve growth factor
N^G-monomethyl-L-arginine (L-NMMA), 242, 297, 303–304
Nicardipine, nitroxidergic nerve stimulation and, 242–243
Nicotine, 68, 241, 242
Nitric oxide
  hypothesis. *See* Nitric oxide hypothesis
Nitric oxide (NO)
  activation, by nitroglycerin, 123–128
  central sensitization and, 82
  CGRP release and, 75
  characteristics, 41, 82
  donors
    endogenous, 247
    exogenous, 247
  formation, 41, 288, 297
  functions, physiologic, 41, 43
  mediation, of CGRP-induced cerebral vessel dilation, 49
  in migraine pathophysiology, 291–292
  pain processing and, 82–83
  release
    in cortical spreading depression, 283
    in migraine initiation, 142–143
  vasodilation, 49, 61
Nitric oxide-cyclic guanosine monophosphate pathway (NO-cGMP)
  activation, supporting evidence for, 256–260
  antimigraine drug mechanisms and, 256, 260–261
  calcium channels and, 262
  products, in primary headache, 256, 303–306
  stimulation, 256, 261–262
Nitric oxide donor migraine
  endothelium-dependent mechanisms, 291–292
  cell adhesion molecules and, 292–293
  proposed scheme for, 294–295
  nitric oxide synthase in, 287–290

SUBJECT INDEX

Nitric oxide hypothesis
  antimigraine drug mechanisms and, 256, 260–261
  basis for, 255–256
  NO-cGMP activation and, 256–260
  NO-cGMP pathway stimulation and, 256, 261–262
  temporal relationships and, 304–305
Nitric oxide synthase inhibitors. *See also specific nitric oxide synthase inhibitors*
  dose response, in healthy volunteers, 248–249
  for histamine-induced headache, 249–251
  for pain reduction, 82–83
  for spontaneous migraine attacks, 251–253
Nitric oxide synthase (NOS)
  acetylcholine and, 74
  in cerebral vessels, inhibition by 5–HT_1 agonists, 297–300
  CGRP vasodilation and, 49
  endothelial-derived, 17–18
  inhibition
    histamine-induced headache and, 249–251
    for spontaneous migraine attacks, 251–253
  isoforms, 247
  in migraine, 287–290
  nitric oxide formation and, 41, 75
  types, 297
L-Nitroarginine, 49
Nitroglycerin
  calcitonin gene-related peptide release and, 237
  in cluster headache, 150
  nitric oxide activation, 123–128
  pressure pain threshold and, 305
  provocation of cluster headache, 259–260
  vasodilation and, 123, 241
7-Nitroindazole, 41
Nitro-L-arginine (L-NNA), 67
Nitroxidergic nerve
  definition of, 242
  stimulation, 244–245
    Ca^{2+} channel inhibitors and, 242–243
    comparisons of, 244
    sumatriptan and, 243–244
NKA. *See* Neurokinin A
NK_1 antagonists, 236
NMDA receptors
  central sensitization and, 91–92, 134
  glutamate and, 139, 142
L-NMMA (N^G monomethyl-L-arginine), 242, 297, 303–304
L-NNA (nitro-L-arginine), 67
nNOS (neuron nitric oxide synthase), 247
NO. *See* Nitric oxide
NO-cGMP. *See* Nitric oxide-cyclic guanosine monophosphate pathway
Nociceptors
  anatomy, 89–90
  cutaneous, 79
  meningeal, activation of, 95
  sensitization, chemical mediators of, 80–82
  sensitization of, 79
Noradrenaline
  cerebrovascular adrenoceptors and, 25
  co-localization with neuropeptide Y, 22–23
  interaction with neuropeptide Y, 26, 27
  intraventricular perfusion, 32–33
  modification, by serotonin receptor agonists, 153–154
  nocturnal migraine and, 140
  omental vessels and, 178–179
  release, 28
  valproate and, 156
  vasoconstriction, 73–74
  vasodilation, 73
Norepinephrine
  in cluster headaches, 149, 150
  endothelium-dependent contraction and, 68
  in rostral ventromedial medulla, 101–102
  in tension-type headaches, 146–147
NOS. *See* Nitric oxide synthase
NPY. *See* Neuropeptide Y
Nucleus raphe dorsalis, 8

O

OFQ, 103
Omental vessel α-adrenoreceptors, variability of, 177–179, 188
Opioid peptides, endogenous. *See also* Dynorphin; β-Endorphin; Met-enkephalin
  classification, 193, 194
  distribution, 193–194
  measurement, 194–195
  during migraine
    in cerebrospinal fluid, 196–197
    in immune cells, 197
    in plasma, 195–196
  off-cell activation, 101
  in rostral ventromedial medulla, 102–103
Oxygen therapy, for cluster headache, 261
Oxymetazoline, 25
Oxytocin, 125–126, 127

P

PACAPII receptor (pituitary adenylate cyclase-activating peptide II receptor), 39
PACAP (pituitary adenylate cyclase-activating peptide), 39
PAG-RVM system (periaqueductal gray matter-rostral ventromedial medulla pain modulating network), 99–101
Pain
  detection threshold, glyceryl trinitrate and, 273–276

Pain (contd.)
  modulation
    forebrain and, 103
    by periaqueductal gray matter and rostral ventromedial medulla, 99–101
    by rostral ventromedial medulla, 101–102
  neural plasticity and, 89–90
  non-nociceptive vs. nociceptive, 93
  physiological vs. clinical, 89
  processing, neurotransmitters in, 131–135
  tolerance threshold, glyceryl trinitrate and, 273–276
Parasympathetic nerves
  anatomy, 202
  cranial, anatomy of, 37
  neurotransmitters, 202. See also specific neurotransmitters
  multiplicity of, 74
Paroxetine, for tension-type headache, 146, 148
Peptide histidine isoleucine (PHI), 38
Peptides
  nonopioid. See Neuropeptides
  opioid. See Opioid peptides, endogenous
Periaqueductal gray matter-rostral ventromedial medulla pain modulating network (PAG-RVM system), 99–101
Peripheral sensitization, 90–91
Perivascular nerve stimulation, cerebral vasodilation induced by, 241–242
Peroxynitrite, cerebral arteriolar dilation and, 67
Phenoxybenzamine, 25, 29
Phentolamine, 25, 29, 32
Phenylephrine, cerebrovascular adrenoceptors and, 25
PHI (peptide histidine isoleucine), 38
Phonophobia, NOS inhibitor 546C88 for, 251–253
Phorbol ester, protein kinase C-activated, 63
Photophobia, NOS inhibitor 546C88 for, 251–253
Pial artery
  diameter, spreading depression-induced NO release and, 283–285
  regional blood flow, spreading depression-induced NO release and, 283–285
  vascular receptors, variability of, 173–176, 188
Piperoxane, 25
Pituitary adenylate cyclase-activating peptide II receptor (PACAPII receptor), 39
Pituitary adenylate cyclase-activating peptide (PACAP), 39–40, 74
Pizotifen, 261
PKC (protein kinase C), 91, 300
Posterior cerebral artery, 3
Post-traumatic headache, 260
Potassium channel activation, in basal blood flow regulation, 67
Practolol, 25

Prodromes, scintillation scotomas, 117
Prolactin release
  in *m*-chlorophenylpiperazine-induced headache, 183–185, 187
  in fenfluramine-induced headaches, 187
  in induced-migraine, 142
Prophylactic drugs, 155–157
Propranolol, 25, 33, 261
Prostacyclin
  endothelial synthesis, 62
  functions, 62–63
  headache induced by, 262
  vasoconstriction and, 75
Prostaglandin
  H_2, 68
  I_2. See Prostacyclin
Protein kinase A, 300
Protein kinase C (PKC), 91, 300

R

Radial artery dilation, in reactive hyperemia, 267–270
Radioimmunoassay (RIA)
  with mass spectrometry, 12–14
  neuropeptides, 11–12
Rat
  brain, Fos protein expression in, 123–128
  sensory nerve fibers, neurotransmitters in, 50–52
  tail-spinal cord preparation, ATP neuronal activation in, 111–116
Rauwolscine, 25
Reactive hyperemia, radial artery dilation in, 267–270
Receptor autoradiography, of $CGRP_1$, 230–232
Red wine-induced headache
  characteristics, 142, 143
  serotoninergic receptor stimulation and, 279–280, 281
Referred pain, from intracranial vessels, 3–4
Reserpine-induced headache, 262, 279, 280
Retinal artery stimulation, vs. cerebral and temporal artery stimulation, 244
Reverse phase high-performance liquid chromatography (RP HPLC), of neuropeptides, 12
Reverse transcriptase polymerase chain reaction, 224, 230
Rheumatoid arthritis, 133
RIA. See Radioimmunoassay
Ritanserin, for chronic headache with depression, 146, 148
Rostral ventromedial medulla (RVM)
  neurotransmitters, 104
  pain-modulating circuits, 101–103
    forebrain and, 103–104
    with periaqueductal gray matter, 99–101

S

Scintillation scotomas, 117
SD. *See* Cortical spreading depression
Sensitization
  central. *See* Central sensitization
  chemical mediators of, 80–82
  peripheral, 90–91
Sensory nervous system, neurotransmitters, redundancy of, 74
Serotonin (5–hydroxytryptamine; 5–HT)
  in cluster headache, 148, 150
  cranial artery blood flow and, 6, 7
  endothelial-dependent contractions and, 68
  in migraine, 140–142
  modification by serotonin receptor agonists, 153–154
  pial artery response and, 188
  release, red wine and, 279–280
  in tension-type headache, 145–146, 147
  as trigger, 142
  valproate and, 156
Serotonin receptor agonists
  mechanism of action, 134–135
  for migraine, 153–155
Serotonin receptors
  excitation of trigeminovascular system and, 161
  stimulation of, 281
  vasoconstriction and, 188–189
Sex headache, 17
SKF525A, 66
Sodium valproate. *See* Valproate
Somatostatin
  in cluster headache, 205–206
  endothelium-dependent contractions and, 68
  immunoreactivity, 24
Spreading depression. *See* Cortical spreading depression
Subarachnoid hemorrhage, 203
Substance P
  calcitonin gene-related peptide and, 74, 75
  in cluster headache, 205
  expression, after inflammation, 94, 95
  histamine release in dura mater and, 167–171
  in human cerebral arteries, 55–56
  immunoreactivity, 24
  individual response variability, 175
  localization, 167
  in migraine
    with aura, 204
    without aura, 204–205
  in pain conditions, 236
  pial artery response and, 188
  in rat sensory nerve fibers, 50–52
  in sensory nerve fibers around cerebral vessels, 47–48
  tension-type headache and, 145, 146

  trigeminal ganglion stimulation and, 203
  vasodilation and, 117
Sulpiride, for tension-type headache, 146, 148
Sumatriptan
  blockage of trigeminal ganglion stimulation, 203
  CGRP blood levels and, 121
  CGRP-induced histamine release and, 168–169, 170, 171
  for cluster headache, 150
  effects, on brain monoamines, 154
  injection, cranial artery blood flow and, 6
  mechanism of action, 153, 260
  for migraine, 153–155
  nitric oxide synthase inhibition, in guinea pig cerebral arteries, 297–300
  nitroxidergic nerve stimulation and, 243–244
  pial artery response and, 188
  SP-induced histamine release and, 170
  for tension-type headache, 146, 148
Superficial temporal artery, serotonin in, during cluster headaches, 148
Superior cervical ganglia
  excision, bilateral, 32
  stimulation of, 27–28
Superior cervical ganglionectomy, 24
Superoxide anion
  induction, of cerebral arteriolar dilation, 67
  vasodilation, 67
Sympathectomy, 23
Sympathetic nerves
  anatomy, 22, 202
  in cerebral circulation regulation, 21
  choroid plexus function and, 31–33
  control of cerebrovascular capacitance, 73
  effects, on cerebrovascular bed in situ, 33
  neurotransmitters. *See* Neuropeptide Y; Noradrenaline
  stimulation
    autoregulation and, 30–31
    species differences in, 28–29
Sympathicoplegia, in cluster headache, 149, 150
Sympathomimetic agents, cerebrovascular adrenoceptors and, 25

T

TEA (tetraethylammonium), 66, 67
Temporal artery
  $endothelin_B$ receptors in, 219–222
  stimulation, *vs.* cerebral and retinal artery stimulation, 244
Tension-type headache (TTH)
  amino acids in, 146–147, 149
  catecholamines in, 146–147, 149
  drug therapy, 146, 148
  pain threshold for, 95

Tension-type headache (TTH) (contd.)
  pathophysiological mechanisms, 145
  serotonin in, 145–146, 187–188
Tetraethylammonium (TEA), 66, 67
Tetrahydrobiopterin, 68
Thrombin, 62, 63
Thromboxane A_2, 68
TNC (trigeminal nucleus caudalis), c-fos
  expression, 119–120, 161–164
Transient ischemic attacks (TIAs), 3
Transmural nerve stimulation (TNS), 68
Trigeminal ganglion
  activation, 203
  stimulation, neuropeptide changes and,
    203
Trigeminal ganglionectomy, 48
Trigeminal nerve
  afferent fibers, neurotransmitter release from,
    47
  anatomy, 202
  electrical stimulation
    c-fos induced by, 119
    CGRP release and, 229
    method of, 118
  neurotransmitters. *See* Calcitonin gene-related
    peptide; Neurokinin A; Substance P
  pain fibers, 7
Trigeminal neuralgia, thermocoagulation for,
    203
Trigeminal nucleus caudalis (TNC), c-fos
  expression, 119–120
  m-chlorophenylpiperazine and, 161–164
Trigeminovascular system, 95, 169
Triggers, 7, 140, 142, 143. *See also specific
    triggers*
trkA receptors, 83, 86, 93–94
Tryptophan, for migraine prevention, 142

TTH. *See* Tension-type headache
Tyrosine, in cluster headaches, 149

V

Valproate (valproic acid)
  γ-aminobutyric acid and, 155–156
  cortical spreading depression and, 120
  dopamine and, 156
  excitatory amino acids and, 156
  for migraine prophylaxis, 155–157
  noradrenaline and, 156
  serotonin and, 156
Vascular headache. *See also specific types of
    vascular headache*
  causes, 260
  migraine as, 3
  nerve growth factor and, 86
Vasoactive-intestinal peptide (VIP)
  characteristics, 38–39
  in cluster headache, 205–206
  immunoreactivity, 24
  in migraine
    with aura, 204
    without aura, 204–205
  receptors, 39
  vasodilatory action, 74
Vasopressin, 125–126, 204–205
Ventriculocisternal perfusion technique, 32
Verapamil, 303
Vertebral artery, 3
Vigabatrin, 157
VIP. *See* Vasoactive-intestinal peptide

Y

Yohimbine, 25